General Surgery for Nurses

Harold Ellis D.M. M.Ch. F.R.C.S.
Professor of Surgery,
Westminster Hospital

Christopher Wastell M.S. F.R.C.S.
Hon. Consultant Surgeon and Reader
in Surgery, Westminster Hospital

General Surgery for Nurses

Including contributions by
Paul Aichroth on Fractures and Orthopaedics
E. H. Miles Foxen on Ear, Nose and Throat
Patrick D. Trevor-Roper on Ophthalmology

Second Edition

Blackwell Scientific Publications
Oxford London Edinburgh Melbourne

© 1976, 1980 by
Blackwell Scientific Publications
Editorial offices:
Osney Mead, Oxford, OX2 OEL
8 John Street, London, WC1N 2ES
9 Forrest Road, Edinburgh, EH1 2QH
214 Berkeley Street, Carlton,
    Victoria 3053, Australia

First published 1976
Second edition 1980

DISTRIBUTORS

USA
    Blackwell Mosby Book Distributors
    11830 Westline Industrial Drive
    St Louis, Missouri 63141

Canada
    Blackwell Mosby Book Distributors
    86 Northline Road, Toronto
    Ontario, M4B 3E5

Australia
    Blackwell Scientific Book
    Distributors
    214 Berkeley Street, Carlton
    Victoria 3053

British Library Cataloguing in Publication Data
Ellis, Harold, b.1926
    General surgery for nurses. — 2nd ed.
    1. Surgery
    I. Title II. Westell, Christopher
    617'.002'4613   RT65
    ISBN 0-632-00532-7

Photoset, printed and bound in Malta by
Interprint Limited.

Contributors

Paul Aichroth M.S. F.R.C.S.
Consultant Orthopaedic Surgeon,
Westminster Hospital, London S.W.1

Harold Ellis D.M. M.Ch. F.R.C.S.
Professor of Surgery,
Westminster Hospital, London S.W.1

E. H. Miles Foxen F.R.C.S. D.L.O.
Honorary Consulting Ear, Nose and Throat Surgeon,
Westminster Hospital, London S.W.1

Patrick D. Trevor-Roper M.A. M.D. B.Chir.(Cantab) F.R.C.S. D.O.M.S. (Eng)
Consultant Ophthalmic Surgeon,
Westminster Hospital, London S.W.1 and
Moorfields Eye Hospital.

Christopher Wastell M.S. F.R.C.S.
Honorary Consultant Surgeon and Reader in Surgery,
Westminster Hospital, London S.W.1

Contents

Introduction

The surgical nurse today faces the difficult task of coping not only with the heavy responsibilities of the care of seriously ill patients but also with the rapidly expanding corpus of Medical knowledge. New operations, drugs and techniques of treatment constantly appear on the scene, yet as a member of the surgical team, she must be fully aware of these advances and, indeed, play a vital part in their success.

This new text-book attempts to present the essential facts of modern surgical practice in a readable and reasonably compact form. The contributors are actively concerned with lecturing to nurses in training and we have endeavoured to put forward our current teaching into its pages. It has been designed with the S.R.N. and the S.E.N. Diplomas in mind.

We have been greatly assisted in this task by many discussions over many years with the sister tutors at the Wolfson School of Nursing at Westminster Hospital.

Copious illustrations have been used and these have all been specifically selected for the student nurse. Both the figures and the text emphasise the common entities which are seen in hospital today. Much less space has been allowed for the many 'classical' conditions like tuberculosis of bone and joint and poliomyelitis, once so common, but now fortunately almost eliminated from our surgical wards.

We would like to thank our colleagues among the medical and nursing staff at Westminster for their help and to express our appreciation for the encouragement we have received from Mr Per Saugman and his staff at Blackwell Scientific Publications.

The need for a second edition has enabled us to carry out a careful revision and updating of both text and illustrations.

H.E., C.W.
Westminster Medical School
1979

Chapter I. Infections

Mona Powell

INTRODUCTION

For the whole of our lives we are surrounded by micro-organisms, many of which are capable of gaining entry to the body and causing an 'infection'. Bearing this in mind it is perhaps surprising that significant infection does not occur more commonly. Micro-organisms can be classified as follows:

1. *Viruses*—these are not often concerned with infections of surgical significance but the viruses of measles and mumps can both cause abdominal pain. The latter virus may cause pancreatitis, oophoritis and generalised lymphadenitis. They are too small to be seen by the conventional microscope.

2. *Bacteria*—these are the most common agents in surgical infections and in general may be divided into bacteria that are round, for example streptococci and staphylococci (Figs. 1.1 and 1.2) or rod-like (for example *Escherichia coli*). Bacteria may be seen, after having been suitably stained, using a microscope. They are further sub-divided depending on their staining properties into, for example, gram positive or gram negative groups and beyond this point other more complex culture procedures are required to differentiate between the different types. The diseases they may be associated with are listed in Table 1.1.

3. *Fungi*—these are relatively large organisms composed of branching filaments which may be seen using a microscope. An example of this type of organism is candida, which is responsible for the infection known as thrush.

4. *Protozoa*—these are single-celled organisms and include plasmodium (responsible for malaria), entamoeba (responsible for amoebic colitis), trichomonas (Fig. 1.3) lamblia and toxoplasma.

Fig. 1.1 Culture of *Staphylococcus aureus* on blood agar.

For centuries man has searched for specific remedies for specific infections and the whole of art and literature is full of his failure to achieve this goal. In the early 1930's, however, specific chemotherapeutic agents were manufactured which had the effect of interfering with the metabolism of certain bacteria whilst not poisoning the patient. The first of these agents were the sulphonamides, originally produced by May and Baker and for that reason for a long time they were known as 'M & B'. The truly significant departure that these compounds resulted in was the 'systemic' treatment of infection. It was an early observation in 1928 by Dr. Alexander Fleming (later knighted) however, which produced the most profound ecological change the human race has ever seen when he noted inhibition of the growth of *Staphylococcus aureus* on a blood agar plate produced by the mould Penicillium notatum. After some studies on this agent, Fleming concluded that the substance producing this inhibition was so unstable as to defy extraction. It was the work of Professor Florey in Oxford, immediately before the

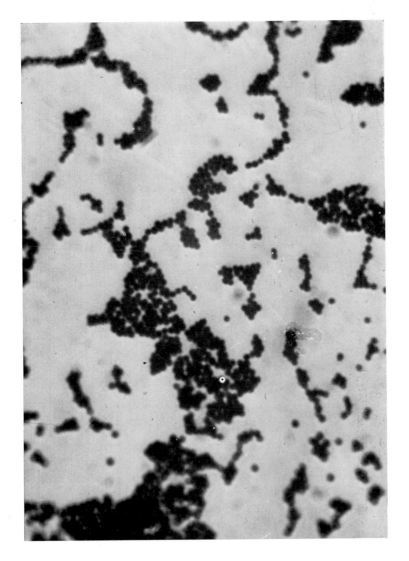

Fig. 1.2. Microphotograph of *Staphylococcus aureus*. These organisms have been stained with gram stain and appear dark blue under the microscope.

second world war in 1939, which resulted in the drug penicillin being extracted in therapeutic quantities. The effect of this work is far-reaching when one realises that, for the first time, man had achieved a significant advantage over the micro-organisms of his environment which had all too often swept millions to their death during pandemic infections, such as the great plagues.

The antibiotics, as they become known, are all produced as a result of metabolic processes in micro-organisms, generally fungi but also in bacteria. There is now a large selection of antibiotics, all with specific activities and varying toxic effects. It is perhaps remark-

Fig. 1.3. *Trichomonas vaginalis*; a single-cell organism with flagellae which allow it to move.

able that penicillin still remains one of the most generally useful antibiotics that we have.

Two definitions

Two terms will repeatedly occur in this chapter and should therefore be defined. The first of these is *pus*, which is defined as 'a collection of dead and alive white cells together usually with dead and alive organisms suspended in serum'. The second is an *abscess*, which is simply 'a collection of pus'.

Mechanisms of infection

Since we are surrounded by micro-organisms, the establishment of an infection depends upon some upset in the balance between our protective mechanism and the infecting organism. If a patient is in a generally reduced state of health by virtue of some other disease, the liability to infection is increased. An example of this is seen in the patient with an advanced malignant disease who dies of bronchopneumonia. The opposite situation also occurs in which a normal patient meets an unusually virulent organism against which he has no protection. The epidemics of Asian 'flu are an example of this phenomenon. Another reason for an infection gaining a foothold is damage to the tissues of the body. If the skin is lacerated, bacteria, such as the staphylococcus, normally resident on the skin, gain entry to the exposed tissues of the body and can multiply. It is also possible for bacteria circulating in the blood to be deposited in tissue damaged by trauma.

One of the general rules of the body is that if a block occurs to a duct, with resulting failure of drainage, infection is likely to occur in the static secretion. Examples of this mechanism are seen in bronchitis when bronchioles are blocked by mucus, upper urinary tract infections which follow obstruction to a ureter or cystitis following obstruction to the urethra.

THE SIGNS OF INFECTION

Local. Infected tissue becomes inflamed. This means that the tissue appears to be red and feels hot because of the increased blood supply to it. It is swollen because of oedema fluid resulting from the increased blood supply to the area. There is usually pain due to the increase in tension within the tissues, which is also due to the oedema fluid. Because the tissue is swollen and painful there is also interference with the normal function of the infected part. These changes are visible when the infection is close to the skin but obviously cannot be seen externally in the case of a deeply placed abscess.

General. The temperature of the patient is raised. The type of pyrexia is often characteristic. When an abscess is present the temperature rises in the evening and falls to normal by the morning; this is known as a 'swinging pyrexia' (Fig. 1.4). Infections of the

Fig. 1.4. Temperature chart exhibiting a swinging pyrexia due to the presence of an abscess. Drainage on the fifth day resulted in rapid resolution of the fever.

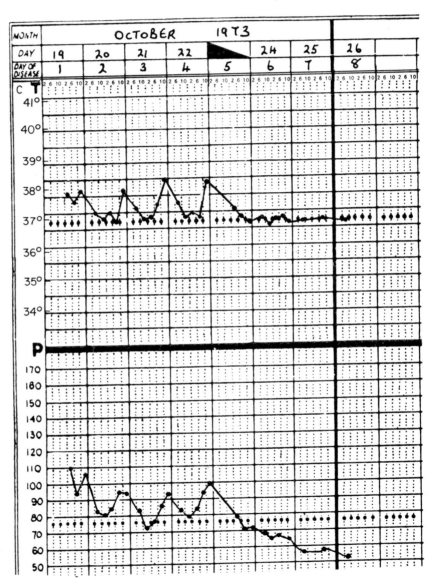

kidney (pyelonephritis) and liver (hepatitis) or of the hepatic ducts (cholangitis) and of the blood (septicaemia), often result in very high fever, up to 39° or 40°C associated with a 'rigor'. When a patient has a 'rigor' he shakes uncontrollably. Usually there is an initial subjective impression of coldness. Typhoid fever results in a slowly rising pyrexia over a period of one to two weeks. Pyrexia with a temperature rise of greater than 0.5°C is always significant and unless the cause is known should never be ignored.

Together with the pyrexia the pulse rate also increases. There are no absolute levels above which a pulse rate indicates an infection; it is the day to day change in pulse rate which indicates the course of the infection. A falling pulse rate in a previously infected patient indicates that the infection is getting better.

If a blood count is made during an acute infection a rise in the number of white cells is detected. The first cells to be affected are the polymorpho-nuclear leucocytes, which can be shown to be of the recently formed variety by the small number of lobes on their nuclei. In some chronic infections, for example tuberculosis, the lymphocyte count is raised. It is characteristic of infections by the helminthes (worms) for the eosinophil count to be raised in the peripheral blood.

Measurement of the plasma proteins will indicate a rise in the gamma globulin fraction, which starts approximately ten days after the onset of infection. This is due to the development of antibodies to the infecting organism. One secondary result of this change in the proteins is that the erythrocyte sedimentation rate (E.S.R.) is raised. The E.S.R. may be used as an index for the patient's improvement following infection and is useful in those who have tuberculosis.

Protecting mechanisms

There are two main groups of protecting mechanisms. The first of these are the white cells circulating in the blood; they are capable of ingesting invading bacteria and so destroying them. They have been likened to the policemen of the body, always on duty and ready to deal with trouble. Their response is rapid and they collect in huge numbers around an infected tissue.

The white cells thus mobilised then ingest the bacteria, a process known as phagocytosis. One white cell is able in this way to dispose of many bacteria, which usually are digested and killed, but the white cell itself may be killed. Thus, at the site of an infection there are many white cells, some alive and some dead, bacteria, some of which are also alive and some dead, together with the serum that has exuded into the area: this is *pus*. Pus may assume several characteristics: staphylococcus—yellow; *E. coli*—faecal smelling; pseudomonas—green; streptococcus—watery, and actinomycosis—watery containing yellow flecks known as 'sulphur granules'.

The second is the production of antibodies. These are gamma globulins produced in lymph nodes and other lymphocyte-rich tissues, for example, the spleen. They have the characteristic of combining with the proteins of the invading organism which has itself stimulated their production. Antibodies are highly specific and to give an example, the antibody to the measles virus will protect against other invasions by that organism but not against other viruses. Whereas the protection afforded by the white cells is immediate, antibodies usually take between 10 and 14 days to be developed. Once a patient has produced antibodies to an organism, subsequent infection with that organism produces an antibody response which is more rapid and of greater magnitude.

Incubation period

The time, in days, from the entry of an infecting organism to the development of the signs of infection is known as the incubation period. This is usually the time taken for the organism to begin multiplying effectively within the body. In general, viruses have an incubation period of between 7 and 21 days. Larger organisms, for example, streptococcus, staphylococcus and other bacteria have a shorter incubation period of 1 to 3 days.

PRINCIPLES OF TREATMENT

The infected part is put to rest. Thus, if a limb has an infection, movement is minimised by means of a splint and a sling. The causative organism is identified and, at the same time, the sensitivities to a wide range of antibiotic agents is determined by culture. If it is necessary to treat the infection before the sensitivities have been established (this usually takes 2 days), then the appropriate antibiotic will have to be deduced. An example of this is in the case of peritonitis for which ampicillin, known to be effective against most intestinal organisms, is used. It is quite wrong in most cases, however, to treat an infection with a 'broad spectrum' antibiotic without accurate knowledge as to the type of organism being treated. If pus has formed, then surgical drainage is required. The old dictum: 'Let not the sun go down on unopened pus' still holds good and antibiotics are totally ineffective in the treatment of a pus-filled cavity. If the duct draining a cavity is blocked then drainage either along the duct or by some alternative route has to be secured.

There is an important general principle in treating acute infections anywhere in the body: antibiotics are invaluable when the

Table 1.1. A list of some bacteria with some of their associated diseases and some of the antibiotics that may be used in their treatment.

Bacteria	Disease	Antibiotic
Staphylococcus aureus	Boils, abscesses wound infections	Penicillin, Ampicillin, Cloxacillin
Streptococcus pyogenes	Cellulitis, lymphangitis	Penicillin, Ampicillin, Cloxacillin, Co-Trimoxazole, Cephalexin
Streptococcus pneumoniae	Lobar pneumonia	Penicillin
Clostridium tetani	Tetanus	Penicillin
Clostridium perfringens (*B. welchii*)	Gas gangrene	Penicillin
Escherichia coli	Some wound infections from intestinal source, urinary infection	Ampicillin, Cephaloridine, Cephalexin, Gentamycin, Co-Trimoxazole
Pseudomonas aeruginosa (*Pyocyanea*)	Infection of burns	Gentamicin
Mycobacterium tuberculosis	Tuberculosis	Streptomycin, Rifampicin

infection is spreading through the tissues (e.g. cellulitis, pneumonia, peritonitis, septicaemia) but drainage is essential when abscess formation has occurred.

The most efficient form of prophylaxis against infection is by the stimulation of antibody production. This method has been highly successful in such infections as poliomyelitis, smallpox, tetanus, whooping cough, typhoid, yellow fever and now measles. Some protection can be afforded by the giving of an immune serum, for example in the case of a pregnant woman who has come into contact with German measles and who requires protection for some weeks. Prophylaxis by antibiotics is not so effective, although it is extensively used for patients with chronic bronchitis and in patients undergoing major arterial or cardio-thoracic surgery. One form of prophylaxis which has been shown to be effective is the instillation of antibiotic powder such as ampicillin into operation wounds and there is no doubt that this reduces the incidence of wound infection.

SOME SPECIFIC TYPES OF INFECTION

BOILS

A boil results from the infection of a hair follicle. At first the skin around it is red and painful and then, as pus develops, the hair follicle appears yellow and the pain increases. As soon as the overlying epidermis ruptures with the release of pus, the pain disappears and the boil is cured. Usually no specific treatment is required. Hot compresses are often soothing and can accelerate the formation of pus. Magnesium sulphate suspension is time honoured when the boil has burst; in reality it probably provides a convenient type of bland dressing more than a specific 'drawing' action. Extraction of the hair with release of tension and pus is the most positive treatment and is always effective.

ABSCESSES

An abscess is a localised collection of pus. It may occur in almost any site in the body. Depending on the tissue involved, an abscess will cause at least some damage and the longer the process is allowed to continue, the greater this will be. For example, a breast abscess can result in considerable destruction of breast tissue unless treated promptly.

Clinical features

Usually, at least in this country, abscesses form for some identifiable reason: in a fresh surgical wound that has become infected, or around an inflamed organ such as the appendix, Fallopian tube or gall bladder.

There is generally associated pain and a swinging pyrexia develops. The patient usually feels ill. If the abscess is close to the skin a mass may be palpable and if the overlying skin is actually involved, it will be red and oedematous. As an abscess develops and enlarges, the skin becomes stretched over it with the result that the surface of the skin becomes smooth and shiny. If the swelling then regresses the surface of the skin is thrown into small wrinkles. The white cell count is raised.

Treatment

This depends on the site and causation. Superficial abscesses should be drained by having an incision made into the wall, the patient being suitably anaesthetised, usually under general anaesthetic. If the cavity is large, a piece of corrugated latex rubber is inserted so as to ensure free drainage for any pus. Some of the pus is collected on a bacterial swab which is immediately sent to the bacteriology laboratory. Identification of the organism is then undertaken by means of culture for 24–48 hours or more, by staining and other tests. In addition to identification, the bacteriologist is able to measure the effectiveness of a range of antibiotics against that particular organism. All this important work is made impossible if the swab is allowed to dry or if it is left in the refrigerator overnight. Provided that the abscess is draining, no further treatment is required beyond suitably frequent dressing. Generally, antibiotics should never be used once an abscess has become established. If a broad spectrum antibiotic (that is, one effective against a wide range of organisms, a good example being ampicillin) is given, there will be an initial reduction in the surrounding inflammation, which will deceive the attendant into believing that a cure will soon be obtained. Inevitably, however, the process of abscess formation will continue, only having been temporarily slowed down. The reason for identifying the organism is to be able to treat the infection if it spreads generally, beyond the abscess itself.

For abscesses in specific areas, see the appropriate chapters (e.g. breast abscess, page 389, appendix abscess 221).

LYMPHANGITIS

This is an inflammation of the lymphatic channels but the term is reserved for those cases in which the inflammation in the overlying skin can actually be seen. The infecting organism is usually a β-haemolytic streptococcus. The condition is most commonly seen when some part of the hand or forearm is injured and subsequently becomes infected.

Clinical features

There is pain in the infected part, and the pain then extends proximally. When the arm is examined a red line is seen to extend from the wound along the anterior aspect of the forearm to the medial side of the elbow and thence to the axilla. It does occur, although less commonly, in other parts of the body as well.

Treatment

This is with the appropriate antibiotic, which is usually penicillin.

LYMPHADENITIS

This occurs when lymphangitis reaches the lymph nodes. It may be due to the streptococcus, although a very wide range of infecting agents will produce it without first resulting in obvious lymphangitis.

Fig. 1.5. Cellulitis of the arm due to β-haemolytic streptococcus.

CELLULITIS

If an infection gains access to connective tissue, for example beneath the skin or in the pelvis, and then spreads, this is known as cellulitis (Fig. 1.5). The most common organism to cause this is again the haemolytic streptococcus, although other organisms, especially staphylococcus, can produce it.

Clinical features

These include pain in the affected part, a raised temperature, pulse rate and white cell count. It is unusual for pus to be formed as a discrete collection, at least in the early stages.

Treatment

The appropriate antibiotic is used. It is unusual to be able to culture the causative organism and the agent used, therefore, should be appropriate for the site. In pelvic cellulitis for example, ampicillin is usually effective.

WOUND INFECTION

One of the complications which may attend any surgical operation is infection of the wound. This is more common when the operation is carried out in an infected area, for example, when the interior of the colon is opened. Usually, wound infections resolve after several days or weeks without causing too much trouble. Occasionally they can be disastrous, particularly in cardiac surgery, orthopaedic surgery, in any surgery that has resulted in the implantation of foreign material within the body or when immuno-suppression is being used in association with organ transplantation. In general abdominal surgery most wound infections resolve without specific treatment, except that if pus is formed deep to the healing skin then free drainage must be encouraged with removal of one, two or three skin sutures. One of the complications of wound infection as it affects the abdominal wall is the later development of an incisional hernia.

TETANUS

Tetanus is an extremely dangerous condition which results from the infection of ischaemic tissue by *Clostridium tetani*. This organism is a gram positive rod and is found in soil and the intestine. Once the organism gains a hold it begins to multiply locally in the tissues and an exotoxin (which is a poison manufactured by the organism) is produced. This rapidly becomes fixed in the nervous system and when this has occurred it cannot be removed by treatment.

Clinical features

The incubation period after injury varies from one day to three weeks. The first symptoms consist of a spastic rigidity in the muscles of the back and neck and also in the muscles of the face and jaw (hence the name 'Lock-jaw'). A curious feature of this disease is that occasionally it is regional; that is, it may affect one group of muscles or one limb, generally the limb that is the site of the infection. If the infection continues unabated, eventually all the muscles become affected and violent spasms with convulsions occur; death then follows because of respiratory failure.

Prophylaxis

Active. It is possible to provide protection against tetanus by injections of tetanus toxoid. This is prepared from cultures of *Clostridium tetani* which are treated so that whilst the exotoxin they produce is rendered non-harmful it retains its capacity to stimulate the production of antibodies. Three injections of toxoid are given at intervals of approximately 4 weeks and confer immunity for a period of 5 to 10 years.

At the time of injury. When an injury is sustained which results in devascularised tissue, the risk of tetanus can be virtually removed by correct care. This includes excision of all dead and devitalised tissue; giving penicillin which is effective against clostridium tetani and for those who have been previously immunised, by giving a booster dose of tetanus toxoid. If previous immunisation has not been given, a full course of toxoid is administered.

Treatment of an established case

Treatment will depend on the severity of the symptoms. In general, the shorter the time from the introduction of the infection to the development of the symptoms, the more severe the attack will be. In all cases an injection of tetanus toxoid is given.

The wound

A swab for culture and identification of the organisms is taken. All dead and devitalised tissue is excised under general anaesthetic and large doses of penicillin are given by intramuscular injection.

The symptoms

If only minor muscle spasms are present, with stiffness of facial and neck muscles, these can be controlled with barbiturates (phenobarbitone 60–200 mg i.m. 6 hourly if necessary) and a tranquillizer such as diazepam.

As the condition progresses, more and more muscles become involved in the spastic process until the patient becomes fixed, with back arched (when all muscles go into spasm the position of joints is determined by the strongest muscle groups—in the case of the trunk this is the extensor muscles of the back) in a position known as opisthotonos. When this horrifying stage is reached breathing becomes impossible and respiratory failure ending in death is the result. The treatment now becomes a question of inducing general anaesthesia with intravenous barbiturate (Pentothal) and giving muscle relaxants. So as to maintain respiration, tracheostomy and artificial ventilation is required, a mechanical ventilator being used. Patients have been maintained in this way for 3 weeks, until the effects of the exotoxin on the central nervous system has worn off, after which full recovery has occurred.

GAS GANGRENE

Gas gangrene is due to infection by *Clostridium welchii*, a gram positive rod which grows in anaerobic conditions and produces an exotoxin. The organisms are found in soil and in the intestine.

Clinical features

The incubation period varies from 2 to 7 days. The situation that may result in gas gangrene is the implantation of soil or faecal material in a wound that contains tissue whose blood supply has been damaged, for example, a compound fracture.

The main feature of this infection is spreading death of cells with the formation of bubbles of gas. When the infected area is palpated the typical 'crepitations' of small bubbles of gas in tissue are felt. This gas contains hydrogen sulphide and results in the characteristic 'bad eggs' smell associated with this condition. The patient is usually extremely ill, with a rapid pulse rate and high temperature, and if the infection continues unchecked results in death, sometimes within a few hours.

Prophylaxis

The main element here is the recognition and correct care of a wound likely to result in gas gangrene. Thus if tissue has had its blood supply removed then it should be surgically excised under general anaesthetic and all contaminating material removed by washing and swabbing. A bacteriological swab is taken so that any clostridia can be identified. Clostridia are sensitive to penicillin, and a prophylactic course is given to patients with compound fractures and those undergoing major limb amputations.

Treatment

The first treatment that should be carried out is with hyperbaric oxygen at 3 atmospheres for 2 hours. This will stop, dramatically, the further multiplication of the infecting organism. The only other therapeutic agent which there is time to give is a large dose of penicillin (2 mega-units). Following the initial treatment with hyperbaric oxygen, the patient is taken to the operating theatre where all gangrenous tissue is excised. Following this the patient receives a total of seven 2 hour sessions in the hyperbaric chamber at 3 atmospheres and the course of penicillin is continued for a period of 7 days.

TUBERCULOSIS

The organism *Mycobacterium tuberculosis* is responsible for this disease. There are two principal types of organism. The first is the human type and the second is the bovine type. The bovine type is capable of infecting human beings, the usual route of infection being via milk. This type of infection has been virtually eradicated in this country now, due to the rigorous policy of attestation of milk herds. The usual method of infection with the human organism is by droplet from an infected person with pulmonary disease.

In this country, therefore, when a person first comes into contact with tuberculosis it is usually by inhalation of infected droplets. The small infected area in the lung, commonly the right upper lobe, forms a small area of caseation (an abscess that contains tuberculous pus, fancifully likened to Swiss cheese). The regional lymph nodes at the hilum of the lung become enlarged. In the majority of children and young adults so affected, the infection is contained and both the lung lesion and the lymph nodes become calcified. These changes are visible on X-ray and are known as a 'primary' or 'Ghon' focus. In a few patients the infection is not contained and the disease spreads throughout the body to produce miliary tuberculosis.

Primary tuberculous infection results in hypersensitivity to soluble products from cultures of the organism (tuberculin). This is the basis of the tuberculin skin tests for tuberculosis. The two most commonly used are the Mantoux and the Heef tests. A small quantity of dilute tuberculin is injected into the skin with a syringe or special perforating device and if within 48 hours the skin becomes red and swollen, the test is described as positive and the patient is therefore known to have had primary tuberculosis.

The identification of tuberculosis is sometimes difficult. In general the organism is looked for in sputum, urine or tissues (Fig. 1.6) by a stain, carbol fuchsin, which renders the mycobacteria red. This stain has the almost unique characteristic of being acid resistant or 'fast'. Culture of the living organism is difficult; it is carried out on Loewenstein egg/malachite green medium and takes 6 weeks. Another method of culture is to inject infected material into a guinea pig (an animal with no resistance at all to tuberculosis) and then to kill the animal 6 weeks later and examine its organs for signs of infection.

The surgical significance of tuberculosis lies in:

1. Pulmonary disease when one or two lobes become hopelessly damaged. Providing the disease has been localised, the affected lobes are removed.

It is also important to recognise pulmonary tuberculosis when it exists in patients who are undergoing surgical operations. This is one of the reasons that chest X-rays must always be carried out before operations because it is possible for anaesthetic equipment to become infected and so transmit the infection to other patients.

2. Urinary tract infection. The kidney ureter, bladder, seminal vesicles and epididymis may become infected. Once again, if the

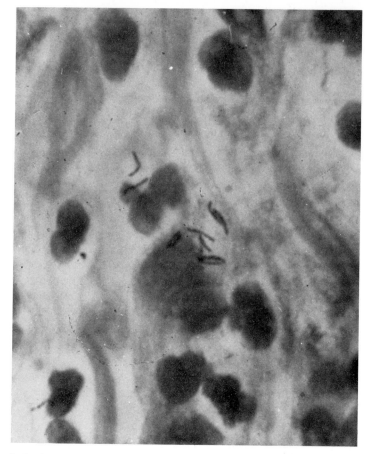

Fig. 1.6. *Mycobacterium tuberculosis* in the tissues.

infection is localised to one kidney or one epididymis then the infected and damaged tissue is removed.

3. Tuberculous peritonitis is an acute condition in which the peritoneum becomes covered with miliary tubercles (that is, whitish spots like millet seeds). In this case the condition presents with generalised abdominal pain and can be confused with all the other causes of abdominal pain.

Prophylaxis

It is possible to vaccinate a person who is tuberculin negative with a vaccine prepared from an attenuated bovine strain (Bacille Calmette-Guerin or B.C.G.). This is not considered worthwhile, because of the slight risk attached, in well-developed countries except for subjects in high-risk areas, for example doctors and nurses. In under-developed countries primary tuberculous infection occurs at an early age and B.C.G. vaccination is worthwhile at as early an age as possible to prevent subsequent clinically significant infection.

Treatment

Streptomycin, para-amino salycilic acid (PAS), isonicotinic acid hydrazide (INAH) and rifampicin are the drugs of choice. The organism is killed only by prolonged treatment which, if started, should continue for at *least* 2 years. In order to prevent resistance developing, the drugs are used in rotation.

ACTINOMYCOSIS

Clinical features

This is an infection produced by the fungus *Actinomyces israeli*. It is contracted by contact with infected material, usually of soil origin.

The common place for infection to occur is in the region of the jaw and side of the neck, the infection usually entering the tissues via carious teeth. The infected area is characteristically very hard and indurated. Eventually it breaks down to discharge a thin pus containing yellowish granules. Several sinuses then tend to form within the indurated area with considerable tissue destruction.

Treatment

This is by incision and drainage of all abscess cavities, with curetting of sinuses. This local treatment is aided by high doses of penicillin to which the organism is partially sensitive.

CANDIDIASIS

This is the commonest fungal infection in man. *Candida albicans* is a normal inhabitant of the digestive tract and vagina. Occasionally the balance between candida and other micro-organisms becomes upset—for example, by the administration of broad spectrum antibiotics—in favour of the former; clinical 'thrush' is the result. In the mouth and vagina the mucosa becomes inflamed and covered with whitish spots due to the colonies of fungi.

Treatment

This is by the antibiotic nystatin applied topically as a lozenge when the infection involves the mouth and as a pessary when the vagina is affected.

Fig. 1.7. *Echinococcus granulosus.* The two eye-like structures are suckers and the head has two rows of hooks around it. The caudal segment contains eggs. The adult worm is between 5 and 6 mm in length.

This condition is due to infection by the platyhelminth *Echinococcus granulosus* (Fig. 1.7). This is the tapeworm whose host may be dogs, wolves, coyotes and related animals. The adult tapeworm produces eggs which are excreted in the faeces of the dog. If these are deposited on vegetables which are then eaten by the human without being washed, the eggs develop in the intestine into larvae which burrow through the wall to enter the portal bloodstream. In this way the larvae are distributed to the liver, lungs or rarely any of the tissues of the body. They then develop into cysts which may reach a large size. The cyst is lined with a germinal epithelium which produces numerous daughter cysts each capable, if liberated, of independent existence.

Clinical features

The condition should be suspected in any patient living in an area in which the disease is known to exist (for example around the Mediterranean and in some parts of South Wales), who develops a mass in the liver or lungs. Blood count may reveal an eosinophilia. The final confirmation is by the finding of a positive complement fixation test in the patient's serum.

Treatment

If symptoms are being caused by the cyst then a surgical operation is required. The cyst is exposed, some of the fluid is carefully aspirated, making sure that no spillage occurs as it may contain daughter cysts which can become implanted and develop in adjacent tissue. The aspirated fluid is replaced with 2% formalin which will destroy the lining of the cyst together with any contained daughter cysts. After the formalin has been left within the cyst for 10 minutes, the contents of the cyst are removed. There is no need to remove the wall of the cyst which may be deeply imbedded in, for example, the liver.

AMOEBIASIS

Clinical features

This is due to infection with the protozoa *Entamoeba histolytica*. This is an organism which is very similar in appearance to the amoeba found in ponds. It is contracted by the ingestion of cysts existing in contaminated food and water. Intestinal amoebiasis results in the development of inflammation of the distal part of the colon, the symptoms of which are diarrhoea with the passage of mucus and blood. Extra-intestinal infection is also possible as the organism may spread beyond the confines of the large bowel to infect the tissue around the caecum and the liver (amoebic hepatitis).

Diagnosis is made by the examination of a fresh specimen of stool when the amoebae will be seen moving in their characteristic way.

Treatment

Intestinal amoebiasis may be treated with tetracyclines combined with emetine. Recently metronidazole (Flagyl) has been shown to be valuable. Hepatitis is more difficult to treat and may require the drug chloroquine combined with emetine.

Chapter 2. Care of the surgical patient

PRE-OPERATIVE CARE

INTRODUCTION

The patient who is admitted for surgery, if normal, will be terrified. Calm and sympathetic handling at this stage will often make the difference between a co-operative patient and one who creates difficulties throughout his stay. Anxiety on the part of the patient is often manifest by aggressive behaviour with apparently trivial complaints; for example, patients may object to the form filling that is required, to the food, to members of staff and so on. Sympathetic listening is often the best method of handling such behaviour. Aggression must *never* be matched by aggression and indeed the harsh reply is only justified, and that rarely, in order to achieve a definite objective such as to persuade the patient to accept treatment.

The precise nature of the pre-operative 'work-up' depends on what operation will be performed, but certain general rules apply.

The consent form

Informed consent, which consists of a reasonable explanation of the nature and intended purpose of the operation, is required. It is strongly advised that consent be obtained in writing and witnessed by a member of the medical staff, although this is not a legal requirement as situations exist when written consent is impossible to obtain, such as with an unconscious patient.

Over the age of 16 all patients of sound mind can consent for a procedure to be carried out. It is usual to obtain the consent of the legal parent or guardian for all patients between the age of 16 and 18 as the patient is still a minor. Below the age of 16 the consent of the legal parent or guardian must be obtained. An important element in the question of consent is the effectiveness of treatment. If, for some reason or other, consent cannot be obtained for a minor because, for example, the parents cannot be contacted, the administration of life-saving treatment is paramount and delay, simply because the form has not been signed, should not be allowed to occur.

Certain religious sects object to the administration of blood transfusion. A patient who is not a minor is perfectly competent to refuse blood if the refusal is dictated by conscience. In the eyes of the law, therefore, the giving of blood without the patient's consent constitutes an assault. In the case of a minor it is possible, if circumstances justify, for the patient to be taken under the care of the Local Authority (Children's Department) by Magistrate's order and the Authority will then decide whether to consent to blood transfusion and any other necessary procedures.

Labelling the patient

Most hospitals now have a system whereby a label is placed around the wrist of all patients on admission giving name and hospital number. This prevents the wrong patient being given the wrong blood, for example, particularly when the patient is unconscious.

The surgeons

Some patients will wish to know which surgeon will perform the operation. Discriminating patients will also wish to know which anaesthetist will give the anaesthetic. Whilst it is true that all patients undergoing an operation are *under the care* of a Consultant (and this is what the term Consultant means) no undertaking is implied or given that he will actually, personally do the operation. In fact the operation may be carried out by the Registrar, S.H.O. or House Surgeon.

Nutrition and Diet

Clearly this is of fundamental importance if wounds are to heal. Ideally the patient should be in a normal nutritional state at the time of operation. Four categories of patients exist in which this may not be so. These are:

1. The elderly, who may be short of all food constituents, including particularly vitamin C and iron.
2. Those with wasting diseases such as carcinoma, intestinal fistulae, uraemia and intestinal abnormalities of absorption such as Crohn's disease or ulcerative colitis.

3. Patients with dysphagia.
4. Severe psychiatric problems. Patients with 'food fads'.

If there is doubt about the level of nutrition, help should be sought from the dietician. Often ridiculously simple things may be at fault particularly in the old, such as ill fitting teeth, difficulty in preparing food due to poor eyesight or degenerative diseases of the joints making movement to and from the kitchen difficult.

The haemoglobin should be normal. If it is not and if there is time it should be restored by giving iron or whichever haematinic is appropriate. In more urgent cases, a blood transfusion may be necessary pre-operatively. Vitamin C 100 mg t.d.s. will restore the body's requirements for this within a few hours.

An outline of special diets for particular patients is listed below:
1. *Patients with jaundice* – low fat diet.
2. *Uraemic patients* – diet low in protein.
3. *Diabetic patients* – carbohydrate restricted diet, details of which should always be carried with the patient.

Pre-operative nursing checks

These always include taking and recording the weight, the pulse rate, temperature, respiration rate and an examination of the urine. This latter test is necessary to exclude previously undiagnosed diabetes, renal disease and liver disease and is carried out with Labstix which tests for the following abnormal constituents: glucose, blood, bile and protein. In addition the pH (acidity) and specific gravity of the urine is measured. Cloudiness, particularly of an alkaline urine (pH greater than 7) is common and is due to insoluble phosphates which will clear if the urine is acidified with acetic acid. The findings are recorded on a chart (Fig. 2.1).

The skin, hair and shaving

An elective operation must be performed through clean skin. If the part to be operated on is hairy, such as the lower abdomen, then shaving of the skin is necessary. But, if the operation cannot reasonably be expected to reach a hair bearing area, shaving is not required. There is no need to perform a pubic shave for operations on the upper abdomen such as cholecystectomy or gastrectomy, providing that an area to at least 3 inches below the umbilicus is clear. Remember that some skin free of hair will be required for dressing and the application of sticking-plaster. If shaving is necessary it must be performed at least on the day prior to operation so that the small ends of hair have time to be cleared from the surface of the skin. Shaving in the

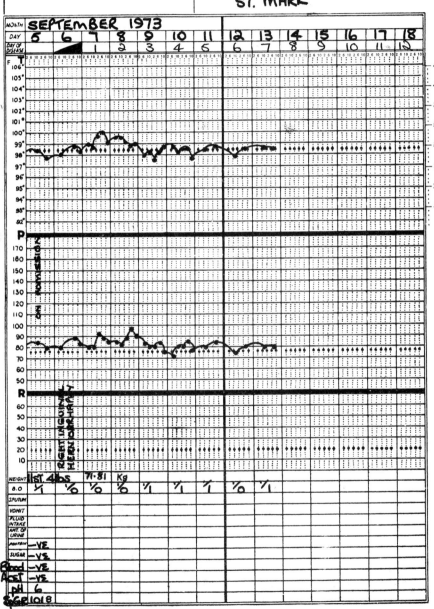

Fig. 2.1. A typical well kept surgical ward chart.

theatre is a disastrous failure of pre-operative preparation because small hairs find their way into wounds and are often the cause of infection.

Operating on the head usually requires the scalp to be shaved. A common exception to this is the removal of sebaceous cysts, when the incision is made with an intact head of hair.

Procedures on the face and neck usually do not require any shaving although parotidectomy will mean the loss of the sideboard on that side. Patients for head and neck surgery should have a well fitting plastic cap applied before going to the theatre to keep the hair out of the operative field.

Cystoscopy does not require a perineal shave and, nor does haemorrhoidectomy.

All patients, for whatever operations, should have a bath on the evening before the operation. It is, of course, quite impossible to sterilise the skin surface and no attempt at this should be made with disinfectants or antiseptics but ingrained dirt from feet and skin should be washed off with ordinary soap and warm water.

For operation on the abdomen the umbilicus should be cleaned and *checked*. This neglected little pit often harbours quite surprising residues of dirt occasionally compacting into an actual lump, called an ompholith or umbolith.

Chest

All patients must stop smoking before operation. It is an extremely interesting observation to ask patients to give just one cough and it is possible on this basis to tell if they are cigarette smokers or not. The larynx, trachea and bronchi are constantly irritated by cigarette smoke and ultimately become irreversibly damaged, giving rise to the husky voice, the productive cough and, in some unfortunate people, cancer of the lung.

In those with a bad chest, physiotherapy will help to clear secretions and will teach patients what is required of them after operation. The sputum should be cultured so that the infecting organism can be isolated and the appropriate antibiotic given if required.

Teeth and other personal effects

False teeth must be removed just prior to the operation and then stored in a cardboard pot marked 'teeth'. If they are wrapped in a paper handkerchief or other unsuitable receptacle they may be thrown away by the ward maid.

With an elective operation attention to dental hygiene is important. Loose, broken teeth should be extracted and the sound remaining teeth cleaned. In an emergency it may be necessary to extract loose teeth before the operation, in the anaesthetic room.

Spectacles must be carefully placed in the patient's locker. Contact lenses should be removed and safely stored and false eyes noted. A classic pitfall is to record a fixed, non-moving pupil in a patient recovering from anaesthetic when in reality a very good false eye is the cause!

Artificial legs and arms should be removed and carefully stored.

Rings should either be removed and placed in the safe or should be retained in place with a small strip of elastoplast.

The drugs given as premedication are mainly to allay anxiety. (One of the effective ways of doing this, which should not be neglected, is by sympathetic explanation of the preceding and following procedures). Usually, two types in combination are given, these are opiates or other sedatives such as papaveretum 2 mgm/7Kg body weight with an atropine-like agent, for example, scopolamine 0.4 mg. Scopolamine is particularly useful because, besides blocking the vagus nerve and causing dryness of the mouth and protecting the heart from vagal overactivity which causes undue bradycardia, it is also an antiemetic and a sedative. The actual dose of these agents depends on the anaesthetist and is tailored to the patient's level of anxiety. Over the age of 65–70 premedicant drugs are often not required at all, and one has to beware of the long-continued sedative effect of a too 'heavy' premedicant continuing long after the operation into the early post-operative phase, causing unwanted respiratory depression.

Children pose a different problem and different drugs are used. Up to the age of approximately 18 months no premedication is required. From 18 months to approximately 8 years trimeprazine tartrate (Vallergan) 3 mg/Kg body weight is a useful drug as it can be given orally and is a very effective sedative. Over the age of 8 an adult type of premedication is given with due reference to dose in relation to the child's weight.

No elective operation must be performed with either food or fluid in the stomach. For this reason 6 full hours must be allowed to elapse between the last meal or drink and the onset of anaesthesia. If this is not adhered to there is a danger of the inhalation of gastric contents on induction of the anaesthetic. If any doubt exists it is safer to pass a nasogastric tube and to empty the stomach by this means prior to anaesthetic. This is also the safest way to ensure an empty stomach in emergency operations.

Bowels

A universal finding is that the normal daily bowel rhythm is interrupted on admission to hospital. Most patients, except those for very minor procedures, benefit from the administration of a small disposable enema to clear the rectum and lower colon on the night before operation.

Before colonic surgery the bowel must be rendered as clear as possible of faeces and bacteria. The patient is placed on a fluid diet on admission to hospital. Over the two days prior to surgery Mist. magnesium sulphate 10 ml is given three times a day and the bowel emptied with a daily rectal washout. Neomycin 1 g and metronidazole 200 mgm are prescribed eight hourly. Of course, if the patient is sub-acutely obstructed or loaded with faeces, satisfactory preparation may take longer than 48 hours.

AFTER OPERATION

Recovery from the anaesthetic and pain relief

Nowadays, nearly all hospitals have recovery wards. It is therefore possible to ensure that the anaesthetised patient recovers coughing and eyelid reflexes whilst in the theatre area under continuous care. If the patient is deeply anaesthetised in the recovery room, then he should be nursed in the semi-prone position until the coughing reflex returns. Oxygen, 28% via a Ventimask, should be given for 1–4 hours and the pulse, respiration and blood pressure measured and recorded every 15 minutes. Only when the patient has fully recovered consciousness should he be allowed to make the journey back to the ward. Once in the ward the degree of surveillance can be slackened a little but pulse, respiration and blood pressure should be recorded every 30 minutes until they have become stable. There is frequently a post-operative fall in blood pressure which is physiological and providing that the extremities are warm and well perfused with blood this should cause no anxiety. It is difficult to provide an absolute lower permitted level of systolic blood pressure but in general this should remain above 100 mmHg.

At first, for 1–2 hours, the patient should be nursed flat but, as recovery proceeds, a sitting up position should be arranged as soon as this can be managed without difficulty. This allows easier breathing and coughing with better aeration of the bases of the lungs.

It is at this stage that the patient usually first becomes aware of pain. The pain which results from an operation can be extremely intense and adequate relief is essential. The typical drugs used to secure this are papaveretum 20 mg or pethidine 100 mg (for an average sized adult). Both these drugs result in some respiratory depression and to some extent adequate analgesia is a compromise with not too profound depression of breathing. Generally 4 hourly intramuscular injections of either of these drugs for up to 3 or 4 doses will be sufficient to make the patient comfortable.

Some anaesthetists will ensure a controllable area of local anaesthesia by the use of an epidural catheter. This nylon catheter is introduced to the outside of the spinal dura mater and lignocaine can be injected down it to spread for a limited distance up and down the outside of the emerging spinal roots. By siting the tip of the catheter at just the desired level and by varying the volume of lignocaine injected so can the area of anaesthesia be controlled. This technique is particularly applicable to thoracic operations or operations on the abdomen when it is essential that there is no inhibition of breathing and coughing, because of pain, for example in patients with very bad chests.

Usually by 24–48 hours after operation little in the way of pain relief is required.

The post-operative care of the chest

Pre-operative physiotherapy should have ensured a clear chest by the time the operation is performed. Smoking before and after operation is banned. After operation the physiotherapist will carry out deep breathing exercises and encourage coughing but it is the duty of every member of the medical and nursing staff to help the patients get rid of their retained sputum. Coughing is essential to clear the bronchi of any plugs of mucus. It is a useful manoeuvre to teach the patient to hold the incision with his hand during coughing in order to minimise jerking of the wound with consequent pain. If these mucus plugs are allowed to remain, the lung distal to them is no longer aerated and will become infected. This is the origin of the post-operative pulmonary collapse and pneumonia which is so commonly seen in cigarette smokers.

Inhalation of steam with tinct. benz. co. is helpful or if the mucus is very tenacious the detergent properties of Alevaire used as an inhalation are useful.

Fluids and the care of 'drips'

For a procedure that does not involve an intestinal anastomosis or an abdominal operation, oral fluids can be allowed directly on recovery from the anaesthetic. All patients are thirsty and will tend to drink too much if allowed. This often results in abdominal distension, nausea and vomiting. Therefore, at first, plain water in small quantities in the range of 30 ml hourly should be given. As the effects of the anaesthetic wear off the volume of fluid allowed can be increased rapidly.

If the operation has been on the abdomen with opening of the peritoneal cavity, there will be a post-operative paralytic ileus. In this case fluid will not pass from the stomach to the duodenum and small bowel and will not be absorbed. Even so, sips of water are allowed to keep the mouth moist and comfortable.

In the absence of peritonitis, paralytic ileus recovers within 48 to 72 hours. On listening to the abdomen with a stethoscope bowel sounds will then be heard. Patients often complain of cramping 'wind pains' at this stage. The most satisfactory indication that all is well with the bowel is the passage of flatus per anum. When this happens the intravenous infusion may be taken down and oral feeding progressively increased towards normal.

Generally the fluid intake in the absence of renal failure should be such that at least 1,000 ml of urine are produced in a 24 hour period. For the first 24 hours therefore, in an average man, as much as 4,000 ml of intravenous fluid may be required. Some of this will go to make up the deficit that will have resulted from the pre-operative deprivation of fluids; some will be secreted into the small bowel where it will be sequestered away and where it will not be available until the paralytic ileus recovers, and some will be used for the normal daily fluid requirement. For a patient with normal kidneys, lungs and heart (which includes the majority of surgical patients), an excess of water and sodium is an advantage as the kidney excretes the excess and the metabolic processes of the body are thus well supplied with the raw materials for maintaining normal acid-base relationships and serum electrolytes. A typical fluid balance after major abdominal surgery is shown in Table 2.1.

On a more practical level, intravenous infusions or drips must be constantly maintained. If they are allowed to stop then the blood in the needle or the catheter in the vein will thrombose. In this case it is often possible to restart them by flushing out the needle with normal saline (which must be suitable for intravenous injection). Some intravenous fluids are more prone to produce damage to the vein endothelium than others with consequent venous inflammation and thrombosis. For example, concentrated solutions such as 30% or 40% laevulose and solutions of amino-acids and carbohydrates tend to produce venous thrombosis in the superficial vein into which they are placed and the patient will actually experience pain while the fluid is being infused. These solutions have to be given into a

Table 2.1. Typical fluid balance for the 1st 24 hours after a major abdominal operation, a nasogastric tube having been left in place.

IN		OUT	
Oral sips only	100 ml	Urine	1,000 ml
Intravenous—N. Saline	2,000 ml	Faeces	nil
Dextrose Saline	2,000 ml	Gastric aspirate	100 ml
		Insensible loss	1,000 ml
Totals	4,100 ml		2,100 ml
Positive balance 2,000 ml			

Notes A. The apparently large positive balance will be distributed between (1) The deficit that resulted from the pre-operative fluid deprivation, and (2), the fluid pooling in the small bowel due to paralytic ileus.
B. Oral sips of water are allowed in spite of the paralytic ileus to keep the mouth moist and comfortable.
C. Insensible loss is made up of water vapour in the breath and sweat from the skin. It increases in fever and in hot weather.

large vein so that they rapidly become diluted by the blood. For this purpose a long plastic catheter may be threaded through a peripheral vein into the superior vena cava (see Fig. 3.1).

Skin and pressure areas

Patients may not be able to move after an operation because of pain. Because of this, many hours may be spent in one position. The whole of the body's weight is then transmitted through four areas; the two heels and the two buttocks. If the patient is simply allowed to lie without movement, pressure sores will develop. The heels and buttocks will become sore and eventually the skin will break down to form a pressure sore (Fig. 2.2). Therefore the patient must be moved every 2 hours from one position to another.

Even in patients who have undergone quite major abdominal procedures it is an advantage for them to stand out of bed during bed-making. In old patients this encourages the maintenance of balance and righting reflexes that can so easily be lost for ever.

Drains

Drains are left in wounds for one of four reasons:
1. To drain a potential space; for example following splenectomy or resection of any other intraperitoneal organ.

Fig. 2.2. A buttock bedsore.

2. To provide a track to an anastomosis that may subsequently leak; for example, colonic anastomoses.

3. To drain away fluid which it is known will otherwise collect, for example the lymph which appears beneath a mastectomy incision.

4. To drain a pus-filled cavity, e.g. after incision of an abscess.

Drains used in the abdomen are commonly of the corrugated plastic type and should have a radio-opaque stripe so that their position can readily be identified on x-ray (Fig. 2.3). They require suitable dressing externally so that any serum or blood can be absorbed as it is discharged onto the surface of the skin. It is unwise to leave most drains in place for more than 5 to 7 days and they should be gradually withdrawn over a period of several days. They do not cause pain even when they are being removed.

Drains used to provide a track should remain in place for 5 days and then be withdrawn. To prevent the tip of the drain causing pressure necrosis of underlying bowel it should be withdrawn by one inch on the second day.

Chest drains are dealt with later, as are 'T' tube drains of the common bile duct and suction drainage following mastectomy (see Fig. 17.12).

Urethral catheters

Urethral catheters are of two main types. The first of these is a plain tube, usually plastic, which is inserted into the bladder and after all the urine has drained, is removed. The second type is the self-retaining catheter and the most common of these is the Foley balloon

Fig. 2.3. Wound drains. A corrugated, B Penrose and C plastic tube.

catheter (see Fig. 15.38). When a self-retaining catheter has been placed in the bladder it should be connected to a plastic drainage bag, using full sterile precautions. Once the system has been set up it must be left undisturbed and the tube must *never be disconnected* as this is the point at which infection so commonly enters the bladder and urinary tract. Most plastic urine bags now have a tap whereby they can be emptied, thus obviating the need for disconnection of the tubes (see Fig. 15.34).

A plastic Foley catheter can be left in the bladder for 2–3 weeks at a time. When this situation obtains it is essential to ensure that no infection is allowed to enter the urine and all patients should therefore receive a suitable antibacterial agent such as sulphadimidine or ampicillin.

If the catheter is left in place for several weeks or if it is permanent then it should be changed regularly (every 2–3 weeks) because deposits tend to form on it.

Wound care

A clean wound, properly dressed in the operating theatre, is probably best left alone. If, however, the dressing becomes soaked with blood or serum it will need to be changed. A wide variety of dressings are available as well as those made up by nurses consisting of gauze and adhesive tape. The main function of a dressing is to prevent the wound from suffering physical trauma—although it should in addition be bacteriologically sterile when applied, it is impossible to provide a complete bacteriological barrier since bacteria live in the depths of the skin at the edge of the wound.

Wound healing is a complex process that proceeds for many months. Sutures are removed when they are no longer required to hold the edges of the skin together. The length of time for this varies with the particular skin incision. In the case of the abdomen and limbs, sutures should be left for 10 days. If there is any tension, such as in mastectomy scars, they may be left for considerably longer; up to 21 days. On the face and neck, sutures should be removed much earlier to prevent ugly cross scarring. In this case the wound is sewn up with deep sutures which result in the skin edges staying together almost without skin sutures at all. Alternate sutures are removed on day 2 and the rest on day 3. Naturally sutures are only removed if the wound edges appear to be safely united.

Different methods are used to secure wounds. The most usual is with a simple through-and-through suture using black silk or monofilament nylon. Very long wounds, such as those resulting from operations to peripheral arteries, are often sewn up with a single continuous suture. Wounds in babies can be sewn up with subcuticular sutures in which the edges of the skin are held together with a suture placed just beneath the surface. This suture may be of monofilament nylon, which will have to be removed on day 10, or it may be of catgut or polyglycolic acid (Dexon), in which case removal is not required. Some wounds can be sewn up with catgut, for example incisions in the scrotum, the stitches being allowed to fall out spontaneously after about 2 weeks.

Even though sutures are removed on the 10th day, the wound as a whole has very little strength at this stage, being united mainly by epithelial cells; immature collagen and fibrin. Patients with laparotomy wounds should be advised not to strain for another month and thereafter to increase gradually the stress applied over another period of 3 months. Then at 6 months from the operation the strength of the scar approximates fairly closely to the pre-operative state.

A common question after operation is 'When is it safe to drive a car?' Experiments conducted with a simulator indicated that 2 weeks should be allowed to elapse from the time of the operation in the majority of cases; providing the car is no more than a small family saloon the average patient should be able to handle it satisfactorily at this stage.

Swimming beyond the depth of the patient should not be permitted until 3 months from operation.

Wound infection

Operations can be divided into 'dirty' and 'clean'. In dirty operations known contamination of the wound occurs and cannot be prevented.

then the heparin must be immediately discontinued and the anti-dote, protamine sulphate, given intravenously in the dose of 1 ml of a 1% solution for each 1,000 units of heparin.

Ligation of the major veins is a procedure which very rarely has to be performed when recurrent episodes of pulmonary embolization occur in spite of adequate anticoagulant therapy. The heparin must be continued after ligation, otherwise further clots form above the site of venous interruption.

Pulmonary embolus

This occurs when a clot from a vein in the lower limb or the pelvis detaches and becomes lodged in the pulmonary arterial tree.

Clinical features. A massive embolus obstructs the right heart output and causes rapid death from heart failure. Less severe cases present with shock, breathlessness and cyanosis, often accompanied by pain behind the sternum. Still milder episodes present with pleural pain, (which is felt in the chest wall and is aggravated by taking a deep breath), dyspnoea and frequently haemoptysis.

If the patient survives the embolus, then dissolution of the clot will occur and the patient can make a complete recovery even after a most serious episode.

It may be difficult to differentiate between a pulmonary embolus and a chest infection or a post-operative coronary thrombosis. A chest x-ray in the early stages is often quite normal although within a few hours patchy shadowing of the affected segment of the lung takes place. An E.C.G. may help in differentiating between an embolus and a coronary thrombosis. In the former, there will be the changes of right heart strain.

It is important to know that a pulmonary embolus may occur without any preceding warning signs of thrombosis in the leg. This applies to the great majority of fatal emboli. Indeed, once there are obvious clinical features of deep vein thrombosis, detachment of an organized and adherent clot from the limb is unlikely, provided that anticoagulant therapy has been commenced so that fresh clot formation is inhibited.

Treatment. Morphia is given for the pain, oxygen administered and heparin treatment commenced if the patient is not already on anti-coagulants. It will be obvious that this regime will do no harm even if a coronary thrombosis has been misdiagnosed as a pulmonary embolism.

In some selected cases in special cardiac units, embolectomy may be performed to remove the obstruction in the pulmonary trunk with the assistance of a heart-lung by-pass machine.

Wound dehiscence

Very occasionally a wound bursts. If the wound is a laparotomy wound this is disastrous because the abdominal contents are forced out. Often the first indication that such an event is about to occur is the escape of a small quantity of bloodstained fluid from the wound (the 'pink fluid sign'). A minor strain, such as moving in bed or coughing, is then the final act which results in rupture of all the layers of the wound.

Certain conditions are associated with poor healing and these are:
1. Disseminated neoplastic disease, especially in the presence of jaundice and anaemia.
2. Uraemia.
3. Scurvy (Vitamin C deficiency).
4. Poor general nutrition.
5. High doses of steroids.
In patients with any of these conditions special precautions must be taken. Pre-operative care should be designed to return the patient to as normal a state as possible. At the operation, deep-tension sutures, which are those that are placed through all layers of the abdominal wall, may be required. If there is any doubt as to the healing of the wound it is wise to leave sutures in place and only to remove them cautiously, perhaps a few at a time.

If an abdominal wound bursts, the intestines literally pour into the bed. The first aid in this situation is to wrap the intestine gently in a sterile towel against the abdomen. Arrangements are then made for the immediate resuture of the abdominal wall in the operating theatre. Amazing as it may seem patients rarely come to harm and the abdomen then heals well.

Visiting

There was a time when visitors were considered to be a nuisance. In these more enlightened days it is realised that a patient's family is of paramount importance to his return to full health. There is absolutely no need to exclude children rigidly from an adult ward. The main consideration is the mental trauma that children may suffer when confronted with sick people. However, children are more resilient than we tend to think and are well able to assimilate what is, in fact, a part of life. It seems foolish to protect children against all such sights and sounds and smells and there is no doubt that a mother, father or grandparent can have the vital strength to recover revivified by the visit of a beloved small child.

After operation there is no reason why a close relative should not visit briefly only an hour or two after the completion of the procedure. What relatives sometimes do not appreciate in this circumstance is that a patient at such a time does not remember anything of the visit. From day one onwards visiting is best organised to fit in with the routine of the ward. Relatives should be encouraged to visit often for short periods of time, say only 10 minutes at first. Undoubtedly long visits can be exhausting and very difficult for a patient to terminate whilst still preserving the social graces.

Telling the patient

This subject always engenders much discussion. In general terms patients should be told precisely, in a way that they can understand, what is wrong with them, what operation they should have or have had and what the likely outcome will be. The exception to this simple rule is in the case of a cancer. If a patient is told bluntly that he has cancer, English usage being what it is, this is equated with a sentence of death and removal of hope is an unkind and usually unnecessary act. Other synonyms such as a 'growth' or 'tumour' do not carry the same connotation and can therefore be used with caution. Complete frankness is necessary with relatives, whose co-operation must be sought in this aspect of the management of the patient.

Certain patients must be told of impending death for their peace of mind. These include devout Roman Catholics, priests and nuns. In these people this information usually produces a state of great calm.

Rehabilitation

This is the single most important part of being in hospital. It is the point of the whole exercise of becoming better. With minor procedures such as hernias or varicose veins, little difficulty will be experienced. With more major operations, however, patients are often extremely anxious and fearful of their capacity to perform their job. If a man is off work for a year there is a considerable risk that he will never be fit for employment again.

For physical defects, such as follow amputation, departments of rehabilitation are available to advise as to suitable occupations and to help with appliances that aid the patient. A good example of a device in use for many years in patients who have undergone amputation of the hand, is the simple forked hook with which many patients become extremely dextrous.

Often the thing that counts most is the counsel of the bedside conversation with a wise and experienced nursing sister. Many patients owe their re-establishment into their lives to such an informal talk.

Chapter 3. Shock

Shock is of extreme importance to the surgeon. One of the reasons for the reduction in operative mortality in major surgical procedures in recent years is our greater knowledge of the aetiology and management of this condition. Most major hospitals now have Intensive Therapy Units which are primarily concerned with the treatment of shocked patients.

Clinical features

Shock is the term used to describe a very typical clinical state which comprises:
1. Pale, cold, and sweating skin with peripheral cyanosis.
2. Rapid, low volume pulse. As the shock state progresses the pulse may become impalpable at the wrist.
3. Low blood pressure. This is a relatively late feature and indicates serious failure of the body's compensating mechanism.

In severe cases there may also be dyspnoea, thirst, nausea or vomiting. The patient may be confused and restless.

Aetiology

Shock is produced by a wide variety of circumstances, all of which result in a state in which there is a failure of perfusion of the tissues with blood.

In the pump mechanism that makes up the cardiovascular system, it is obvious that three basic circumstances can produce this state of affairs:

1. Loss of fluid to prime the pump; this is termed *hypovolaemic shock*
2. Dilatation of the peripheral vessels. This increases the capacity of the vascular tree, and so reduces the effective blood volume available for tissue perfusion; this is termed *normovolaemic shock*.
3. Heart failure, which reduces the effectiveness of the cardiac pump; this is *cardiogenic shock*.

Hypovolaemic shock

Hypovolaemia is the condition which occurs when fluid is lost from the circulation and is not replaced; it simply means that there is insufficient blood to fill the vascular system. It occurs in severe haemorrhage, or when large quantities of plasma leak from the skin as the result of severe burns, or when water and electrolytes are lost in profuse vomiting or diarrhoea.

When the blood volume is reduced, the following chain of events will take place. There will be a reduction in the amount of blood returning via the veins to the right side of the heart; the pressure in these veins (that is the *central venous pressure*) falls. Since it is obvious that the heart can only pump the blood that arrives to it from the veins, there will be a reduction in the amount of blood pumped into the peripheral arterial circulation and there will therefore be a fall in the cardiac output. At first this is compensated for by constriction of the peripheral arteries of the body, which is partly a sympathetic reflex mechanism, and partly due to the secretion of adrenalin and noradrenalin from the adrenal medulla. These hormones produce peripheral arterial constriction and acceleration of the heart rate. This combination of sympathetic over-action and adrenal secretion is the explanation of the cold, pale, sweating extremities and rapid pulse seen in patients with hypovolaemic shock. This mechanism at first maintains the blood pressure and therefore the blood flow to the vital organs, but progressive fluid loss eventually reaches the stage at which compensation can no longer be maintained, and the blood pressure then falls.

A continued low blood pressure may produce a series of irreversible changes, so that the patient may die in spite of later fluid replacement. The oxygen lack affects all the vital organs; there may be damage to the brain, the heart may fail due to inadequate coronary perfusion, there may be tubular necrosis of the kidney resulting in renal failure, and there may be damage to the liver and the adrenals. In the tissues themselves inadequate blood flow may produce capillary paralysis and dilatation, so that copious fluid loss occurs into the interstitial spaces.

Normovolaemic shock

In this condition the blood volume is normal, but the capacity of the blood vessels is increased. This may be seen in the *vasovagal syndrome*, which is the simple faint which may follow severe pain or emotional disturbance. The mechanism of this is a reflex dilatation of the blood vessels in muscle together with vagal cardiac slowing. This syndrome may be recognised because the shock picture is accompanied by slowing of the heart and responds to the simple measure of lying the patient flat with the legs elevated.

In surgical practice normovolaemic shock may be seen in septicaemia (particularly when caused by gram-negative organisms). Here the picture may be complicated because, in addition to dilatation of peripheral vessels, there may also be fluid loss from vomiting, etc., and the effect of chemical or bacterial toxins on the heart.

Cardiogenic shock

If the heart is unable to pump blood around the body, obviously adequate tissue perfusion with blood becomes impossible. Such a situation may arise following a large myocardial infarct due to coronary artery occlusion, or may occur in an extensive pulmonary emobolism.

STAGES OF SHOCK

These are divided into the following:
1. Early.
2. Reversible.
3. Refractory.
4. Irreversible.

In early shock, although some of the signs described above are present, they are rapidly corrected by prompt treatment.

Reversible shock means that the patient can be returned to normal, provided that rapid adequate restoration of the circulation is secured.

In refractory shock careful and skilled handling is required if the patient is to recover, and there are often complications, such as renal tubular necrosis, which require management over several weeks before full recovery is achieved.

Irreversible shock, as its name implies, means that prolonged and severe impairment of tissue perfusion has produced irreversible changes in vital organs so that, even though adequate tissue perfusion is eventually restored, the patient succumbs.

The treatment for the shocked patient obviously depends on diagnosis.

Where haemorrhage is the cause of the shock, further bleeding must be arrested; this may require direct pressure to a wound, the application of an artery forceps to a spurting vessel in a laceration, or surgical exploration where continued bleeding is the result of a peptic ulcer haemorrhage, a ruptured spleen, or an ectopic pregnancy.

Hypovolaemic shock requires rapid restoration of the blood volume. The appropriate fluid should be replaced; blood in the case of haemorrhage, plasma in severe burns, and saline in profuse vomiting and diarrhoea. In severely shocked patients it is useful to set up a caval drip; a long (60 cm) nylon catheter is introduced into the superior vena cava via one of the veins in the arm. This catheter serves a double function. The first of these is to introduce the appropriate fluid as quickly as possible into the circulation, and the second is to allow measurement of the central venous pressure (Fig. 3.1). In hypovolaemic shock, the central venous pressure is low, but as the transfusion of fluid becomes adequate it will rise and should be maintained at a level of between + 2 and + 8 cm of water, measured from the upper border of the heart. This is marked by the junction between the sternum and the manubrium (the angle of Louis), when the patient is in the lying position. The measurement of the central venous pressure protects the patient against over-transfusion and therefore cardiac failure.

In order to measure the effects of treatment, it is essential to make frequent recordings of pulse, blood pressure, the central

Fig. 3.1. Diagram of a central venous pressure catheter. This is passed into the superior vena cava via an arm vein. The manometer is filled with saline; the C.V.P. is the height in centimetres of the water level in the manometer above the base line, which is taken as the junction of the sternum and the manubrium.

venous pressure, urinary output, and the general appearance of the patient. Often the most sensitive index of recovery will be the return of colour to the periphery together with a rise in skin temperature. If the skin is pink, dry and warm, then it is likely that adequate tissue perfusion is taking place.

In order to measure urinary output a self-retaining catheter is introduced into the bladder, and the volume of urine secreted each hour is measured. As a rough guide this should be equal to, or more than, 1 ml per minute

Relief of pain by means of an injection of morphia is necessary where pain is a marked feature. Obviously, any fracture should be splinted to reduce pain from this source, as well as to prevent further injury.

Excessive warmth should be avoided; this produces vasodilatation of the skin vessels, thereby diverting available blood from vital organs. Oxygen is not usually required since the arterial blood is fully oxygenated, unless there is an associated chest injury or respiratory depression due to a head injury.

When a patient is extremely ill, and multiple procedures are being carried out rapidly, it is important to chart precisely when therapy is started, what is given, and to note the patient's general condition, as well as recording pulse, blood pressure, central venous pressure, and urinary output. Quite apart from absolute values, the trend of the patient is often of importance in judging response to treatment.

Treatment of septicaemic shock

The measures outlined for the patient with hypovolaemic shock should all be carried out in this condition, with the difference that the infecting organism must be eliminated with the appropriate antibiotic. The condition can be extremely confusing in its early phase because peripheral vasodilatation takes place, so that often the periphery is warm, in contrast to the usual picture of cold, pale, extremities seen in the more common hypovalaemic shock. Diagnosis is confirmed by blood culture, and while waiting for the result to come back, a broad spectrum antibiotic, such as ampicillin or gentamicin, is commenced, although the drug regime may have to be altered when the sensitivity of the organism has been checked by the bacteriologist.

Plasma or dextran is given by drip in order to fill the increased capacity of the dilated vascular system.

In long continued stress due to shock it may be necessary to give hydrocortisone 100 mg 6 hourly intravenously to combat failure of the adrenal cortex.

Chapter 4. Burns

Major burns still present serious problems for the surgical and nursing team. The mortality of extensive deep burns remains high, with infection still the commonest ultimate cause of death. The patient presents a unique problem in nursing care, quite different from other emergency situations. He is often the causative factor in his own catastrophe—the few exceptions in peacetime being the innocent victims of air disasters and road crashes. From being a normal healthy person he is suddenly converted into someone faced by an illness which may last for many months and which he knows may produce extensive disfigurement. He is often unable to help or feed himself. He is smelly, unclothed, isolated, subjected to frequent painful (or at least uncomfortable) surgical and nursing procedures and he makes slow progress, often beset by setbacks. A great part of his burden must be shouldered by a sympathetic, knowledgeable and skilled nursing staff.

PATHOLOGY

Burns are classified into partial or full thickness, depending on whether or not the deep germinal layer of the skin is intact or destroyed (Fig. 4.1).

A partial thickness burn may be quite superficial, the skin being erythematous (reddened) due to capillary dilatation. If rather more severe, areas of blistering are produced by exudation of plasma beneath coagulated epidermis. The underlying germinal layer of the epithelium is intact and complete healing takes place within a few

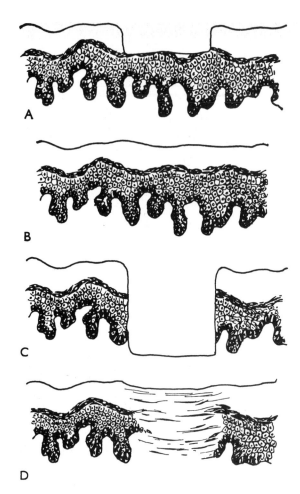

A

B

C

D

Fig. 4.1. A partial thickness burn (A) leaves part or whole of the germinal epithelium intact and therefore complete healing takes place (B). However, a full thickness burn (C) destroys the germinal layer and therefore heals by scar tissue (D).

days. Deeper partial thickness burns extend down to the germinal layer and may partially destroy it. There is intense blistering, which is followed by the formation of a slough. This scab separates after about 10–17 days, leaving healthy newly formed epithelium.

Full thickness burns completely destroy the epithelium. There may be initial blistering, but this is soon replaced by a coagulum or slough; more often, this is present from the onset in an intense deep burn. Unlike more superficial burns this slough separates only slowly over 3 or 4 weeks, or longer, to leave an underlying surface of granulation tissue (Fig. 4.2). Unless grafted, this will heal only by dense scar tissue, with consequent contractures and deformity (Fig. 4.3).

Fig. 4.2. A full thickness burn of the buttock undergoing excision three weeks after the accident. As the slough is cut away with scissors the underlying granulation tissue is revealed.

Fig. 4.3. The gross deformity produced by the contracting fibrous scars of a full thickness burn.

As well as local tissue destruction, the following general phenomena may be present in the extensively burnt patient:

1. *Pain*

This is due to the stimulation of numerous nerve endings in the damaged skin. It is more severe in superficial burns and, indeed, deep burns may be relatively painless because the nerve endings are to a great extent destroyed as they lie beneath the germinal epithelium.

2. *Plasma loss*

The damaged capillaries in the burnt skin allow plasma to exude through their walls, especially during the first 24 hours of an injury. This loss ceases by the time a coagulum has formed over the burn, a process which takes about 48 hours. As a direct result of this plasma loss from the blood stream, the circulatory volume falls and, in an extensive burn, the patient passes into oligaemic shock with rapid pulse and low blood pressure (see chapter 3). Since shock is a direct result of plasma loss, it is therefore proportional to the surface area of the body which is burnt. The loss of the plasma fraction of the blood is demonstrated by a rapid rise in the haematocrit reading of the blood, which is estimated by spinning down a blood sample in the centrifuge. The blood from a severely shocked burnt patient will have a much higher haematocrit level than normal, due to the increased proportions of red blood corpuscles compared with the plasma.

3. *Anaemia*

This results partly from destruction of the red cells within involved skin capillaries and partly from toxic inhibition of the bone marrow if infection of the burnt area takes place. It is therefore particularly marked in deep, infected burns.

4. *Stress reaction*

The body shows the typical stress reaction which follows any severe injury and which is due to an excess secretion of hormones from the adrenal cortex. There is comparative retention of water and sodium chloride, together with an excess breakdown of tissue protein and loss of potassium in the urine. Occasionally stress ulcer of the stomach and duodenum may develop (*Curling's ulcer*), with perforation or haemorrhage.

5. *Toxaemia*

This is a combination of factors which include biochemical disturbances, plasma loss and infection (the latter sometimes complicated by septicaemia). It is rather less common now that burns are treated adequately.

The principles underlying the treatment of burns are:

1 *General*, to mitigate the more widespread effects of burns listed above.

2 *Local*, to prevent infection and to promote healing of the epithelium, either spontaneously or by skin grafting.

General treatment

1. *Pain* is relieved with morphia, and this is best given initially by slow intravenous injection.

2. *Oligaemic shock due to plasma loss.* This is treated by replacement with either plasma or plasma substitutes such as dextran. The amount of plasma to be given and its rate of administration depend on careful and repeated assessments of the patient. If the patient is being overtransfused there may be congestion of the neck veins, cyanosis and a fall in the haematocrit reading below normal, showing that too much haemodilution is taking place. Too little replacement is suggested by a rapid thready pulse, a low blood pressure, low urinary output and a high haematocrit level. During transfusion the patient must therefore be kept under strict observation, on a quarter or half-hourly chock chart, the urinary ouaput must be carefully charted (if necessary a catheter is inserted in the bladder) and the haematocrit level is estimated our-hourly or at even more frequent intervals. As a guide to the amount of fluid replacement 'the rule of nine' is helpful. The body is divided into zones of percentage of surface area as follows (Fig. 4.4):

$$
\begin{aligned}
&\text{Head and neck} &&- 9\% \\
&\text{Each arm} &&- 9\% \\
&\text{Each leg} &&- 9\% \times 2 = 18\% \\
&\text{Front of trunk} &&- 9\% \times 2 = 18\% \\
&\text{Back of trunk} &&- 9\% \times 2 = 18\% \\
&\text{Perineum} &&- 1\%
\end{aligned}
$$

As a rough rule, the patient's hand is approximately 1% of his surface area. In adults, as a guide, 1 litre of fluid is required for each 9% of the body affected per 24 hours.

In children special charts are available which equate size of the patient with area of burn and amount of fluid replacement required. If the burns are full thickness, approximately one third of the fluid replacement may be given as blood in order to restore the extensive red cell destruction within the affected area. Subsequent anaemia, if present, may also require blood transfusion.

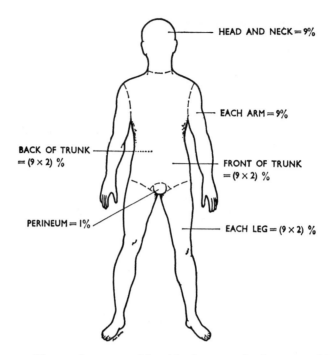

HEAD AND NECK = 9%

EACH ARM = 9%

BACK OF TRUNK
= (9 × 2) %

FRONT OF TRUNK
= (9 × 2) %

PERINEUM = 1%

EACH LEG = (9 × 2) %

Fig. 4.4. 'The rule of nine', a useful guide to the estimation of the area of a burnt surface.

These rules are useful guides but must be interpreted in the light of the patient's response to transfusion.

Local treatment

A burn at the moment at which it is sustained is sterile—our duty is to try and keep it so. The immediate first aid treatment of a burn is to wrap the area in sterile dressings during transfer to hospital. The treatment of major burns may be either by the *open* or the *closed* method. Sometimes a combination of the two is required.

The open or exposure method

This is based on the principle that bacteria cannot grow on the dry coagulum which rapidly forms over the exposed burn surface. The patient is therefore completely exposed in a warm isolated room. Elevation is used wherever possible to reduce oedema. It is excellent for the face, the limbs (apart from the fingers), or where only the front or the back of the trunk is involved. It is obviously a difficult technique to apply to circumferential burns of the trunk outside special burns units, and is best avoided for burns of the fingers. It has the advantage of simplicity and comparative freedom from discomfort for the patient (Fig. 4.5).

Fig. 4.5. Exposure treatment for severe burns of the face, chest and arms.

The closed treatment

This aims at excluding bacteria from the burnt areas by means of sterile dressings which are supplemented by antibiotics or chemical antiseptic agents. The burn is cleaned with a mild detergent, covered with an antibiotic cream, Vaseline gauze and thick layers of sterile dressings, which must be changed if they become soaked with plasma (Fig. 4.6). Recently a sulphonamide preparation termed maphenide acetate in a water soluble cream (sulphamylon) has been introduced with good results. It requires twice daily application, but unfortunately it is painful and drug sensitivity may occur. Gentamycin sulphate as a 1% cream may also be used but, again, toxic reactions may occur and some strains of pseudomonas are resistant to this antibiotic. Silver nitrate as a half per cent aqueous solution is relatively painless to use with no local sensitivity, but it has to be repeatedly applied as wet dressings which require re-soaking every 2—4 hours and it is not effective in the treatment of infected burns. The silver stains normal skin and the sheets, as well as pretty well

Fig. 4.6. Closed treatment of burns using topical antibiotic and bulky sterile dressings.

everything else with which it comes into contact. Recently silver sulphadiazine cream has been introduced, which eliminates some of these disadvantages.

At the end of about 10 days in both methods of treatment the slough will separate from superficial burns to leave an underlying healthy healed pink epithelium and no further local treatment is then required. In contrast, the slough over a full thickness is still adherent and attempts to remove it will produce bleeding (see Fig. 4.2). Full thickness burns are therefore excised at about 14 to 17 days and covered with split skin grafts (Fig. 4.7).

Fig. 4.7. Extensive full thickness burns of the buttocks which have been excised and grafted with split skin. (A later stage in the treatment of the patient shown in Fig. 4.2.)

Chaper 5. Tumours; principles of radiotherapy and cytotoxic therapy

INTRODUCTION

The word 'tumour' literally means a swelling, but for practical purposes the term is now used to describe a new growth or neoplasm. All the cells in the body, apart from the nerve cells within the central nervous system, are undergoing reproduction throughout life and in some organs, especially the bone marrow, the epithelia of the skin, alimentary canal and the reproductive organs, this is occurring very rapidly indeed. In a normal person this cell division merely keeps pace with the wear and tear of the tissues; under some circumstances there may be sudden very rapid bursts of cell division, for example in a healing wound or in the rapid growth of a fetus within the uterus, yet such growth is controlled and is in response to some need of the organism. In complete contrast to this, a tumour may be defined as 'an uncontrolled new growth of tissue' and it is a characteristic feature of such growths that they develop without any relationship to the requirements of the body. Indeed often their development may be harmful or even lethal.

CLASSIFICATION OF TUMOURS

Tumours are divided into *benign* and *malignant* and it is to this second group that the term 'cancer' is applied. It should be noted that some tumours are intermediate in their behaviour between benign and malignant neoplasm (a neoplasm means literally 'new growth') and that sometimes malignant change can take place in a benign tumour.

The pathological terms used to describe tumours at first sound complicated but, in fact, in the majority of cases, the technical name of the tumour tells us its tissue of origin and whether or not it is benign or malignant. Throughout, the termination '-oma' means 'some sort of tumour'. Next, tumours are divided according to their tissue of origin, depending on whether they arise from epithelium (skin, the lining of the alimentary canal and its associated glands, the kidney and the genito-urinary tract), or from the connective and supporting tissues of the body (bone, cartilage, muscle etc.).

Epithelial tumours

Benign epithelial tumours are termed *papillomas* when they derive from a simple epithelium, for example a papilloma of the bladder, but the term *adenoma* is used for benign epithelial tumours which arise from glands or a gland-bearing epithelium; for example a benign tumour of the pancreatic ducts would be termed a pancreatic adenoma. All malignant tumours arising from epithelia are termed *carcinomas*, to which is added the organ in which they originate; thus we talk about a carcinoma of the stomach or a carcinoma of the rectum where we mean a malignant tumour arising from the epithelial lining of these organs.

Supporting tissue tumours

Benign tumours of connective and supporting tissues are designated by the suffix 'oma' preceded by the name of the cell of origin. Thus 'lipoma' means a benign tumour of fat, 'chondroma' a benign tumour of cartilage. Malignant tumours have the suffix 'sarcoma' preceded by the name of the cell of origin—'liposarcoma' and 'chondrosarcoma' are thus malignant tumours of fat and cartilage respectively. Sometimes, two or more types of cell are found in the same sarcoma thus a fibro-liposarcoma contains elements of both fibrous tissue and fat.

Not all tumours fall into this neat classification and a number of special groups exist. Among the more common of these are the tumours of lymphoid tissue termed the *lymphomas*, which include Hodgkin's disease and lymphosarcoma, the *leukaemias*, which can be thought of as malignant disease of the white cells, the *melanomas* (both benign and malignant) which originate in the melanin-producing cells (melanocytes) of the skin and elsewhere, and the *teratomas* which are derived from a number of different cell types, which occur particularly in the testis and ovary and which may contain bone, glandular tissue, muscle and other structures in conglomeration.

Differentiation between benign and malignant tumours

As a general rule malignant tumours grow faster than benign neoplasms and this is mirrored in their microscopic appearance. A benign tumour shows only an occasional cell undergoing division and its appearance is very similar to that of its parent tissue (Fig. 5.1A). In contrast, a highly malignant tumour viewed under the microscope will show numerous cell divisions and the malignant cells themselves are often grossly abnormal, with large nuclei and relatively little cytoplasm. Instead of having the microscopic appearance of their tissue of origin, malignant tumours may simply show sheets or columns of rapidly dividing cells spreading through the parent organ (Fig. 5.1B).

A

B

Fig. 5.1. (A) A well differentiated and (B) a poorly differentiated (anaplastic) carcinoma of the large intestine viewed under the microscope.

Fig. 5.2. (A) A benign tumour compresses and pushes aside surrounding tissues. (B) A malignant tumour invades surrounding structures.

Fig. 5.3. Benign epithelial tumours tend to become pedunculated (A) whereas the malignant surface tumours tend to be sessile (B).

Although both benign and malignant tumours grow without regard to the needs of the body, they have very different behaviour in their relationship to surrounding tissues. A benign tumour simply compresses and pushes aside surrounding structures as it enlarges and these tissues may become compressed to form a fibrous capsule around the tumour. In contrast, a malignant growth invades its surrounds as a result of which no capsule is formed (Fig. 5.2). The tumour will grow along the paths of least resistance, easily tearing through soft connective tissues but halting for a time when it encounters bone or large blood vessels, although these in turn may eventually be invaded and destroyed. Cartilage is relatively resistant to tumour invasion so that, for example, when cancer deposits occur in the vertebral column the bones themselves may be almost destroyed but the cartilaginous intervertebral discs remain intact. This invasion is very typical of malignancy and indeed the word 'cancer' literally means 'crab', and describes the crab-like processes which the malignant growth sends into adjacent tissues (Fig. 5.2B).

Benign epithelial tumours tend to project outwards and often to develop a pedicle. Only when they reach a very large size will such pedunculated tumours ulcerate. Epithelial carcinomas, in contrast, usually form a flat mass, to which the term 'sessile' is applied (Fig. 5.3). Such a tumour rapidly outgrows its blood supply and often undergoes ulceration (Fig. 5.4). All malignant tumours possess the properties of local invasion. Many, in addition, have another feature which differentiates them from benign tumour, this is the ability to spread elsewhere in the body with the formation of *secondary deposits* or *metastases*. This spread may occur along the lymphatics to regional lymph nodes, a property which is possessed by carcinomas but not by sarcomas. However, both carcinomas and sarcomas may invade through the blood stream to produce deposits, which are especially likely to be found in the liver, lungs, the skeleton and the brain (Fig. 5.5). For some mysterious reason they are rare in the spleen and the heart.

Carcinomas within the chest and abdominal cavities may seed and spread over these pleural and peritoneal surfaces, a process termed *transcoelomic spread*. Pleural effusion and ascites are the usual clinical manifestations of this phenomenon (Fig. 5.6).

Very few things in nature fall into neat classifications and it is a general rule that most natural phenomena show a gradation from one end of a continuous spectrum to the other. Tumours are no exception. At each end of the scale are undoubtedly benign and undoubtedly malignant growths, but in the middle are those which have a rather untidy intermediate behaviour. Adenomas of the parotid gland, for example, do not have a well defined capsule and if

A   **B**   **C**

Fig. 5.4. As tumours enlarge they tend to outgrow their blood supply and therefore ulcerate. Note that this explains the usual raised and everted edge of a malignant ulcer.

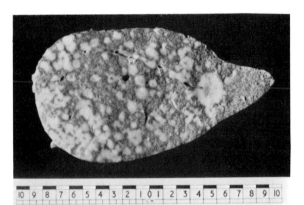

Fig. 5.5. Metastases in the liver from a patient dying of carcinoma of the breast. These secondaries result from blood stream spread.

Fig. 5.6. Chest X-ray showing a large left pleural effusion in a patient with breast cancer. This results from transcoelomic spread in the pleural cavity.

simply enucleated by the surgeon they tend to recur locally in the operation wound; moreover, long-standing tumours may undergo frank malignant change. Papillomas of the urinary tract may deposit on other parts of the lining epithelium, may seed into the surgical scar when removed at operation and may also eventually turn into a typical carcinoma.

Obviously a malignant tumour which spreads throughout the body may harm and eventually kill the patient. The majority of benign tumours are little more than a nuisance but it should not be thought that this is always so and there are situations where benign tumours may be just as dangerous as a malignant growth. For example, a small benign growth within the rigid framework of the skull may produce fatal brain compression, or a benign tumour within the bowel or urinary tract may cause serious haemorrhage or obstruction. Adenomas of the endocrine glands may produce excessive and harmful hormone secretion; examples are Cushing's syndrome which results from an adenoma of the cortex of the adrenal gland, or hypoglycaemia produced by excessive secretion of insulin from an adenoma of the islet cells of the pancreas.

There is little doubt, also, that benign tumours occasionally undergo malignant change. This may occur in melanomas of the skin, adenomas of the bowel and urinary tract and even occasionally in the commonest benign tumour of all, the subcutaneous lipoma which very rarely becomes a liposarcoma.

THE CLINICAL FEATURES AND DIAGNOSIS OF MALIGNANT DISEASE

There are three ways in which a malignant tumour may draw attention to itself:

1. *By the effects of the primary tumour*; for example, a woman may feel a lump in her breast and this proves to be a carcinoma, or a man coughs up blood from his lung cancer.

2. *By the effects produced by secondary deposits*; for example, the woman with the carcinoma of the breast may have overlooked the lump itself, but comes to the doctor because of back pain due to the presence of secondary deposits in her vertebrae, or the patient with the lung cancer may report because he has noticed a mass above the clavicle which is a clump of secondarily involved supraclavicular lymph nodes.

3. *By the general effects of malignant disease*; these patients report with loss of weight, loss of appetite, anaemia and general debility (Fig. 5.7). In its most advanced stages, this is termed *malignant cachexia*.

It should be noted that a patient may present with features which fall into one, two or all three categories—for example, a patient with a carcinoma of the stomach may complain of having noticed a lump in his abdomen (the primary tumour), and of having become jaundiced (from the secondaries in his liver), and may also have noticed that he has become pale and has lost a considerable amount of weight (the general effects of the tumour).

Now it is a general rule that the diagnosis of any condition in the whole of medicine and surgery follows three logical steps. First, a history is taken, then the patient is examined and then, if necessary, certain special investigations are carried out in the laboratory and X-ray department.

Let us now apply these three steps to the diagnosis of a cancer, bearing in mind the three ways in which a tumour may present that we have already mentioned. As an example, let us take the commonest killing cancer in this country, carcinoma of the lung:

Fig. 5.7. Malignant cachexia in a patient with an advanced carcinoma of the stomach. Note that the abdomen is distended with ascites.

The history

(a) *The primary tumour* may present with cough, haemoptysis, breathlessness or chest pain.
(b) *Secondary deposits* may bring the patient to the doctor with the complaints of enlarged glands in the neck, back pain or pathological fractures due to bone deposits, headaches or drowsiness from cerebral metastases, or jaundice from liver deposits.
(c) *General effects of malignant disease*—the patient may present with lassitude, anorexia, loss of weight or anaemia.

Examination

(a) *The primary tumour* may produce physical signs in the chest which can be detected by percussion or by auscultation through the stethoscope.
(b) *Secondary deposits* may cause enlarged lymph nodes, enlargement of the liver or obvious bony deposits.
(c) *The general effects of malignant disease* may be suggested by clinical anaemia or cachexia.

Special investigations

(a) *For the primary tumour*—a chest X-ray may reveal a suspicious shadow in the lung, microscopic examination of the sputum may show the presence of malignant cells and the tumour itself may be visualised directly at bronchoscopy, at which time a biopsy of the growth may be obtained for microscopic examination.

(b) *For secondary deposits*—X-rays of the skeletal system may demonstrate secondary deposits in the bones and special radioactive scanning techniques may reveal deposits in liver or brain.

(c) *For general manifestations of malignant disease*—a blood count may reveal anaemia.

This simple scheme can be applied to any of the principal malignant tumours and will be employed throughout this book.

GENERAL PRINCIPLES OF TREATMENT

The majority of benign tumours require simple surgical removal. The patient may not like the cosmetic appearance of the lump and in any case is worried by it. Furthermore, the surgeon cannot be entirely certain of the nature of the lump, even though he suspects that it is benign, and it is safer to have it removed and put it under the microscope. Some tumours may undergo malignant change, so that their removal before this can happen is obviously a wise prophylactic measure. In other situations, the benign tumour may produce unpleasant effects due to obstruction, bleeding, pressure on adjacent organs, or, in the case of the endocrine glands, symptoms due to hormone over-secretion. In all these cases, surgical removal is indicated.

Turning now to the treatment of malignant tumours, these must always be considered under two headings: first, *curative* in which an attempt is made to remove the disease entirely and second, *palliative* where, although the disease is incurable or has recurred after an attempt at curative treatment, steps can still be taken to ease the patient's symptoms.

In this chapter the possible lines of treatment will be dealt with in general and, in subsequent chapters, the management of the main tumours of specific organs will be considered in more detail.

Curative treatment

There are two methods by which at present an attempt can be made to cure a patient of cancer. The first is *surgical excision*, in which the tumour, often together with adjacent draining lymph nodes, is widely excised. The surgeon hopes to diagnose the cancer before metastases have developed, and, by complete excision, prevent the possibility of later dissemination. Typical examples of such a treatment are mastectomy, in which a carcinoma of the breast is removed together with surrounding breast tissue, the overlying skin and the adjacent axillary lymph nodes, or resection of a carcinoma of the colon when the growth is removed together with adjacent bowel wall clear of the cancer and a generous wedge of the mesocolon containing the draining lymph nodes. The second method is *radiotherapy* which is usually employed to destroy tumours which are not readily accessible to surgical removal, for example, cancers of the mouth and pharynx. Later in this chapter the principles underlying radiotherapy will be considered in more detail.

In some circumstances a combination of surgery and radiotherapy is employed.

Palliative treatment

In many cases the patient presents too late for any attempt at cure; by now the tumour has widely disseminated and there are obvious metastases elsewhere in the body which preclude curative treatment. In other instances, the patient returns to hospital after an attempted cure by surgery or radiotherapy carried out months or even years before but has now developed recurrence of the original disease or metastases elsewhere. Although the patient is now beyond cure, a number of measures are available which may prolong life and provide freedom or relief from pain. The types of therapy can be listed as follows:

1. *Surgery.* Even though secondary deposits may be present it may still be worthwhile carrying out a palliative excision of the primary tumour. For example, a patient with an obstructing carcinoma of the colon may be treated by partial colectomy to remove the primary growth even though secondary deposits are already present in the liver. He will be relieved of his obstructive symptoms and may live for many months or even years in comfort before eventually dying of his liver metastases. An inoperable obstructing tumour of the oesophagus or the upper end of the stomach may be intubated by means of a plastic tube so that dysphagia can be relieved. Although the patient is doomed to die of his cancer, at least he will be able to swallow comfortably for the rest of his days (Fig. 5.8).

2. *Radiotherapy.* This is extremely valuable in the treatment of localised irremovable disease, for example, painful secondary deposits in bone, advanced irremovable breast tumours, inoperable lymph node metastases, etc. The principles of radiotherapy are considered in the section below.

3. *Cytotoxic therapy.* A large number of cytotoxic agents are available which may temporarily produce regression of tumours. The principles of this treatment are considered in a section later in this chapter.

Fig. 5.8. Some of the tubes which are available for pallatiave intubation of inoperable carcinomas of the oesophagus and cardia. From above down, these are: A Mousseau-Barbin tube, a short and a long Souttar's tube, and a Celestin tube.

4. *Sex hormone and endocrine surgery.* Two carcinomas, those of the breast and the prostate, are often sensitive to changes in the sex-hormone environment and may respond either to the administration of sex hormones (e.g. stilboestrol) or to removal of the sex hormone secreting glands (the gonads and/or the adrenals) or the pituitary gland which controls their secretion. Further details will be found in the chapters on breast and prostrate.

5. *Pain relief.* This is extremely important in patients with advanced cancer. The judicious use of pain relieving drugs may be supplemented by employing tranquillising agents and anti-emetics, among which chlorpromazine is particularly valuable. Nerve blocks by means of phenol or alcohol may anaesthetise the conduction pathways from a painful inoperable tumour.

6. *Maintenance of morale and nursing care.* An essential part of the nursing treatment of patients with advanced cancer is a kindly understanding and yet cheerful attitude of the medical and nursing staff, coupled with the difficult nursing care of a patient who is often bedridden and in pain.

PROGNOSIS IN MALIGNANT DISEASE

One of the most difficult tasks facing doctors and nurses is when the patient who knows he has malignant disease, or his relatives, ask for the prognosis. It must be realised that we can only give the chances, or possibilities, in each particular case. If we say, for example, that the patient has a 90% chance of cure, we must remember that he may be unfortunate enough to fall into the 10% who are to suffer a

fatal recurrence of the disease. In any particular patient we have four main features upon which prognosis depends:
1. The extent of spread of the tumour
2. Its microscopic appearance
3. Its anatomical situation
4. The general condition of the patient.

The extent of spread

The prognosis of any tumour deteriorates in proportion to the extent of invasion and dissemination which has taken place. For example, a cancer of the bowel which is confined to the mucosa has a better prognosis than the same tumour which has invaded through the wall of the bowel and this, in turn, has a better outlook than a tumour which has spread to the draining lymph nodes. Prognosis is worst of all if metastases have spread to the liver or other organs (Fig. 5.9). A woman with a small tumour confined to the breast has, on average, a much better prognosis than a woman of the same age and same type of tumour which has disseminated to the lymph nodes in her axilla, or, worse still, widely to the liver, bones and lungs. Clues about the extent of the spread may be found in the pre-operative examination of the patient, where, for example, enlarged lymph nodes or a nodular swollen liver may be found, or this may be determined at the time of surgical exploration. Finally the microscopic examination of the specimen may reveal involvement of

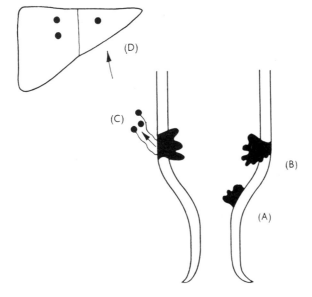

Fig. 5.9. Diagram to show the progressive stages of a tumour of the large bowel. A, confined to the bowel wall; B, penetrating the wall; C, involvement of regional lymph nodes; D, distant spread to the liver. Each stage is associated with progressive worsening of the prognosis.

lymph nodes which had not been detected clinically, or of microscopic extension of the growth to the very edges of the resected specimen with consequent worsening of the outlook for the patient.

Microscopic appearance

The pathologist's examination of a biopsy of the tumour or of the resected surgical specimen is valuable in telling us the degree of differentiation of the tumour. As a general rule, the more actively growing the tumour, and the more primitive its cells (to which the term 'de-differentiation' or 'anaplastic' is applied) the worse the prognosis.

These two factors, the spread of the tumour and its degree of differentiation, should always be taken in conjunction with each other. A small tumour, with no apparent spread, may still have a relatively poor prognosis if it is highly anaplastic, whereas an extensive tumour is not incompatible with long survival if microscopic examination reveals that it is very well differentiated and therefore tends to be slowly growing.

Anatomical situation

The situation of the tumour is of some prognostic significance, because on this may depend whether or not the lesion is easily accessible to surgical removal. A brain tumour located in the frontal lobe may be resected, whereas a similar tumour buried deeply in the brain stem would be a hopeless surgical proposition. An anteriorly placed cancer of the rectum in a male, which is invading into the prostate and bladder base, is usually considered irremovable, whereas a similar state of affairs in the female in which the tumour is invading the posterior vagina is still amenable to abdomino-perineal excision of the rectum in which the posterior wall of the vagina can also be sacrificed.

The general condition of the patient

This is something that must be taken into consideration in giving the prognosis of any surgical condition. Although the tumour itself in a particular patient may be curable, it may, in practical terms, be inoperable because of the poor general condition of the patient. For example, gross congestive cardiac failure may render what is technically an operable carcinoma of the rectum a hopeless surgical risk. In dealing with an elderly, unfit patient the surgeon, in consultation with the anaesthetist, has to weigh up in each case the risks

of the operation against the suffering the patient is likely to undergo if left untreated.

PRINCIPLES OF RADIOTHERAPY

Each year the number of patients attending the radiotherapy departments of our hospitals increases. The nursing care of these often
very sick and very anxious people is a considerable responsibility
and it behoves the nurse to have a clear understanding of the basic
principles underlying radiotherapeutic treatment.

Radiotherapy may be used in the primary treatment of cancer,
especially where the tumour is deeply placed and relatively inaccessible (e.g. the mouth, pharynx, larynx, and for extensive tumours
of the bladder) or it may be used as a pre-operative treatment to
shrink down a tumour and render it more amenable for operation.
In its most widespread use, radiotherapy is employed in the management of inoperable or recurrent cancers in order to give palliative
relief of symptoms.

Three main techniques are currently available:
1. Supervoltage or cobalt beam therapy.
2. Implants into tissues or cavities such as the uterine canal of radioactive materials—for example, radium, caesium or radioactive gold.
3. Radioactive isotopes administered orally or by injection.

X-rays were discovered by Wilhelm Roentgen in 1895 as mysterious
rays of a very short wavelength found to be emitted from the anode
(positive electrode) when this is struck by cathode rays (a stream of
negatively charged electrons) passed through a vacuum tube (Fig.
5.10). These X-rays were found to penetrate human tissues and then

Fig. 5.10. Diagram of an X-ray
tube.

to be picked up on photographic paper—the basis of modern radiology. But powerful X-rays, produced by increasing the voltage applied between the electrodes, also cause tissue damage, which is now harnessed in our therapeutic use of X-rays. Rays of intense penetration are produced by using a linear accelerator at 4 to 6 million volts as the source of the electron beam (Fig. 5.11).

In 1896 Bequerel discovered by chance that photographic plates placed near a mineral called pitchblende, (from which uranium is obtained) become fogged; obviously this contained some 'radioactive' substance. Madame Marie Curie, a Polish scientist working in Paris, succeeded, 2 years later, in the difficult task of extracting a newly discovered element from pitchblende—she named this 'Radium'.

Radium and radioactive isotopes of other elements are unstable and break down with the liberation of radiant energy.

Fig. 5.11. The 4 million volt linear accelerator at Westminster hospital.

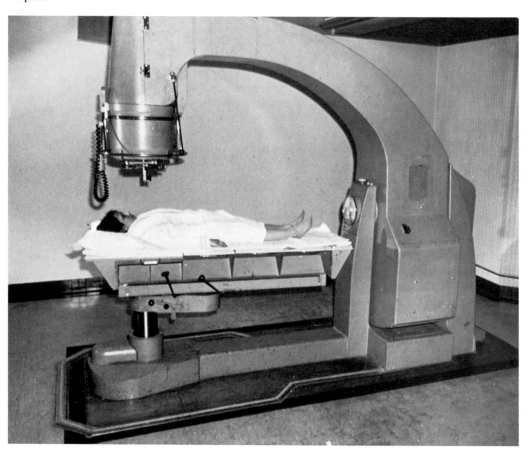

This radiation is made up of three components:

1. *Alpha particles*, which are positively charged helium nuclei. These move at high speed, but are large particles and are readily stopped, for example, by a sheet of paper.

2. *Beta particles*, which are electrons travelling at nearly the speed of light. These can be absorbed by a thickness of lead of about 1 mm, by spectacles, or a 1 cm thick piece of perspex, and can penetrate the body tissues to a depth of about 1 cm.

3. *Gamma rays*, which are short wavelength electro-magnetic waves and which can penetrate several centimetres of lead.

There is no practical difference between X-rays produced in high voltage X-ray machines and the gamma rays emitted by some radioactive elements such as Cobalt 60.

X-ray therapy is now usually employed at very high voltage and short wavelengths (mega voltage X-rays in a range of 2 or more million volts).

Radium is employed in the form of gold or platinum coated needles. The coating filters off the alpha and beta particles, allowing the gamma radiation to be used by implantation of the needles into the tissues (for example, tongue cancer) or else as an intra-cavitory application, for example in the treatment of carcinoma of the cervix or body of the uterus (Fig. 5.12).

Radioactive isotopes may occur naturally, for example isotopes of uranium, or they may be produced artificially by bombarding an element in a nuclear reactor. Radioactive isotopes may be employed in the form of a solution to be injected into the pleural or abdominal cavity to control malignant effusions (radioactive gold, which utilises beta ray emission, is used for this purpose) or as a radioactive implant directly into tissues (e.g. radioactive tantalum wire) or, perhaps most important of all, certain radioisotopes such as Cobalt 60 and Caesium 137 produce extremely powerful gamma radiation which can be used instead of megavoltage X-rays in external radiotherapy.

The effects of irradiation

Electro-magnetic radiation (X-rays and gamma rays) or particulate beams of alpha or beta rays produce their effect by causing ionisation in the living tissues through which they pass. Ionisation is the process in which atoms throw off negatively charged electrons which in turn bombard other atoms to produce more ionisation. Alpha rays, with their small penetration, can only be used in therapy if in direct contact with cancer cells as a surface application. Beta particles produce dense ionisation but only for up to 1 cm penetration into

Fig. 5.12. X-ray of patient who has radium needles implanted into a carcinoma of the tongue.

the tissues, whereas X-rays (particularly supervoltage) and gamma rays can penetrate deeply into the body.

When cells are irradiated, both the nucleus and cytoplasm are damaged so that the cells are killed. This rarely takes place immediately but the cells appear to die after one or more further divisions. Irradiation of sufficient dosage will destroy any tissue but its use in the treatment of cancer depends on the fact that cells are damaged differentially by the irradiation. Those cells which are rapidly growing tend to be far more sensitive than slowly growing cells. When we irradiate a rapidly growing malignant tumour we try to adjust the dosage so that the cancer cells are destroyed without too much damage to surrounding normal structures.

Complications of irradiation

Patients undergoing radiotherapy may develop a number of general and local side-effects. The general complications include *radiation sickness*, in which the patient becomes nauseated or vomits, and complains of lassitude and anorexia. This syndrome is particularly liable to occur when large fields of radiation are used, for example, in the treatment of intra-abdominal or intra-thoracic disease. This phenomenon is seen at its worst in people who have been injured in nuclear explosions or accidents and who have therefore received whole-body irradiation. The most important general effect is damage to the bone marrow; there is a drop in the white cell count, affecting first the lymphocytes and then the polymorphs. The platelet count falls and the patient becomes anaemic. The depressed white cell count (which may fall below 2,000) is accompanied by a low resistance to infection and the fall in platelets produces a bleeding tendency, which may be associated with haemorrhages into the skin and other tissues. The white cell count is quite a sensitive guide to the tolerance of a patient undergoing large field irradiation and regular blood counts are therefore carried out in the radiotherapy department in patients undergoing extensive treatment.

The skin in the area irradiated usually becomes red (erythema) and, following high dose irradiation, often undergoes moist desquamation. This is followed by local pigmentation of the skin, atrophy, or the development of telangiectases. During treatment any irritation of the skin in the irradiated area must be carefully avoided and this includes exposure to sunlight, constricting clothing, soap and water and cosmetics.

Radiotherapy to the brain is followed by loss of scalp hair (depilation); it usually recovers in about 6 months.

The affected skin remains more sensitive than normal for many years; it may break down if subjected to subsequent trauma, producing an area of *irradiation necrosis* and it may not heal well after subsequent surgery. It is dangerous to give further irradiation to a previously treated area because of the risk of skin necrosis. Occasionally malignant change may occur in the skin long after exposure to heavy irradiation.

It should be noted that the problems of skin reaction, which were very serious in the days of conventional X-ray therapy, are less severe now that megavoltage therapy is used. This is because modern high voltage therapy and gamma treatment spare the skin and produce maximal effect in deeper tissues, so that the very badly affected skin that we used to see following irradiation is now seldom encountered.

Irradiation of deep structures may be followed by damage to adjacent tissues, so that, for example, pulmonary fibrosis can result from treatment of the lung and too high a dose of radiotherapy to the pelvis may cause stricture formation or fistula involving the intestine, bladder or ureter.

Modern, accurate supervoltage irradiation has the advantage of sparing skin and of not being differentially absorbed by bone. The cosmetic results of treatment are thus much improved and the morbidity of irradiation greatly reduced. It has become a particularly useful weapon in our armoury in the treatment of cancer.

CYTOTOXIC THERAPY

The word 'cytotoxic' means 'injurious to cells'. The dream of this type of therapy would be the discovery of some drug, completely innocuous to normal cells, which would, however, seek out the cancer cells in the body, enter into their metabolic process and destroy them. This would resemble, let us say, the injection of a dose of penicillin into a patient invaded by streptococci—the bacterial cells are destroyed but the patient's own tissues are unaffected. Unfortunately, at present, an ideal anti-cancer drug is still to be discovered. None of the vast number of substances at present available in the treatment of malignant disease is specifically toxic to tumour tissues, but every one of them attacks all rapidly dividing cells, whether malignant or normal. The latter include specially the bone marrow, the mucosa of the gastro-intestinal tract, the skin and fetal tissues. The inevitable damage to normal cells explains why the use of cytotoxic drugs is so dangerous and so replete with side-effects and complications.

The cytotoxic drugs fall into four main groups:

1. Anti-metabolites.
2. Alkylating agents.
3. Antibiotics.
4. Miscellaneous.

1. *The anti-metabolites* resemble in chemical structure substances which are normally present in cells, or else they compete for metabolites required by the cells for their normal function. In this way essential chemical processes within the cell are disturbed, with lethal consequences. A good example of an anti-metabolite is *Methotrexate* which resembles folic acid, which itself is essential for the enzyme system used in the synthesis of DNA and therefore of cell reproduction. *5-Fluorouracil* is a pyrimidine antagonist and *6-Mercaptopurine* is a purine antagonist; both these substances block the synthesis of nucleic acid by substituting themselves for essential chemicals in its manufacture.

2. *Alkylating agents* are compounds which are capable of replacing a hydrogen atom in another molecule with an alkyl radical. They alter the essential components of cells (nucleic acids, proteins, cellular enzymes), leading to cell death. These drugs include *Nitrogen Mustard, Chlorambucil, Cyclophosphamide, Melphalan* and *Thiotepa*.

3. *Antibiotics*. As part of the search for antibacterial substances produced by bacteria and fungi, a group of substances have been discovered which have anti-tumour activity. These include *Actinomycin D* and *Mithramycin*.

4. *The miscellaneous group* include alkaloids extracted from the periwinkle (*Vinca rosea*) which are termed *Vinblastine* and *Vincristine*. These block mitoses in dividing cells. Other drugs in this ever-enlarging group include *Urethane*, and derivatives of *Colchicine*.

Modes of administration

At present the clinician chooses a cytotoxic drug for a particular case out of this bewildering variety of available substances in a rather arbitrary manner based on previous clinical experience. For example, 5-Fluorouracil seems to be the most useful drug in the treatment of advanced cancer of the large bowel. It may be that in future we shall be able to grow a portion of the particular tumour under treatment in tissue culture and test it against a variety of cytotoxic drugs to see which ones are especially effective against it, just as now the bacteriologist tests organisms in culture for their sensitivity of resistance to a variety of antibiotic agents. In some cases several cytotoxic drugs are used in combination in order to attack the cancer cells from different metabolic aspects. For example, in quadruple therapy, cyclophosphamide, methotrexate, vincristine and 5-Fluorouracil are used sequentially.

Most drugs can be given orally, although some must be given by intravenous injection. Cytotoxic drugs may also be instilled into the pleural or peritoneal cavities in treatment of malignant effusions at these sites. Tumours confined to a limb or to the head and neck may be treated on occasion by perfusion via the feeding artery in order to provide a high local dosage in the tumour area and less effect on normal structures elsewhere.

Indications for use

Cytotoxic drugs are of particular value in the reticuloses— Hodgkin's disease, leukaemia, and disseminated lymphosarcoma. Two solid tumours, chorioncarcinoma of the uterine cavity and Burkitt's lymphoma, a tumour seen particularly in African children, are particularly sensitive to cytotoxic therapy and long-term cures have now been reported. For solid, disseminated tumours results are far less good so that cytotoxics are usually only employed when other methods have failed, but remissions of many months, or occasionally, even years, may sometimes be obtained.

Side-effects

These are very similar to those mentioned under the general effects of radiotherapy, and, indeed they result in the main from the same underlying cause—damage to cells in those normal tissues which are undergoing rapid cellular division. The most important in this respect is the bone marrow; an early sign of toxicity from any of the cytotoxic drugs is a fall in the white cell count and in the blood platelets. If the total white count drops below 3,000, drug treatment must be stopped at once. Other toxic effects are nausea and vomiting, oral and intestinal ulceration due to damage to the mucosa of the alimentary canal, secondary monilial (thrush) infection of the mouth and gut, loss of hair, skin rashes, and haemorrhages into the skin and other tissues, the last resulting from depletion of the blood platelets.

Chapter 6. Chest and lungs

ANATOMY

The chest wall is composed of 12 ribs on either side that articulate posteriorly with the transverse processes and the bodies of the vertebrae. The upper 7 are joined anteriorly to the sternum by cartilaginous joints; 8, 9 and 10 articulate with the cartilage of the rib above and 11 and 12 are free anteriorly, ending in the layers of the abdominal muscles. The ribs are joined together by the intercostal muscles (Fig. 6.1).

Nerves, arteries and veins run beneath each rib from the spinal cord, aorta, azygos and hemi-azygos veins respectively to supply the muscles and the overlying skin. The chest is separated from the abdominal cavity by a muscular and tendinous sheet, the diaphragm. This arrangement permits the cavity of the chest to expand and contract, altering its volume by as much as 2 litres in an adult male.

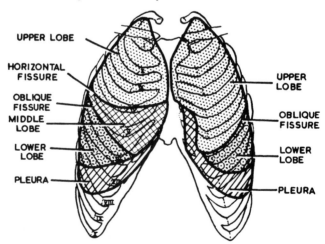

Fig. 6.1. The chest wall, lungs and pleura.

The right ventricle of the heart pumps blood into the lungs. The lungs are elastic structures which allow intimate contact between the oxygen in the inspired air and blood, separated by only one cell. If a lung is removed from the body it will contract down to a small ball of tissue, but it is kept in an expanded state in the thorax by the integrity of the chest wall. The chest is lined by a thin, smooth and shining membrane, which is termed the *parietal pleura*. The *visceral pleura* covers the lungs and the mediastinum in an exactly analogous way to the peritoneum in the abdomen. Thus, during respiration, expansion and contraction of the lungs within the chest is possible without friction.

Air is drawn into the lungs via the pharynx, trachea and left and right main bronchus which then divide into bronchi (Fig. 6.2) which supply the lobes of the lungs (3 on the right and 2 plus the lingula on the left). Each lobe of the lung is further subdivided into segments.

The heart, great vessels (that is aorta and venae cavae) and the root of the lungs occupy a central position in the chest termed the *mediastinum*.

PHYSIOLOGY

Respiration, that is the process whereby blood is oxygenated, requires:
1. Normal inspired air.
2. A clear airway.

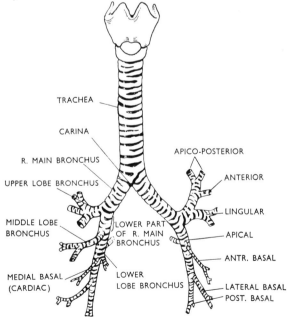

Fig. 6.2. The trachea and main bronchi.

3. Efficient neuromuscular co-ordination to move the chest.

4. An intact chest cavity.

In addition to oxygenation, the lungs are one of the routes for the clearance of carbon dioxide as gas, water as vapour (a mechanism whereby the body is cooled and the most important in the dog) and certain volatile compounds and drugs, for example alcohol and Fluothane.

The nervous control of respiration is a complex function which can be interfered with by certain drugs and by alteration in consciousness. For example, deep surgical anaesthesia depresses respiration to the point at which it will completely cease and an overdose of barbiturate kills the suicide by depressing respiration to the level at which insufficient oxygen and carbon dioxide exchange occurs. On these occasions it is possible to pass a tube through the larynx into the trachea (an endotracheal tube) and inflate the lungs rhythmically with oxygen. This process is called intermittent positive pressure respiration (IPPR). This can be carried on indefinitely mechanically using a ventilator until such time as normal respiratory control is established; the endotracheal tube can then be removed.

FRACTURED RIBS

Normal ribs may be fractured by direct external violence, for example, when the chest strikes the steering wheel in a road accident. They may also be fractured by excessively severe coughing. Ribs that are diseased by, for example, osteomalacia or by malignant deposits may be fractured by slight coughing or moderate external trauma.

The symptoms associated with a rib fracture are pain, which is aggravated by breathing and coughing, and which is localised to the area of the fracture. Compression of the chest wall by the hand will cause intense pain. If a number of ribs are fractured on one side the pain may be so intense as to prevent the patient being able to draw in breath and he may thereby become cyanosed.

STABLE FRACTURES

Treatment

If only one or two ribs are fractured and respiration is satisfactory this is known as a stable fracture and the only treatment required is a suitable analgesic. Strapping of the chest with adhesive plaster is usually not effective and if too efficiently applied will so reduce respiratory movement as to compromise bronchial clearing and may precipitate pneumonia. The ribs are splinted one by the other and will heal quite rapidly if left alone.

Some patients may suffer fracture of the ribs and have some underlying lung disease, such as occurs in chronic smokers. In this case, it is important to establish normal respiratory and coughing movements rapidly. It is possible to achieve complete analgesia by the use of an epidural local anaesthetic; a small catheter is introduced to the side of the spinal dura mater and local anaesthetic can be injected around the posterior nerve roots as they emerge to pass around the chest. This extremely effective and elegant technique is often successful in allowing the patient to be managed without IPPR in a borderline case.

UNSTABLE FRACTURES

If ribs are fractured on both sides of the chest or at both their extremities it is possible for there to be a loose segment of chest wall. This results in a condition known as *'flail chest'*. In this case when the chest expands the flail segment instead of moving out is drawn in. Air is not sucked into the trachea and respiration is thereby interfered with (Fig. 6.3).

Treatment

In this case the patient will require endotracheal intubation with IPPR together with full doses of analgesic, for example morphia 15 mg or pethidine 100 mg and basal narcosis to reduce awareness using such drugs as diazepam to permit tolerance of the tube in the conscious state. After 48 to 72 hours the chest usually stabilizes by clot and fibrin sufficient for the patient to be 'weaned off' the ventilator.

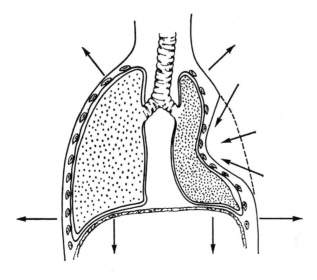

Fig. 6.3. Flail chest. On inspiration the detached segment of the chest wall is sucked inwards, producing paradoxical movement

Pneumothorax is the condition that occurs when air is introduced between the layers of visceral and parietal pleura—the lung on that side then collapses and is not aerated by the respiratory movements. There are a number of causes:

1. By a leak from the lung tissue via the bronchus (bronchopleural fistula). This is a common cause and results when a lung cyst or bulla ruptures. It occurs in young people for no known reason (Fig. 6.4).

Occasionally the leak is associated with a flap of pleura which forms a valve which permits air to enter the pleural space without being able to return to the bronchus. This results in a *tension pneumothorax*. The particular danger of this condition is that the mediastinum is pushed across to the other side of the chest with compression of the other lung. Unless the air is allowed to escape from the pleural cavity, the patient will asphyxiate (Fig. 6.5).

Fig. 6.4. Chest X-ray showing a left-sided pneumothorax. The collapsed lung lies against the left border of the heart; the rest of the left chest is full of air. Note that the heart and mediastinum are pushed over to the right.

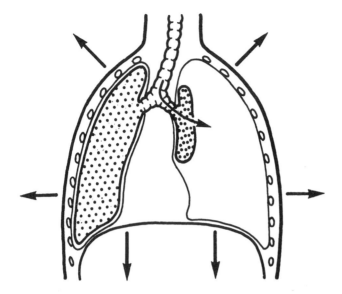

Fig. 6.5. Tension pneumothorax produced by a valvular tear in the lung. Air is sucked into the pleural cavity on inspiration and cannot escape on expiration.

2. By rupture of the bronchus in an accident. This is rare.

3. By an external puncture of the chest wall such as might occur in a stab wound. If the hole in the chest wall is large, air is sucked in and out of the pleural cavity with the movements of respiration. This is known as a *'sucking pneumothorax'*. The puncture may also rupture the lung with a further leak of air.

4. In error when a pleural effusion is tapped. In this case a quantity of air may be allowed to enter the chest.

5. Post-operatively. When operations on the chest wall or the underlying lung are carried out inevitably air enters the pleural cavity and has to be expelled at the completion of the operation.

The diagnosis of pneumothorax is confirmed by chest X-ray.

Treatment

If the pneumothorax is small and the chest wall is intact, the lung can usually be relied on to seal itself and the air will absorb spontaneously from the pleural cavity. No active treatment is required therefore, other than regular surveillance by chest X-ray to confirm that re-expansion of the lung is occurring. If on the other hand there is a persistent bronchopleural fistula or if the chest wall is punctured, then drainage of the pleural cavity via an underwater drain is required. If in spite of this the lung does not re-expand, a pump will have to be applied to the system to draw the air out. Occasionally when the hole joining the pleural cavity to the bronchus is large, operative closure is required.

It is a matter of life and death to treat a tension pneumothorax rapidly. All that is required is for a large bore needle to be plunged into the chest wall through an intercostal space. Following this emergency measure drainage of the pleural cavity via an underwater drain will usually result in cure of the condition (Fig. 6.6).

Haemothorax

This is a collection of blood in the pleural cavity. It is usually the result of trauma or it may occur post-operatively. If the bleeding is only of moderate severity, the treatment is aspiration of the effusion, blood replacement and observation; if the bleeding is severe operative treatment is required to control the source of the haemorrhage.

Hydropneumothorax

This is the condition that obtains when there is both liquid and air within the pleural cavity. Diagnosis is confirmed by chest X-ray and treatment follows the same general lines as for haemothorax.

Fig. 6.6. Underwater seal chest drain in the treatment of a pneumothorax. Air escapes from the pleural cavity on expiration but cannot be sucked back through the water seal on inspiration.

Post-operative pneumonia—see p. 27.

LUNG ABSCESS

This is usually due to one of a variety of causes:
1. Inhaled foreign body, for example a peanut.
2. Infected pulmonary embolus.
3. Failure of pneumonia to resolve.
4. Distal to an obstructing carcinoma of the bronchus.
5. As part of a staphylococcal or other septicaemia.

Clinical features

The symptomatology is that of an abscess anywhere, that is a raised
white cell count, swinging pyrexia, plus local pain in the chest if the
parietal pleura is involved and cough if the abscess communicates
with the bronchus. Diagnosis is confirmed by chest X-ray, with
tomography if required (Fig. 6.7).

Fig. 6.7. Chest X-ray of a patient
with bilateral lung abscesses. Note
that each has a fluid level at the
interface between air and pus in
the abscess cavity (each arrowed).

Treatment

The majority of abscesses point into the bronchus and drain that way. The patient experiences a rush of offensive material which is expelled by expectoration and he soon feels better. In this case all that is required is for the pus to be cultured for micro-organisms and their sensitivities determined. The patient is then tipped by the physiotherapist so as to encourage drainage via the bronchus. Antibiotics are usually unnecessary. The underlying condition that caused the abscess in the first place must be treated; e.g. if a foreign body is present it must be removed.

An important complication of a lung abscess is rupture into the pleural cavity and production of an empyema which is a collection of pus in this space. It will then require external drainage.

PULMONARY TUBERCULOSIS

A few years ago most people in this country contracted a primary tuberculous pulmonary infection. This was usually overcome by the defences of the body and left no more than a slight trace at the apex of one or other lung visible on X-ray. Nowadays with control of the infection in the population and in the milk supplies, this primary infection is not so common.

If a virulent mycobacterium infects a person who has no previous experience of the disease, a generalised pulmonary infection may result. The chest X-ray in this case shows the lung fields to be covered by a multitude of small white spots (Fig. 6.8). This condition of miliary tuberculosis, if left untreated, is rapidly fatal after a short period of a wasting disease which lasts for a few days or a few weeks at the most. If treatment is adequate with antituberculous therapy there is a high chance that cure will result.

Usually, however, the infection will become localised to one lobe or segment of a lobe. In this case the lung tissue breaks down and a cavity is formed (Fig. 6.9). The cavity usually drains via the bronchus and results in copious expectoration of sputum. It is very common for such patients to cough up blood, which is bright red and frothy.

Treatment

This is similar in principle to that of any infection but is complicated by the fact that the mycobacterium of tuberculosis takes approximately 6 weeks to culture.

After sputum has been sent for culture the patient is given 'rotating' therapy with streptomycin 1.0 gm daily INAH 100 mg three times per day and PAS. Nowadays there is a tendency in this

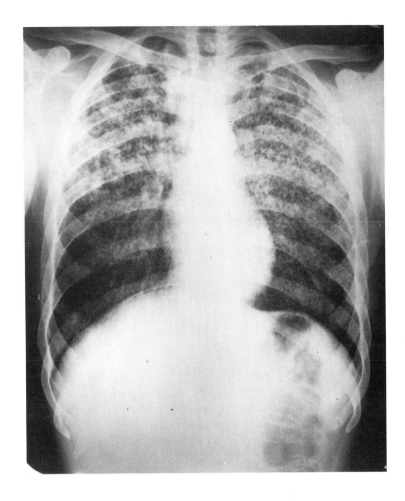

Fig. 6.8. Chest X-ray of a patient with miliary tuberculosis. Note the myriad of small white deposits throughout the lung fields.

country for PAS to be replaced by rifampicin but this has the disadvantage of being more expensive. Six weeks from the onset of treatment the sensitivities of the infecting mycobacterium are known in some cases and therapy can be gauged accordingly. It is unusual to continue with streptomycin for more than six to twelve weeks, rifampicin and INAH being continued for a total period of 2 years. The exact length of treatment is a subject of several trials at the present moment but it is hoped that with the greater use of rifampicin the total length required will be reduced.

If pulmonary tuberculosis is treated prior to the development of cavitation complete resolution of the disease can be expected. If cavitation has occurred then there will be residual damage to the lung tissue. If this is slight no harm will result but if it is gross then there will be some danger of a lingering infection which could be re-

Fig. 6.9. Severe tuberculosis of the upper lobe of the lung, which is studded with small abscesses containing caseous (cheesy) pus (post-mortem specimen).

activated. In this case the severely damaged lobe or segments of the lung are removed (lobectomy or segmental lobectomy).

BRONCHIECTASIS

This is a condition associated with areas of dilatation of the bronchi and may follow such diseases as whooping cough. It gives rise to the production of large quantities of infected sputum and results in a progressive destruction of lung tissue due to the effects of infection which is never completely eradicated. It is also a common cause of haemoptysis.

The most satisfactory method to confirm the diagnosis is by performing a bronchogram in which a radio-opaque solution is injected down the bronchial tree (Fig. 6.10).

Treatment

If the disease is localised to one lobe only of the lung and if it is severe then surgical excision by lobectomy is indicated. The majority of cases however are managed perfectly satisfactorily by postural drainage together with the use of an appropriate antibiotic to cover a phase of significant infection.

Fig. 6.10. A bronchogram of the right lung. This patient has a moderate degree of bronchiectasis of the right lower lobe.

This term means that there is a collection of pus within the pleural cavity. It may be caused in a number of ways:

1. Extension of infection from the lung.
2. By extension of infection from beneath the diaphragm, for example from a subphrenic abscess.
3. By penetrating injuries of the chest wall.
4. Following operations which involve the chest wall.
5. Spread of infection from the mediastinum, for example following rupture of the oesophagus.
6. By blood stream spread.

Clinical features

The patient with an empyema is usually ill with a raised temperature and gives a history consistent with the cause of the empyema. There is usually pain on the affected side of the chest which is aggravated by breathing. The white cell count is raised. Diagnosis is confirmed by chest X-ray which will indicate an effusion within the pleural cavity (Fig. 6.11).

Treatment

The treatment is similar to that for a collection of pus anywhere in the body, that is, the pus has to be drained. A needle is inserted into the chest under local anaesthetic and the fluid in the pleural cavity is removed. Some of this fluid is sent to the laboratory for culture so that the causative organism can be identified and its sensitivity to antibiotics established. One million units of soluble penicillin are inserted in the pleural cavity through the needle before it is withdrawn. Aspiration is continued on a daily basis so long as it is possible to evacuate completely the pleural cavity. If the pus becomes too thick to aspirate it will then become necessary to insert a drain and this is done by resecting a small portion of rib. The tube that is inserted need not be connected to an underwater drain because the visceral pleura is stuck to the parietal pleura in the region of the empyema, making pulmonary collapse impossible. Thereafter the tube is dressed each day in the usual way. So as to check that the cavity is becoming obliterated, a sinogram is performed at approximately 2 weekly intervals.

Sometimes, particularly in the case of tuberculosis, the visceral pleura becomes covered with a thick layer of fibrin. Normal function will never be established in this case and it is necessary to peel this layer off at operation, a procedure known as *decortication*.

Fig. 6.11. Chest X-ray of a patient with an empyema. Note the opaque effusion in the left pleural cavity.

NEOPLASMS OF THE LUNG AND BRONCHI

These may be either benign or malignant, and the malignant neoplasms may be either primary or secondary. By far the most important group of neoplasms are the primary malignant carcinomas of the bronchus.

Benign lung neoplasms

These are rare and include adenomas of the bronchus and carcinoid tumours, which may produce the hormone 5-hydroxytryptamine, which results in attacks of flushing and diarrhoea.

CARCINOMA OF THE BRONCHUS

Pathology

This is the commonest primary malignant tumour in males in this country and results in 27,000 deaths in England and Wales per year. There is now no doubt that one of the factors involved in its causation is the smoking of cigarettes. The fact that the incidence continues to rise may also be a reflection on atmospheric pollution by industry. It is a condition that is more common in men than women, although the incidence in women is rising and it is suggested that this is due to the increasing number of women who smoke.

In approximately half of those affected the tumour arises in one or other of the main bronchi and in the other cases it arises peripherally. The tumour spreads by infiltration and to the regional lymph nodes at the hilum of the lung as well as disseminating widely in the bloodstream. If the tumour is situated in a main bronchus it can enlarge and eventually block the bronchus with subsequent collapse of the lung distal to the obstruction (Fig. 6.12).

Clinical features

If the tumour ulcerates it very commonly bleeds and this gives rise to one of the most common presenting symptoms, namely, haemoptysis. Other presenting features include cough, shortness of breath,

Fig. 6.12. Specimen of lung showing an extensive carcinoma. The patient was a heavy cigarette smoker.

lung abscess or secondary deposits in distant tissues, for example, the liver which may become enlarged, bones producing pathological fractures, enlarged lymph nodes in the neck, and cerebral metastases with psychiatric presentation. Patients with bronchial carcinoma which has metastasised lose weight and appear to be ill. Some patients may have a silent carcinoma which is only discovered on chest X-ray either of the mass miniature type or being carried out for some other purpose. (See also page 57.)

Special investigations

Diagnosis is confirmed by chest X-ray, which often shows a shadow in the lung (Fig. 6.13) but absolute confirmation of diagnosis is only obtained by bronchoscopy and biopsy of the tumour.

Fig. 6.13. Chest X-ray showing an extensive carcinoma of the right lung.

Treatment

Unfortunately carcinoma of the lung is often one of the most malignant tumours and by the time diagnosis is made in the majority of patients the disease has spread beyond the local confines of the primary tumour. As soon as distant spread occurs surgical excision is no longer possible. Nevertheless the ideal method of treatment in a suitable case is surgical excision of the primary tumour together with the lobe or lobes of the lung which are involved; this is only possible in 1 in 20 of the patients who present with the disease. Of these patients operated on, only 1 in 5 can expect to be alive and free of disease 5 years later.

In the inoperable case radiotherapy is of some help in controlling the local spread of the tumour and in providing palliation for painful secondary deposits, for example, those which occur in bones. Chemotherapy is now being used more often and in some cases produces a good response.

Secondary neoplasms of the lung

These are particularly common from non-epithelial tumours, for example, osteogenic sarcoma of bone and melanoma. Deposits also occur however from other carcinomas of, for example, breast or kidney.

Chapter 7. Heart and great vessels

ANATOMY

The heart is a remarkably effective pump which functions day and night and without attention for 70 or more years, altering its rate and output to the body's requirements. It is made up of striated but involuntary muscle fibres. Essentially it is in two halves, one to deliver oxygenated blood at high pressure to the systemic circulation, and the other to perfuse the deoxygenated blood at low pressure through the lungs.

The heart is irregularly conical in shape (Fig. 7.1) and is placed obliquely in the mediastinum. It is invested in the tough fibrous pericardium and possesses four chambers and four valves. *The right atrium* (Fig. 7.2) receives deoxygenated venous blood from the superior and inferior venae cavae as well as the coronary sinus, which drains the heat muscle itself. It communicates with the *right ventricle* through the tricuspid valve, while the right ventricle empties into the pulmonary trunk guarded by the pulmonary valve. *The left atrium* has the four pulmonary veins opening into it, and communicates with the *left ventricle* via the mitral valve. The left ventricle opens into the aorta, the orifice being guarded by the three semi-lunar cusps of the aortic valve. The openings of the right and left coronary arteries, which supply arterial blood to the heart wall, open immediately above the aortic valve.

The atria are thin walled in contrast to the thick ventricles. The inner aspect of both the ventricles is marked by the presence of a number of irregular muscular elevations (trabeculae carneae) from some of which the papillary muscles project into the lumen of the ventricle and find attachment to the free borders of the cusps of both

A. Anterior aspect.

B. Posterior aspect.

Fig. 7.1 The heart and great vessels. S.V.C. = Superior vena cava, I.V.C. = inferior vena cava, L.A., R.A., = left and right atrium, L.V., R.V., = left and right ventricle).

the tricuspid valve (on the right) and mitral valve (on the left) by means of the chordae tendineae (Fig. 7.3).

The atria are separated from each other by the interatrial septum which contains an oval depression termed the *fossa ovalis*. This represents the foramen ovale of fetal life since, in the embryo, much of the blood returning from the umbilical veins along the inferior vena cava is shunted through this directly into the left side of the heart and hence into the systemic blood vessels, rather than perfusing through the non-functional lungs.

The interventricular septum, which divides the two ventricles, is muscular in its lower part and its upper portion is fibrous. Septal defects are a relatively common congenital abnormality and are specially likely to occur in the region of the fossa ovalis and in the membranous upper portion of the interventricular septum.

PRINCIPLES OF CARDIAC SURGERY

Much of surgery comprises the closing of defects and the relieving of obstructions. It is now possible to carry out these procedures on the heart and great vessels. Operations on the pericardium, the main

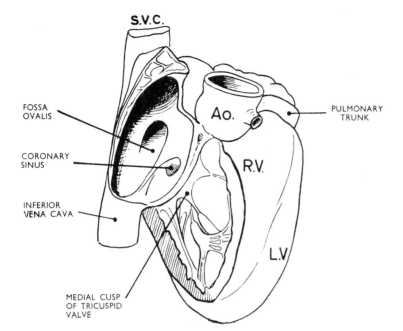

Fig. 7.2. The interior of the right atrium and ventricle

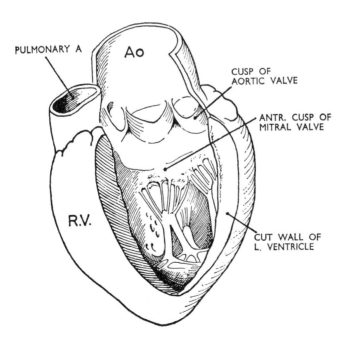

Fig. 7.3. The interior of the left ventricle.

vessels emerging from the heart, and some relatively simple cardiac procedures, such as splitting of the mitral valve for stenosis, can be performed without interruption of the circulation. However, major cardiac surgery can only be carried out in a relatively bloodless field produced by temporary cardiac arrest.

There are two main techniques at present employed, hypothermia and cardio-pulmonary bypass.

Hypothermia

If the circulation is stopped at normal body temperature the brain undergoes irreversible changes after 3 minutes. The liver, heart muscle and kidneys are also extremely susceptible to ischaemia, but may tolerate between 30–60 minutes of cardiac arrest. Hypothermia reduces the metabolic requirements of the tissue and thus allows prolongation of the period of permissible circulatory arrest. At $28°C$ up to 10 minutes of arrest can be tolerated, whereas in deep hypothermia ($10°C$ or lower) arrest can be carried out for periods of up to one hour. Conventional hypothermia is produced by surface cooling of the body whereas profound hypothermia requires the circulation of blood through a heat exchanger.

Cardio-pulmonary bypass

In this technique the heart-lung machine takes over the functions of pumping and oxygenation of the blood. Catheters are inserted into the venae cavae or the right atrium so that blood returning to the heart from the systemic venous circulation is siphoned off and pumped into an oxygenator (Fig. 7.4). There are 3 main types; the blood may be spread over rotating discs as a thin film in an oxygen chamber, or may be passed over the surface of a permeable membrane, or may have oxygen bubbled directly through it.

Once oxygenated, the blood is pumped back into the aorta, either through the femoral artery or directly through the ascending aorta. This technique will perfuse the whole body with oxygenated blood at an adequate pressure while shunting it away from the heart and lungs. If the aorta is cross-clamped it may be necessary, in addition, to perfuse the coronary arteries separately, and to drain the returning blood from the heart by means of a catheter in the coronary sinus.

At present the heart-lung machine is the more commonly used method.

Fig. 7.4. Cardio-pulmonary by-pass ('the heart-lung machine') in diagram form. (I.V.C., S.V.C. = inferior and superior vena cava).

SURGICAL DISEASES OF THE HEART AND GREAT VESSELS

For convenience of further discussion, these can be subdivided into 3 main groups:
1. Diseases of the Great Vessels.
2. Congenital Defects of the Heart.
3. Acquired Cardiac Diseases.

DISEASES OF THE GREAT VESSELS

Diseases of the great vessels include persistent ductus arteriosus, coarctation of the aorta, aortic stenosis and aortic aneurysm.

PATENT DUCTUS ARTERIOSUS

Normally this channel between the aorta and the pulmonary artery closes at the time of birth. If it persists, (Fig. 7.5) blood will be shunted from the high pressure systemic circulation into the pulmonary low pressure circulation, with resultant pulmonary hypertension.

Fig. 7.5. Patent ductus arteriosus.

Clinical features

The patient is often asymptomatic and diagnosis is made because the doctor finds the characteristic machinery-like continuous murmur in the upper chest on routine examination with the stethoscope. If the condition is allowed to persist, the abnormal strain on the heart may lead to cardiac failure.

Any congenital abnormality of the heart or its great vessels may become infected with the *Streptococcus viridans* with resulting *subacute bacterial endocarditis*.

Special investigations

Chest X-ray usually shows enlargement of the left ventricle and increased pulmonary arterial markings.
Angiocardiography will outline the patent ductus.

Treatment

Surgical treatment should be carried out as soon as possible after the age of one year to prevent heart failure and the possibility of infection of the duct. Ligation and division is preferable where possible to mere ligation, because of the possible risk of recanalisation in the latter case.

COARCTATION OF THE AORTA

Pathology

This is a congenital narrowing of the aorta (Fig. 7.6) and is usually in the region of the ductus arteriosus; indeed, on occasions, a patent ductus may also be present. The stenosis is usually extreme, and only a pinpoint lumen remains. Blood reaches the lower aorta through anastomotic channels, but only at grossly diminished pressure. The patient develops hypertension which results not from the blockage of the aorta itself, but in a large part is due to the relatively poor blood supply to the kidneys. Renal ischaemia causes a release of renin, which is a potent hypertensive agent. The danger of coarctation is due to the effects of this raised blood pressure, which may result in cerebral haemorrhage or heart failure. Another risk is the development of subacute bacterial endocarditis.

Clinical features

The diagnosis is usually made because hypertension is discovered in a child or young adult. A characteristic physical sign is absent or diminished femoral pulsations in contrast to the bounding pulses in the upper limbs.

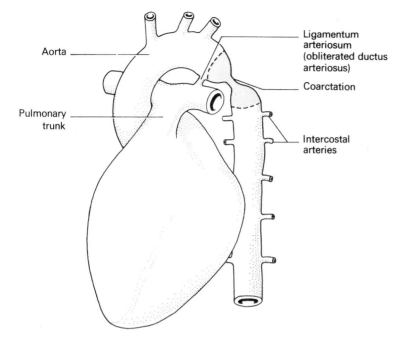

Aorta

Ligamentum
arteriosum
(obliterated ductus
arteriosus)

Coarctation

Pulmonary
trunk

Intercostal
arteries

Fig. 7.6. Coarctation of the aorta. The dotted lines represent the segment which is resected in surgical correction of this condition.

Special investigations

Chest X-ray will demonstrate hypertrophy of the left ventricle and often the ribs are seen to be notched by the large intercostal collateral arteries shunting blood around the stenotic area.

Treatment

The stenotic segment is excised and an end to end anastomosis performed. If the gap is too great, an arterial graft is used to join the two ends.

AORTIC STENOSIS

This may be congenital or may follow rheumatic heart disease. The damaged valve becomes grossly distorted and is liable to calcification.

Clinical features

Because the flow of blood into the aorta is diminished, the coronary blood flow is consequently reduced and the patient experiences angina pectoris. The left ventricle hypertrophies proximal to the stenosis and the patient may develop left ventricular failure with pulmonary oedema.

Attacks of syncope (unconsciousness) are common.

Treatment

Initially dilatation of the stenosed valve was used by a blind technique through the wall of the left ventricle or through the ascending aorta. Nowadays valve replacement is carried out under cardio-pulmonary bypass.

AORTIC ANEURYSM

The subject of aneurysm is considered in Chapter 8, but here we must note that aneurysms may involve the thoracic part of the aorta. These are commonly syphilitic, but may occur in Marfan's syndrome. Arteriosclerotic aneurysms may occur in the descending part of the thoracic aorta, but these are more likely to involve the abdominal aorta.

Dissecting aneurysm is especially likely to occur in the region of the aortic arch.

Direct repair of aneurysms in this region require heart bypass.

CONGENITAL CARDIAC DEFECTS
SEPTAL DEFECTS

Pathology

Congenital defects in the atrial or ventricular septal walls allow blood to shunt from the systemic into the pulmonary circulation. The effect may be negligible with a small defect, but a large one may be associated with considerable flow. As the pressure rises in the pulmonary system (pulmonary hypertension) there may eventually be reversal of flow with deoxygenated blood passing into the left atrium, so that the patient becomes cyanosed. The situation is complicated by the fact that other congenital abnormalities of the heart may coexist, particularly stenoses of valvular outflow tracts.

Clinical features

These vary from the asymptomatic patient, who is found to have a cardiac murmur on examination, to the cardiac cripple with cyanosis and heart failure. The situation may be complicated by infection of the defect (*subacute bacterial endocarditis*).

A chest X-ray may show dilatation of the heart.
Cardiac catheterisation and angiography may be used to demonstrate the size of the shunt, the degree of pulmonary hypertension and whether there are other associated congenital abnormalities.

Treatment

Although small symptomless atrial septal defects may be kept under observation, other defects with considerable shunting of blood require repair by open operation, using either hypothermia or cardiopulmonary bypass (Fig. 7.7).

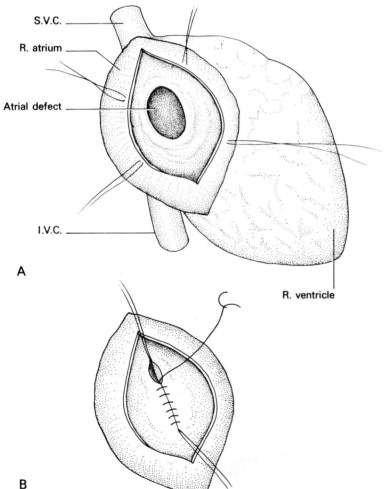

S.V.C.

R. atrium

Atrial defect

I.V.C.

A

R. ventricle

B

Fig. 7.7. Surgical closure of an atrial septal defect.

This is a relatively common congenital cardiac lesion (Fig. 7.8) which is associated with cyanosis. It comprises:

1. pulmonary stenosis.
2. a ventricular septal defect.
3. an aorta whose orifice overlies the right as well as the left ventricle.
4. right ventricular hypertrophy, which results from attempts to force blood through the stenosed pulmonary trunk.

The cyanosis results from the aortic blood becoming mixed with venous blood returning to the right heart, and which fails to enter the pulmonary circulation for oxygenation.

Clinical features

Cyanosis is usually present from birth. The child is breathless, is stunted in development, adopts a characteristic squatting position at rest and has clubbing of the fingers and toes. The heart is usually grossly enlarged on its clinical examination and a murmur can be heard at its root.

Special investigations

The chest X-ray confirms the enlargement of the heart, which has a characteristic boot shape.
Cardiac catheterisation and angiocardiography are necessary to delineate the abnormality.

Treatment

A major break-through in the treatment of congenital abnormalities of the heart was the development by Blalock of Boston of his operation in which an anastomosis was made between the left subclavian

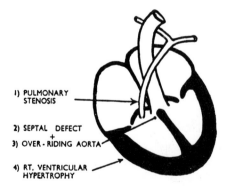

1) PULMONARY STENOSIS

2) SEPTAL DEFECT
   +
3) OVER-RIDING AORTA

4) RT. VENTRICULAR HYPERTROPHY

Fig. 7.8. The tetralogy of Fallot.

artery and the pulmonary artery. This resulted in blood being shunted into the pulmonary circulation beyond the region of the stenosis. Today the condition is dealt with by open heart surgery in which the interventricular defect is closed by suture or graft and the pulmonary stenosis relieved.

ACQUIRED DISEASES OF THE HEART
CONSTRICTIVE PERICARDITIS

Gross fibrosis and even calcification of the pericardium may result from a number of conditions—tuberculosis, rheumatic pericarditis, virus pericarditis, or fibrosis in a previous haemopericardium. The inelastic jacket which results impedes both the cardiac action and venous return to the heart. The patient develops ascites and hepatomegaly.

The chest X-ray may reveal calcification in the pericardium and on screening the pulsations of the heart are seen to be grossly impaired.

Treatment

The thickened pericardium is excised.

MITRAL STENOSIS

Pathology

Mitral stenosis commonly follows rheumatic carditis. The cusps of the mitral valve become thickened, fibrosed, and eventually calcified, so that the orifice of the valve becomes grossly narrowed. There may be associated involvement of the aortic valves.

Clinical features

The condition usually affects patients between the 20th and 40th year, females more commonly than males.

The damming up of blood proximal to the stenosed mitral valve produces pulmonary oedema with breathlessness and haemoptysis. Eventually the right ventricle goes into failure, with resultant hepatomegaly, ascites and oedema.

The complications of this condition include right heart failure, auricular fibrillation, peripheral arterial embolism from thrombus which forms in the dilated fibrillating left atrium, and subacute bacterial endocarditis from infection of the diseased valve.

Treatment

In the absence of mitral regurgitation, calcification of the valves or emboli, the closed operation is used. The original procedure was to insert the finger through the left atrium to split the valve, but it is now more satisfactorily achieved by means of a dilator inserted through the wall of the left ventricle while a finger palpates the valve through the left atrium.

If the valves are calcified, or if there is regurgitation, or if the left atrium is full of clot giving rise to emboli, then open operation is preferable with replacement of the diseased valve by means of a prosthetic (Fig. 7.9) or homograft valve.

ANGINA PECTORIS

Severe angina due to myocardial ischaemia may be treated surgically in selected cases. It may be possible to improve the cardiac blood supply by implantation of the internal mammary artery directly into the heart muscle (*Vineberg's Operation*). In some cases a localised segment of arteriosclerosis in the coronary artery may be removed by endarterectomy or bypassed with a saphenous vein graft from the aorta.

Fig. 7.9. A Starr-Edwards prosthesis for heart valve replacement, with introducer.

The place of cardiac transplantation in the treatment of severe myocardial disease is still the subject of world-wide controversy. At present there seems no doubt that such operations should only be carried out in one or two highly specialised centres where full assessment of the advantages and disadvantages of such a procedure can be assessed.

Chapter 8. Peripheral vascular disease

PERIPHERAL ARTERIAL DISEASE

Introduction

The function of the arteries is to convey nourishment and oxygen to the tissues. If the flow of blood in major arteries supplying a limb is diminished the first tissue to be affected is muscle, since this is the structure within the limb which has greatest demands on oxygen and metabolites, far more than skin or subcutaneous tissue which, in turn, require a better blood supply than relatively inert bone and tendon.

When a muscle is exercised its demand for oxygen and glucose is increased and its production of waste products of metabolism are proportionally higher. If insufficient blood is reaching the muscle, these products accumulate in the tissue and produce pain. This can easily be reproduced on oneself if the arm muscles are vigorously exercised while a sphygmomanometer cuff is applied to the upper arm and pumped up above the arterial pressure. Very soon a severe cramp-like pain is felt in the forearm muscles, which disappears as soon as the cuff is let down. This is because fresh arterial blood sweeps through the forearm muscles and washes away the pain-producing chemicals produced in the course of muscle action. This same pain is experienced by a patient whose major arteries in the lower limb are obstructed. He will complain of severe cramp, particularly in the back of the calf (where the muscles are especially bulky), which comes on after a few yards of walking and which disappears again when he has rested for a time. Such episodes of pain on exercise receive the term *intermittent claudication* from the Latin word Claudicare, which means 'to limp'. Nurses who remember their history will recall that the Emperor Claudius, who ruled in Rome in the first Century A.D., was so called because he had a severe limp, perhaps due to poliomyelitis acquired in infancy.

As the degree of arterial obstruction increases, so the claudication distance correspondingly diminishes and the period of time the patient must rest before the pain disappears becomes longer. Eventually the blood supply to the muscles is insufficient to wash away the metabolic breakdown products produced even when the muscles are inactive; the patient now complains of 'rest pain', often sufficiently bad to prevent sleep at night.

The normal pink appearance and warm feel of the fingers and toes is due to their perfusion by oxygenated blood through dilated arterioles and capillaries. If the amount of blood entering the limb is grossly limited by severe obstruction of the major arteries or if the peripheral small vessels are clamped down in severe spasm as in Raynaud's disease, the digits become cold and pale. If the limb is held dependent, it will demonstrate peripheral cyanosis, since the circulation is so slow through it that blood in the small vessels stagnates, becomes deoxygenated and therefore dark blue in colour. Eventually the blood supply to the skin is so impaired that death of tissue takes place and gangrene supervenes. Often this is precipitated by some very minor trauma. For example, the toe may become gangrenous following a nick produced in cutting the toe nails, or the pressure of the mattress against the heel may produce gangrene of the skin over this region (Fig. 8.1).

Note that the complete loss of blood supply to any tissue must inevitably result in its death, but *gangrene* implies the macroscopic (visible) death of tissue accompanied by infection. If a patient has a severe obstruction of one of the coronary arteries, for example,

Fig. 8.1. Gangrene of the toes in arterial obstruction. Note that there is also an area of gangrene over the lateral malleolus.

the cardiac muscle supplied by that vessel will undergo necrosis and die. This takes place in the absence of bacteria and gangrene of the heart muscle does not supervene. However, whenever the blood supply is cut off in the presence of organisms, these will invade the necrotic tissue. Typical examples are the gangrene which take place in acute appendicitis or in strangulated intestinal obstruction. Similarly, when a finger or toe has its blood supply cut off, inevitably the tissues will be invaded by bacteria entering through minute cracks or cuts in the skin, so that gangrene then ensues.

The causes of impaired limb circulation

There are a large number of conditions which can cause impaired arterial blood flow to the limbs and these include:

1. Injury to vessels by trauma, heat, cold or chemicals.
2. Atherosclerosis with superadded thrombosis.
3. Embolism.
4. Small vessel spasm (Raynaud's phenomenon).
5. Diabetes, either by itself or complicating atherosclerosis.
6. Buerger's disease.
7. Ergot poisoning.

The common conditions seen in this country are, first and foremost atherosclerosis, far outstripping the other conditions, although peripheral embolism and Raynaud's phenomenon are also common. Diabetes frequently complicates atherosclerotic disease.

ARTERIAL INJURY

Peripheral arteries may be injured by closed or open trauma.

Closed injuries may complicate fractures and dislocations, the ones most likely to be associated with arterial injury being supracondylar fracture of the humerus with damage to the brachial artery and dislocation of the knee or fracture of the lower end of the femur implicating the popliteal artery. Arterial injury may also occur from too tight application of a plaster of Paris splint to an injured limb or from a tourniquet which has been left on for more than an hour. Vessel damage from such closed injuries may take the form of spasm, thrombosis, rupture, or, in some cases of comminuted fracture, a direct tear of the artery by a spicule of bone.

Open injuries are not common in civilian practice in this country, although from time to time a butcher will be admitted whose knife will have slipped during the cutting up of a joint and who has stabbed himself in the femoral artery at the groin. In Spain the bullfighter may be damaged in the same place by the bull's horn. In less civilised parts of the world, stab wounds and gunshot wounds are more common. The damaged artery may go into spasm, or undergo thrombosis. It may be divided, and such division may either be partial or complete. Interestingly enough a partial division tends to bleed more furiously than a complete tear because, in the latter case, spasm may completely close the vessel.

Occasionally the damaged wall of the artery gives way to form an aneurysm (see below).

Clinical features

Arterial damage in an open wound is suggested by severe bright red bleeding. In a closed injury there may be the production of a massive haematoma. Major arterial interruption is accompanied by the signs of distal ischaemia which can easily be remembered since they all begin with the letter P:

Pain (due to extreme ischaemia of the muscles of the limb)
Pallor (due to lack of blood flow through the skin capillaries)
Pulselessness (the pulses below the point of injury disappear)
Paraesthesia (pins and needles due to peripheral nerve ischaemia)
Paralysis (due to loss of blood supply to the affected muscles)

Recently a colleague of ours in Dublin added a sixth P to the list— 'Perishing with cold', and certainly the ischaemic limb rapidly cools.

Treatment

Any obvious compression, such as a tight plaster or obstructing tourniquet, is removed. If vascular damage accompanies a closed fracture or dislocation, this must be reduced under a general anaesthetic and the stretched or spastic artery may then return to normal. If this does not occur rapidly, say within the next half hour, the artery must be explored. If found to be in spasm it may respond to the local application of a 2.5% solution of Papaverine, which is the only effective local antispasmodic. If the artery is found to be torn it will require repair, usually by means of a vein graft.

In an open injury associated with arterial bleeding the haemorrhage can usually be controlled by direct pressure and it is rarely necessary to use a tourniquet or pressure on a pressure point. A blood transfusion is arranged and the wound explored in the operating theatre under a general anaesthetic. Small peripheral arteries (below the elbow or the knee) can be treated by ligation but major vessels should be repaired, or, if the ends cannot be brought together, grafted. A suitable vessel to use is the patient's own saphenous vein so that most of us carry our own artery bank with us.

Definitions

An aneurysm is a sac communicating with the lumen of an artery. The following types may occur (Fig. 8.2):

1. *True aneurysm.* This is an actual dilatation of the wall of the artery itself. It may be *fusiform*, when the whole circumference of the artery is expanded, or *saccular*, when one side of the artery is dilated and communicates with the arterial wall through a comparatively narrow neck.

2. *False aneurysm.* This occurs when an artery is perforated by a puncture wound so that a cavity is produced which communicates with the lumen of the artery and which is lined by clot and fibrous tissue.

3. *An arterio-venous aneurysm* is formed by a communication between an artery and a vein. It may be congenital or traumatic in origin.

4. *A dissecting aneurysm* is formed when there is a tear in the inner coat of an artery (almost invariably the aorta) and blood dissects the wall of the vessel to form a second channel. This may either rupture back into the main arterial lumen or else burst through the outer coat of the vessel, with disastrous results.

Aetiology

A wide variety of pathological processes may produce an aneurysm. These include:

1. *Congenital.* The commonest example of this is the berry aneurysm which occurs on the branches of the internal carotid or vertebral arteries within the skull at the base of the brain on the circle of Willis (Fig. 8.3). This may rupture and is a common cause of subarachnoid haemorrhage. Much less common are congenital arteriovenous aneurysms, often multiple, which may occur between major vessels in the upper or lower limb.

2. *Traumatic.* Aneurysms are common in times of war and in areas where stabbings and shootings are everyday occurrences. The wall of the artery may be damaged by a penetrating wound and the weakened area may subsequently distend into an aneurysm. Puncture wounds may produce false aneurysms or, if the injury goes through both the artery and vein, an arterio-venous aneurysm may result.

3. *Inflammatory.* Patients with subacute bacterial endocarditis may develop an infective arteritis in peripheral arteries which leads to aneurysm formation. Syphilis may involve the thoracic part of the aorta but fortunately this once common occurrence is now rare in this country, thanks to early treatment of the disease.

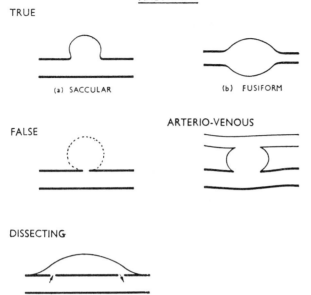

TRUE

(a) SACCULAR

(b) FUSIFORM

FALSE

ARTERIO-VENOUS

DISSECTING

Fig. 8.2. The types of aneurysm.

4. *Degenerative disease*. In modern practice atherosclerosis is the commonest cause of aneurysm. Degeneration of the arterial wall may result in a true aneurysm of the fusiform type and this is especially seen in the abdominal aorta, the iliac vessels, the femoral artery at the groin and the popliteal artery immediately behind the knee. It is also responsible for dissecting aneurysm of the aorta.

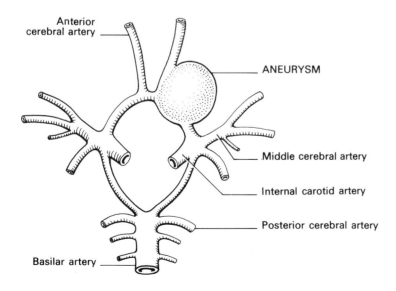

Anterior cerebral artery

ANEURYSM

Middle cerebral artery

Internal carotid artery

Posterior cerebral artery

Basilar artery

Fig. 8.3. A berry aneurysm on the circle of Willis at the base of the brain.

Clinical features

It is usually easy to diagnose an aneurysm. There is a dilatation along the course of an artery, which can be felt to pulsate. Pressure on the artery proximal to the aneurysm may reduce both its size and pulsation and it may also be possible to diminish its size by direct compression. If the entering artery has a narrow orifice, a thrill may be felt if the fingers are gently rested on the aneurysm because of the turbulent flow of blood within it. By the same token, a bruit (a rushing sound) may be heard over it by means of a stethoscope.

The commonest differential diagnosis is from a dilated, tortuous atherosclerotic artery, which is not uncommon in elderly subjects. It may also be mistaken for a highly vascular tumour, which because of its enormous blood supply may be felt to pulsate. In doubtful cases it may be necessary to perform an arteriogram to clinch the diagnosis.

Left untreated, an aneurysm may rupture into surrounding tissues, may thrombose, with impairment of the peripheral arterial circulation, may produce pain from pressure from an adjacent structure or, rarely, may become infected.

Treatment

Small peripheral aneurysms can be excised without endangering the peripheral circulation. More major aneurysms are removed and continuity of the artery restored by means of a graft (Fig. 8.4). In

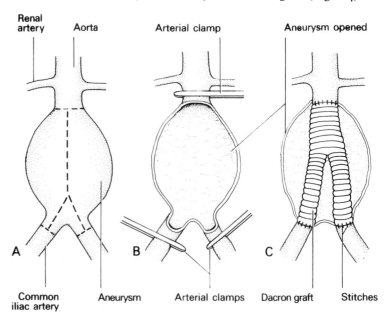

Fig. 8.4. Steps in the excision and grafting of an aortic aneurysm.

some situations the artery is ligatured proximal to the aneurysm sac in order to induce thrombosis and obliteration of the aneurysm; ligation of the carotid artery, for example, may be used to thrombose an intracerebral aneurysm.

ATHEROSCLEROTIC DISEASE

Pathology

Atherosclerosis (arteriosclerosis) is the commonest non-malignant killing disease of modern civilisation. Not only does it affect the peripheral arteries but it also involves the coronary and cerebral vessels which give rise to the potentially lethal complications of coronary and cerebral thrombosis. In spite of considerable research the aetiology of this condition is unknown. Its incidence and severity increase with advancing age and it is especially likely to be found in obese, diabetic subjects who are heavy smokers and who have a high blood cholesterol level.

In the initial stages, there are deposits of fatty material in the artery wall which may then become thickened, calcified and even ulcerate. Actual obliteration of the lumen of the artery is brought about by deposition of platelets on the damaged intima of the artery wall to produce a thrombus (Fig. 8.5).

Clinical features

Many patients with quite severe atherosclerosis of peripheral vessels have no symptoms because sufficient blood is able to reach the periphery through the narrowed arteries themselves, or along the collateral arteries. However, as the disease progresses, and particularly as arteries become completely occluded with thrombus, the deficient blood supply to the leg may first produce symptoms of claudication and, in the most severe cases, gangrene (see above).

Treatment

The treatment of patients with atherosclerotic disease of the legs must be sub-divided into the management of claudication, which is for the most part conservative, and the treatment of gangrene, which often requires surgical intervention.

Claudication

Since the principle disability is limitation of walking because of pain, it is often possible to keep a claudicating patient at work simply by altering his job. For example, a postman may have to change from delivering letters to office employment. If the patient is overweight,

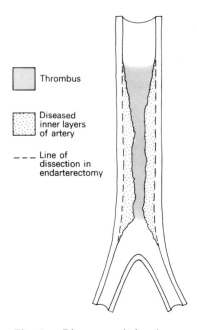

Thrombus

Diseased inner layers of artery

Line of dissection in endarterectomy

Fig. 8.5. Diagrammatic longitudinal section through an atherosclerotic artery. The lumen is obliterated with thrombus. The dotted line demonstrates the plane along which the diseased inner part of the artery together with the thrombus is removed in the operation of endarterectomy.

this must be corrected, since obesity gives added work to the muscles of the leg. It is quite unusual for patients with claudication not to be heavy smokers and it is essential for this habit to stop at once. Cigarette smoking produces spasm of the small blood vessels, increases the tendency for thrombosis to occur and, furthermore, replaces the oxyhaemoglobin in the arterial blood with carboxyhaemoglobin due to the inhalation of carbon monoxide in the cigarette smoke. We tell our patients that while they are smoking, coal gas rather than oxygen reaches the tissues of their limbs!

Careful chiropody is essential since gangrene can commence from the trauma produced by inexpert cutting of the nails or of a corn.

If a patient with atherosclerosis has diabetes it is extremely important that this is satisfactorily controlled since in addition to the impaired circulation due to atheroma, the diabetic is especially likely to develop gangrene, partly as a result of his increased tendency to infection and partly due to the associated diabetic neuritis, which may lead to trophic ulceration in the anaesthetic foot.

Naturally the patient is apprehensive that he is going to lose his leg. He should be told that, provided he carries out the above instructions, particularly with regard to complete cessation of cigarette smoking, he has a 90% chance that the claudication will remain at its present level or even improve; only approximately 10% of patients eventually develop gangrene.

Unfortunately, atherosclerosis is a generalised disease and many of these patients are going to succumb from the other major complications of this condition—coronary or cerebral thrombosis.

Arterial reconstructive surgery should only be considered when claudication is so severe that the patient can hardly walk and can no longer carry on his work. The details of such operations are given under the treatment of gangrene below.

We may summarise the treatment of claudication as follows:

1. Learn to live within the claudication distance and change job if necessary.
2. Lose weight—less effort for the leg muscles.
3. Stop smoking completely.
4. Take care of the feet to prevent minor trauma which may lead to gangrene.
5. Treat diabetes if present.
6. Consider reconstructive surgery if symptoms are severe and do not respond to conservative treatment.

GANGRENE

Once the patient has severe pain in the leg even at rest or has developed an area of gangrene on the foot, the intensity of the symptoms usually forces the surgeon to consider more active treatment. Provided that the patient's general condition is reasonable, an arteriogram is carried out in order to determine whether some sort of reconstructive operation is possible. If the popliteal artery and its branches are blocked then reconstruction is virtually impossible, but if the x-rays show that there is a good 'run-off' beyond the block in the iliac or femoral artery then an attempt can be made to shunt blood from above to below the obstruction (Fig. 8.6).

Two main types of operation may be carried out:

1. *Thromboendarterectomy.* In this the surgeon cores out the inner part of the diseased artery together with its contained thrombus, either through one long incision or through several small openings in the artery using a special ring stripper (Fig. 8.7). The incisions

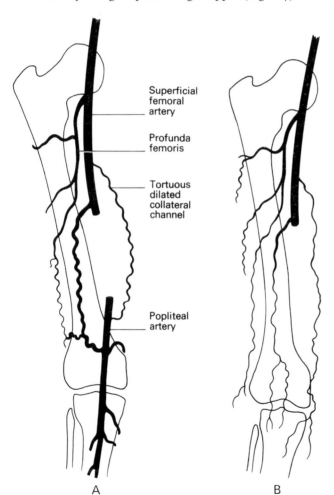

Superficial femoral artery

Profunda femoris

Tortuous dilated collateral channel

Popliteal artery

A

B

Fig. 8.6. Tracings of arteriograms which demonstrate, A, an example of good 'run-off' with a patent popliteal artery; this is suitable for reconstructive surgery. In B, however, the main arterial tree is obliterated and reconstruction cannot be carried out.

may be some association with sex hormones as a considerable proportion of female patients complain of discomfort in their veins just before menstruation and many women develop varicose veins during pregnancy which then regress after delivery. Although this may represent a hormonal effect, another contributory factor could be that the venous pressure in the lower limbs is raised due to the presence of the pregnant uterus pressing against the iliac veins.

The most common complaint of patients with varicose veins is their unpleasant appearance. As the veins become more dilated the patient may then complain of aching and heaviness of the limb during prolonged periods of standing; doctors and nurses often complain of their veins, possibly for this reason. As the veins become progressively worse, the venous circulation of the legs becomes more abnormal, and swelling of the ankles occurs.

Treatment

There are three possibilities, some or all of which may be appropriate to the particular patient. These are:

1. Surgical treatment.
2. Injection treatment
3. External support, for example by the use of elastic stockings.

1. *Surgery.* When a patient has incompetence of the valves in the long saphenous vein just as it joins the femoral vein, surgery is required. The saphenous vein is exposed at the groin through a small incision and is tied and disconnected together with all its tributaries at its junction with femoral vein (Trendelenberg operation). The operation of stripping of the long saphenous vein is no longer performed except in the rare instance of an incompetent mid-thigh perforator, when the long saphenous vein is stripped down to, but not below, the knee.

There are other methods of surgical treatment, such as multiple ligations, but the same effect is achieved much more simply by the use of injection sclerotherapy.

It must be explained to a patient undergoing a Trendelenberg operation that the visible varicosities in the leg will persist, but the origin of the increased pressure in the veins has been removed and if she wears an elastic stocking for approximately six weeks, the varicosities will tend to regress, particularly if there are no other incompetent communicating veins in the leg. Six weeks after operation, if there are any remaining varicosities these are treated by injection.

2. *Injection treatment.* (Fig. 8.14). This involves the injection of a sclerosant solution (the most commonly used is a 3% solution of

A

B

C

Fig. 8.14. Injection treatment. The veins are marked out (A), injected at the sites of perforation into the deep veins (B) and firm compression is then applied (C).

sodium tetra-decyl-sulphate, S.T.D.) at the points where the varicosities drain into the deep veins as they come through the deep fascia, a technique introduced by Professor George Fegan of Dublin. The principle is to inject the visible vein at the point at which the communicating vein emerges from the deep fascia. A fine needle is inserted into the vein, the leg is then elevated so that the vein is emptied, the segment of vein to be injected is isolated between fingers and 0.5 ml of S.T.D. is injected. This injection site is then kept in a compressed state so that the vein is kept empty by means of a bandage and a rubber pad. The S.T.D. is an intense irritant which damages the lining of the vein so that thrombosis occurs and scar tissue forms within it, thus producing obliteration of the varicosity and of the communicating vein. In order to be effective, the vein must be kept empty during the period of fibrous tissue formation, and this is achieved by firm compression bandaging maintained for a period of six weeks. A firm elastic stocking is worn over the bandage which holds the pad in place, and the patient is instructed to walk for at least three miles each day of the treatment period.

It is quite common for there to be pigmentation of the skin over a varicose vein. A successful injection of a varicose vein usually results in brown pigmentation in the line of the vein. This is usually stated by the patient to be bruising, this however is not the case. It is due to the deposition of blood pigments in the skin after a successful, therapeutically induced, thrombosis.

3. *External support.* In elderly or unfit patients a firm, full-length elastic stocking will compress the veins, give relief from the aching experienced by the patient on prolonged standing and reduce the oedema of the leg. As previously mentioned, when the pressure in the varicosities has been reduced by Trendelenberg operation, the wearing of an elastic stocking will assist the regression of the veins. If a patient has a tendency to varicose veins it is a good idea to wear elastic tights during the later stages of pregnancy.

Apart from the above, the main place of external support is in the treatment of a varicose ulcer which is described below.

The complications of varicose veins

There are three important and common complications:
1. Haemorrhage.
2. Thrombophlebitis.
3. Ulceration.

1. *Haemorrhage.* This usually follows some quite trivial injury. The dilated vein is close to the skin surface, thin-walled and contains blood under high pressure, when the patient is in the upright position or if the leg is hanging down.

Treatment: emergency treatment is extremely simple; the patient lies flat on the back with the leg elevated and a pressure bandage is applied, although the bleeding will stop if the tip of the thumb or finger is applied to the correct place. There is a recorded case of a woman patient who bled to death after one of her chickens pecked her varicose vein. This sad outcome would have been prevented had she not panicked and had simply applied a little pressure over the bleeding point.

Once the emergency is over, the varicose veins should be treated either by injection or by operation.

2. *Thrombophlebitis.* Thrombosis may occur spontaneously in the stagnant column of blood within a varicose vein or may be secondary to trauma of the leg. Thrombosis is intentionally induced, of course, by the sclerosing fluid used in the injection treatment of varicose veins. The affected segment of vein becomes tender and hard and the overlying skin may be red and hot. There is often a mild pyrexia

and malaise. This is not an infective condition but is due simply to the tissue reaction to the segment of blood clot within the vein. Bacterial infection is only seen when an infected injection or intravenous infusion has been given into the vein.

Treatment: since this is a chemical and not a bacterial reaction, there is no indication at all for antibiotic therapy. The patient requires bed rest if the condition is very severe, with the foot of the bed elevated and a mild pressure bandage applied to the leg. Generally, however, the condition is not sufficiently serious to require bed rest and will respond to the use of an elastic stocking and a suitable analgesic, for example Paracetamol. Anti-coagulant therapy is never indicated because the thrombus is adherent to the wall of the vein and there is no risk of its detachment with the formation of a pulmonary embolus.

3. *Ulceration.* An ulcer may be defined as an area where epithelium has been lost, and the commonest ulcer by far is the so-called varicose ulcer. A better name is a 'gravitational ulcer' since this includes the concept of the cause of the condition as the high venous pressure within the leg veins. The immediate precipitating factor which may result in an ulcer is a trivial injury to the affected skin (Fig. 8.15).

A rare complication of a long-standing ulcer is malignant change in its edge with the result that this becomes raised above the surface (Marjolin's ulcer).

Treatment: the high venous pressure within the incompetent veins and the superficial venous system can be abolished by putting the patient to bed with the foot elevated. Under these circumstances the venous abnormality is corrected and tissue health is improved. However, this simple treatment is not always a practical one as quite often the patients are elderly and prolonged recumbency will carry with it the dangers of venous thrombosis, pressure sores and chest infection. The other way to abolish the high venous pressure is to use elastic bandaging of the leg from the toes to the knee. This acts by emptying the superficial dilated veins, thus enabling the muscles of the leg to pump the venous blood back towards the heart. There is absolutely no need to place exotic ointments on the ulcer and antibiotics should at all costs be avoided; indeed, all that is required is some bland dressing to apply to the ulcer itself in order to prevent the Elastoplast from sticking to it. The most commonly used dressing is Viscopaste, although other preparations are available if this does not suit the patient. If the skin of the patient is badly affected by varicose eczema, Icthopaste may be used or if there is an extensive scaly eruption of the skin, coal tar paste is the dressing of choice. The technique involved in dressing the leg is

Fig. 8.15. An extensive varicose ulcer.

important. The bland bandage dressing is applied without wrinkles and then over the top of this Elastoplast is applied in smooth circular sweeps so that an even and firm pressure is applied to the whole of the leg and foot to the level of the knee (Fig. 8.16).

Once the elastic bandage has been applied to the leg, the patient should be advised to sleep with the foot of the bed elevated to encourage venous return, and should also walk about as much as possible to encourage muscle pumping. The first bandage is removed after a week, because there will often have been considerable oozing through the dressing. Once this has ceased, the next bandage can be left on for two or sometimes three weeks and progressive healing will be seen to take place. Small ulcers will heal in a few weeks, although larger ulcers will take several months of patient dressings before epithelialisation is complete.

Occasionally, very extensive ulcers may require skin graft and

Fig. 8.16. Steps in the bandaging of a varicose ulcer. A sterile gauze dressing is placed over the ulcer and the eczematous skin is protected with a Viscopaste bandage (A). Elastoplast bandaging is commenced distally (B) and continued to below the knee (C).

now and again ulceration is so extensive with destruction of the underlying tissues and fixing of the ankle joint that patients are advised to submit to below-knee amputation.

Other causes of ulcers of the leg

Gravitational ulcers account for 9 out of every 10 ulcers seen in this country. The most important of the others is the ischaemic ulcer due to impaired arterial blood supply. This should be diagnosed if the foot is felt to be cold and pale, the patient complains of intermittent claudication on walking and the peripheral pulses are absent. An ulcerated tumour may be a breaking-down melanoma or a squamous carcinoma of the skin, but this often arises in a pre-existing chronic ulcer. A gumma in advanced syphilis used to be common, but it is now only rarely seen. Ulcers may complicate some medical diseases including ulcerative colitis, rheumatoid arthritis and acholuric jaundice. From time to time we see self-inflicted ulcers on the leg, and this should be suspected if the ulcer has a peculiar shape such as an exact square and also if the patient has an unusual psychological make-up.

Chapter 9. The lymphatics and lymph nodes

INTRODUCTION

The lymphatics are fine, thin walled tubes which ramify through all the tissues of the body with the exceptions of the central nervous system and cartilage. They are concerned with the circulation of tissue fluid, which passes into the lymphatics and is then shunted into the venous system. In addition, lymphatics can take up fine particulate matter and this is of particular importance in the intestine, where the bulk of fat is absorbed in this manner into the lymphatics of the gut wall. The lymphatics filter through the lymph nodes, which number approximately 800, and which are found particularly in the neck, axillae, groin, the mesenteries of the alimentary canal and in the mediastinum. The lymph drains back into the blood stream principally via the thoracic duct, which opens into the commencement of the left innominate vein at the root of the neck, and the smaller lymph ducts, which open in the major veins (subclavian and jugular) on the right side of the neck.

The lymph nodes serve the following functions:

1. As filters for bacteria and other foreign particles, including cancer cells.

2. As the sites of production of lymphocytes.

3. As centres which respond to foreign proteins (*antigens*) to produce *antibodies* from the plasma cells and to develop sensitised lymphocytes. These two processes are the fundamentals of the immune response to any foreign proteins, which include bacteria, viruses, transplanted tissues, such as kidneys, and probably also cancers.

The particulate material which may be taken up by the lymphatics includes bacteria, and these organisms may produce an acute inflammation of the lymphatics draining an infected area (*acute lymphangitis*). This is especially likely to occur with streptococcal infection and is characterised by the appearance of red streaks along the skin which correspond to the lymphatic channels. At the same time, the draining lymph nodes become swollen and tender (*acute lymphadenitis*) and these may indeed suppurate, with abscess formation.

Treatment

This condition, once extremely serious, can now be treated very satisfactorily with antibiotic therapy. Rapid resolution takes place, provided that the organism is sensitive to the antibiotic employed. The wound itself or the regional nodes, if either or both are the site of abscess formation, will require surgical drainage.

Fig. 9.1. Congenital lymphoedema of the right leg and the scrotum.

LYMPHOEDEMA

Obstruction of the lymphatic flow from any cause results in the accumulation of fluid in the affected region, for which the term *lymphoedema* is applied. The common causes of lymphoedema are:

1. *Congenital abnormality of the lymphatics of the lower limbs*
Lymphoedema in these patients may be present at birth but usually develops early in adult life. Females are more affected than males, and the conditions may run in families (Fig. 9.1).

2. *Post-inflammatory*
Repeated attacks of acute lymphangitis may result in obliteration of the lymphatics by fibrous tissue.

3. *Filariasis*
A tropical disease due to the nematode worm Filaria bancrofti which is transmitted by the mosquito. The filaria infects the lymphatics with consequent fibrotic lymphatic obstruction. This results in gross lymphoedema, especially of the lower limbs and the genitalia. Chylous ascites may also complicate this condition—the peritoneal cavity becoming filled with milky lymphatic exudate.

4. *Following radical surgery*
Extensive removal of the lymphatics, for example block dissection of the groin or the neck in the treatment of malignant disease, may be followed by lymphoedema.

Fig. 9.2. Lymphoedema of the arm. The patient has had a previous mastectomy and radio-therapy and has now developed recurrent tumour in the axilla and supraclavicular fossa. All three have combined to destroy or obstruct the lymphatic drainage of the arm.

5. *Post-irradiation fibrosis*

Heavy irradiation in the treatment of malignant disease may obliterate the lymphatics in the treated area, and this state of affairs may be aggravated by previous radical surgery. Lymphoedema of the arm, for example, may be seen after an extensive radical mastectomy, in which the axillary lymph nodes have been removed, and which has then been followed by a full course of irradiation.

6. *Malignant disease*

Extensive secondary deposits in the lymph nodes frequently produce sufficient lymphatic obstruction to result in lymphoedema. Late oedema of the upper limb after mastectomy is often indicative of massive recurrence of tumour in the axilla, occluding any residual lymphatic pathways (Fig. 9.2).

Differential diagnosis

There are, of course, many other causes of oedema apart from disturbance of lymphatic drainage. Increased venous pressure, either from venous obstruction or from congestive cardiac failure, causes transudation of fluid into the tissues as a result of high pressure in the capillary vessels. Conditions which lower the plasma protein (starvation, the nephrotic syndrome, cirrhosis, etc.) produce a lowered osmotic pressure of the plasma which results in decreased fluid take up of tissue fluid through the capillaries.

Treatment

The treatment of lymphoedema naturally depends to a great extent on its aetiology. Conservative treatment comprises elevation of the affected limb and the use of elastic compression by means of either an elastic bandage or stocking. Gross cases of congenital lymphoedema may be treated surgically by excision of the oedematous subcutaneous tissue. This will restore the contour of the leg, but leave it with considerable scarring.

The massive brawny arm or leg that is seen in late cases of malignant obstruction of the lymphatics is a serious and intractable condition which can only be helped slightly by limb elevation, elastic bandages and analgesic drugs.

THE LYMPHADENOPATHIES

This is a convenient term for the group of conditions characterised by enlargement of the lymph nodes, the causes of which can be classified as follows:

1. Acute infection.
2. Chronic infection.
3. Neoplastic—due to secondary spread of tumour.
4. The reticuloses.
   (a) Hodgkin's Disease
   (b) Lymphosarcoma and reticulum cell sarcoma
   (c) Lymphatic leukaemia.

Enlarged lymph nodes may also be seen in sarcoidosis and rheumatoid arthritis.

The acute infective causes may be due to some local infection. The commonest example of all is the cervical lymphadenopathy secondary to tonsillitis, which nearly everybody has experienced at some time. But lymph nodes draining any area where there is an acute infection may become inflamed.

A generalised infection associated with enlarged lymph nodes is *glandular fever* (infective mononucleosis) which is a viral infection associated with enlarged lymph nodes, fever, a sore throat, a rash, and sometimes enlargement of the spleen. The blood film shows a raised total count, in the region of 15,000 white cells, the majority of which are monocytes.

Of the chronic infections, *tuberculosis* is the commonest and is considered below. Enlarged lymph nodes are found in the area draining a primary syphilitic chancre and a generalised enlargement of lymph nodes may occur in the secondary stage of syphilis.

Neoplastic nodes are hard and, as they enlarge, may become matted together and eventually ulcerate through the skin. Common examples are the enlarged axillary nodes found in carcinoma of the breast or the cervical nodes associated with cancer within the oral cavity.

The reticuloses usually produce rubbery enlarged nodes, frequently affecting more than one anatomical site. The liver, spleen and other organs may be involved and enlarged.

TUBERCULOUS LYMPHADENITIS

With a general decline in tuberculosis, this once common lesion (mainly of children) is now quite unusual in this country. However, the incidence has shown some rise recently, particularly among immigrants. The cervical nodes are most commonly involved, the bacilli having entered via the tonsil. The organisms may be human or bovine, the latter due to the ingestion of milk contaminated with tubercle bacilli. Occasionally enlarged cervical nodes are found in elderly patients who usually have active tuberculosis of the lung apex.

It is quite common on routine X-rays of the chest and abdomen to

Fig. 9.3. A tuberculous 'cold abscess' of the neck.

see calcified nodes in the mediastinum or mesentery. These represent burnt out tuberculous disease resulting from a previous pulmonary inoculation in the case of the mediastinal nodes, or the ingestion of bovine organisms in contaminated milk with subsequent take-up by the intestinal lymphatics in the case of the mesenteric nodes. Tuberculous lymphadenitis in the neck commences as a group of small discrete painless nodes, usually found in the upper part of the neck in the carotid triangle. As they enlarge they become matted together, break down into a tuberculous abscess, which then bursts through into the subcutaneous tissues. This is a chronic abscess and, unlike the usual acute affair, there is very little pain and although the skin may be reddened it does not feel hot to the touch. For this reason the term 'cold abscess' is applied to this lesion (Fig. 9.3). Left untreated, the abscess will discharge spontaneously onto the skin with the formation of a chronic tuberculous sinus. Fig. 9.4 shows diagrammatically the stages of the progression of this condition.

Solid nodes must be differentiated from acute lymphadenitis, from secondary deposits or from one of the reticuloses. At the stage of a breaking down abscess the differential diagnosis is from a branchial cyst. Diagnosis is assisted by an X-ray of the neck, because usually the chronic tuberculous nodes show flecks of calcification, which are not seen in other causes of lymph node enlargement.

Treatment

If the patient is seen at an early stage, before abscess formation has occurred, it is possible to excise the enlarged node. If the patient presents with an abscess already present, the pus is evacuated and the underlying breaking down tuberculous nodes evacuated by curettage. Once the diagnosis has been confirmed by pathological examination of the node and bacteriological study of the pus, a full course of anti-tuberculous chemotherapy is commenced. This normally comprises an initial three months of triple therapy with streptomycin, PAS and INAH followed by a further nine months in which the latter two drugs only are administered. In addition, the patient's general condition is improved by a full diet and fresh air.

SECONDARY CARCINOMA

One of the commonest causes of enlarged lymph nodes is the presence of secondary deposits from a primary carcinoma which lies in the area of lymphatic drainage of that particular group of nodes. Thus nodes in the groin may derive from a tumour situated anywhere

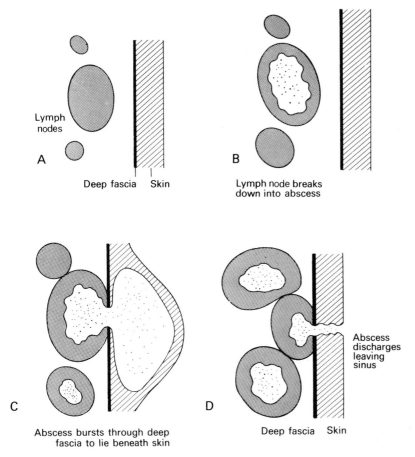

Fig. 9.4. Tuberculous infection of cervical lymph nodes leading to a 'cold abscess' and eventually a chronic sinus.

along the leg, buttock, lower abdominal wall, external genitalia, or lower part of the anal canal; axillary nodes may be involved from a primary of the upper limb or breast, and enlarged cervical lymph nodes may be secondary to a primary growth of the face, the mouth, larynx, pharynx, oesophagus, bronchus, breast, or thyroid. The cervical nodes may also be involved via the thoracic duct from the primary tumour situated in the breast, stomach, large intestine, or the testis (Fig. 9.5).

Treatment

The treatment of secondarily involved lymph nodes in the common tumours is dealt with in the appropriate sections, but here we may sum up by saying that, as a rule, enlarged superficial nodes which are mobile may be removed by block dissection provided that the

Fig. 9.5. Secondaries in cervical lymph nodes following a mastectomy for carcinoma of the left breast.

Fig. 9.6. Hodgkins' disease affecting the right cervical lymph nodes.

primary tumour is either operable or can be treated effectively by radiotherapy. For example, a patient with a carcinoma of the tongue may have this treated by a radium implantation, following which block dissection of a group of enlarged but mobile nodes in the neck may be carried out. If the primary tumour is inoperable because of fixation and invasion, or if the nodes themselves have now reached the stage where they are matted and fixed to surrounding structures, then obviously radical surgery is out of the question, and usually palliative radiotherapy is employed. A frequent cause of death in such circumstances is ulceration of the lymph nodes, leading to lethal haemorrhage from invaded adjacent blood vessels.

THE RETICULOSES

Primary tumours of lymphoid tissues are termed the reticuloses or malignant lymphomas. The most important of these are:
1. Hodgkin's Disease.
2. Reticulum cell sarcoma.
3. Lymphosarcoma.
4. Chronic lymphatic leukaemia.

These conditions usually present with lymph node enlargement, particularly the cervical nodes, but any group or groups of lymph nodes may be affected, including the mediastinal, abdominal or retroperitoneal groups. Spread from one lymph node group to another frequently occurs, and there may be involvement of spleen, liver, bone marrow and other tissues. Males are more often affected than females. Hodgkin's disease particularly affects young adults, whereas the other reticuloses are more often seen in more elderly patients (Fig. 9.6).

The differential diagnosis between the various types depends on the microscopic examination of a lymph node taken at biopsy.

Hodgkin's disease is characterised by replacement of the normal lymph node architecture by pleomorphic tissue made up of mononuclear cells, giant cells (containing several nuclei), lymphocytes, eosinophils and fibrous tissue, although there is wide variation in the microscopic appearance of this condition.

Reticulum cell sarcoma is made up of undifferentiated cells which, on special staining, show interspersed reticulin fibres.

Lymphosarcoma is made up of darkly staining lymphoid cells. Chronic lymphatic leukaemia gives the same histological picture as lymphosarcoma, but is characterised by the presence of large numbers of abnormal lymphocytes in the blood, the count rising to between 30,000 and 300,000.

Treatment

Some examples of localised lymphoma, for example, Hodgkin's disease confined to one group of superficial nodes, or a lympho-sarcoma localised to a segment of intestine, may be treated by surgical excision. In the main, treatment depends on radiotherapy and/or cytotoxic therapy.

Chapter 10. The central nervous system

HYDROCEPHALUS

The circulation of the cerebro-spinal fluid (C.S.F.)

Hydrocephalus is gross distension of all or part of the ventricular system of the brain by cerebro-spinal fluid. It is therefore essential to understand the production, circulation and absorption of C.S.F. if the mechanism and treatment of this condition is to be understood.

C.S.F. is produced by the choroid plexuses of the lateral, third and fourth ventricles (Fig. 10.1). These plexuses are made up of vascular folds derived from the lining epithelium of the ventricles. The fluid escapes from the 4th ventricle through a mid-line and two lateral foramina into the subarachnoid space surrounding the brain. About four fifths of the fluid is reabsorbed via the arachnoid villi; these are minute projections of the arachnoid mater which pierce the dura covering the venous sinuses to lie immediately

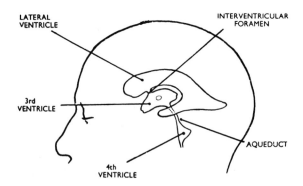

Fig. 10.1. The ventricular system within the brain.

beneath their endothelium and pump C.S.F. back into the venous blood stream. The remaining one fifth of the C.S.F. is absorbed by the arachnoid villi in the spinal segment of the dural sheath or else escapes along the spinal nerve sheaths to be absorbed in the lymphatics.

The C.S.F. itself is a water-clear fluid containing electrolytes similar to those in the blood plasma together with glucose.

The total quantity of C.S.F. in the adult is about 150 ml and approximately 500 ml of this fluid is produced daily.

Obstruction anywhere along the C.S.F. pathway produces a rise in pressure and then dilatation within the system proximal to the block. This resulting hydrocephalus can be divided into:

1. *Obstructive.* Here the fluid cannot escape due to blockage within the duct system. This may be produced by a congenital abnormality, a chronic abscess, scarring from previous trauma, or by pressure from a tumour. One form of congenital stenosis is the *Arnold-Chiari malformation* which is a congenital downward protrusion of the cerebellum through the foramen magnum of the skull. There is consequent occlusion of the foramina of the 4th ventricle, and hydrocephalus ensues. Frequently this condition is associated with spina bifida.

2. *Communicating.* C.S.F. can escape from within the brain but absorption via the villi is prevented by obliteration of the subarachnoid channels. This may be the result of meningitis, birth trauma, or perhaps congenital failure of development of the arachnoid villi.

Clinical features

From the clinical point of view hydrocephalus may be sub-divided into two important groups: the first comprises the congenital type, and the second the acquired variety which present with features of raised intracranial pressure as described later in the chapter.

Congenital hydrocephalus is usually of the communicating type but may be produced by congenital stenosis within the ventricular system of the brain of the Arnold-Chiari malformation (see above).

The enlargement of the head may occur before birth and may be a cause of obstructed labour. After birth rapid enlargement of the head takes place and produces a typical clinical picture (Fig. 10.2). The head is large, the fontanelles are wide, tense and fail to close at the normal times, the skin is stretched over the skull and dilated cutaneous veins are present over the scalp. Typical of the condition is the downward displacement of the eyes, and the brow overhangs

Fig. 10.2. Congenital hydrocephalus. Note the dilated cutaneous veins over the enormous skull.

Plastic catheter
shunts C.S.F.
from hydrocephalic
lateral ventricle
into cisterna magna

Dilated
lateral
ventricle

Skull

Fig. 10.5. Ventriculo-cister-
notomy for obstructive hydrocephalus (Torkildsen operation).

3. An intracranial tumour—today by far the commonest cause.
Other causes are rare in this country, although from time to time
curiosities such as hydatid cyst or a syphilitic gumma are encountered.

Clinical features

A space-occupying lesion may produce raised intracranial pressure
and/or localising signs in the central nervous system.

Raised intracranial pressure

A mass within the skull produces raised intracranial pressure, partly
by its actual presence within the enclosed space of the cranium,
partly by surrounding oedema, and sometimes by impeding the
circulation CSF with the production of hydrocephalus (see page
132). If the rise in pressure within the skull is slowly progressive,
the following features may be found:

1. *Headache*. This is severe and is often present when the patient wakes from his sleep; it is aggravated by straining or coughing.

2. *Vomiting*, which typically is often without preceding nausea.

3. *Papilloedema*—the raised pressure produces swelling of the optic disc of the fundus seen through an ophthalmoscope. This may be accompanied by blurring of vision and may even progress to blindness.

4. *Mental deterioration*—the patient may undergo a marked personality deterioration, become demented, or drowsy and eventually lapses into coma.

Localising signs

Localising signs will depend on the situation of the tumour. Severe personality change suggests frontal lobe involvement, spastic hemiplegia points to involvement of the internal capsule and defects in the visual field indicate pressure on the optic pathway, whereas cerebellar lesions are associated with inco-ordination, dizziness and often nystagmus (a flickering of the eyes on lateral deviation).

CEREBRAL ABSCESS

There are three common causes of brain abscess:

1. *A penetrating wound* of the skull, which allows direct access of bacteria into the brain.

2. *Direct spread* from an infection of the middle ear, the mastoid, or the frontal nasal sinus.

3. *Blood-borne spread*, especially from a lung infection (e.g. lung abscess or bronchiectasis).

Clinical features

The patient may present with features of the underlying cause, for example, a mastoid infection or a penetrating brain wound, followed by evidence of the development of an intracranial space-occupying lesion. During the early stages there may be marked toxaemia, fever and meningeal irritation. However, once the abscess is walled off, the general manifestations of infection may not be evident and the features we have already listed—headache, vomiting, papilloedema and mental deterioration—may dominate the picture.

Accurate localization of the abscess may require special investigations, including an electro-encephalogram, computerised tomography (CAT scan), gamma scan, and cerebral angiography.

Treatment

Once the abscess is localised it should be aspirated by means of a brain needle passed through a burr hole. The pus is replaced with antibiotic together with a radio-opaque solution, which enables subsequent X-ray studies to be made (Fig. 10.6). The aspirations may require to be repeated and systemic antibiotics are given depending on the bacteriology report on the pus.

Occasionally the abscess fails to respond to aspiration, and its capsule must then be excised surgically.

INTRACRANIAL TUMOURS

It is a fascinating fact that the only cells in the human body that never give rise to tumours are the nerve cells of the C.N.S. This is because although all other tissues are constantly being replaced at a greater or lesser speed throughout life, no new brain cells form once our basic quota is established in fetal life—a thought that can give rise to a great deal of interesting philosophical discussion. Primary intracranial tumours can therefore only develop from the supporting framework of connective tissue cells (neuroglia) or from the numerous structures which surround the brain—the meninges, cranial nerves, the pituitary and pineal glands, blood vessels and the skull. Added to this it is important to remember that secondary deposits in the brain are very common. In specialised neurosurgical units they account for only about 15% of the cases seen, but many patients dying of widespread metastases have intracranial deposits and these do not usually come under specialist neurological care.

Fig. 10.6. Cerebral abscess shown by injection of radio-opaque dye following aspiration of the pus through a burr-hole.

The incidence of the various intracranial tumours encountered at a neurosurgical unit is approximately:

Glioma—45%
Meningioma—15%
Metastases—15%
Acoustic Tumours—5%
Pituitary Tumours—5%
All others—15%

Gliomas

The gliomas arise from the neuroglial supporting cells and are responsible for about 45% of intracerebral tumours (Fig. 10.7). They are classified according to the principal cell component and details of this highly complex field of neuropathology can be obtained in larger text books than this. The tumours vary considerably in their histological differentiation and invasiveness from highly anaplastic and rapidly destructive tumours to relatively benign, cystic, slowly growing lesions.

Meningioma

These account for 15% of intracranial tumours and arise from the dura mater, to which they are almost invariably attached. Typically they occur in middle-aged patients. The majority are slowly growing and do not invade the brain tissue, but involve it only by expansion

Fig. 10.7. A highly malignant glioma. Note the compression and displacement of the lateral ventricle by the tumour.

and pressure, so that they may eventually become buried in the brain. The tumour may invade the overlying skull producing a hyperostosis which may occasionally be enormous.

Acoustic tumours

Cranial nerve tumours arise from the cells of the nerve sheaths. The great majority arise from the 8th cranial nerve (the auditory nerve) and this accounts for 5% of intracranial tumours. It is usually found in adult patients.

As the acoustic tumour enlarges it stretches the adjacent cranial nerves, especially the 5th (trigeminal) and 7th (facial), as well as pressing on the neighbouring cerebellum and the brain stem. Initially, damage to the auditory nerve itself produces unilateral nerve deafness with giddiness and ringing in the ear (tinnitus). Pressure on the 5th and 7th nerves produces facial numbness and facial paralysis respectively, while compression of the cerebellum results in nystagmus and motor inco-ordination. Eventually features of raised intracranial pressure become evident.

Pituitary tumours

These account for about 5% of intracranial tumours. They have two special features—their endocrine disturbances and their relationship to the optic chiasma.

Pituitary tumours are classified by the staining reaction of their cells into chromophobe adenomas, whose cells are non-granular, eosinophilic tumours, whose cells have granules which stain with eosin, and basophilic tumours whose cell granules stain with basic dyes.

Chromophobe adenoma is the commonest pituitary tumour. As it enlarges it compresses the optic chiasma, producing blindness in both temporal fields (Fig. 10.8). It is a non-secretory tumour which gradually destroys the normally functioning pituitary. In childhood there is arrest of growth and in adults there is loss of sex characteristics. As the tumour extends there may be involvement of the adjacent hypothalamus with diabetes insipidus and obesity.

Eosinophil adenoma secretes the pituitary growth hormones. If it occurs before puberty it induces gigantism. After puberty acromegaly results (Fig. 10.9).

Basophil adenoma is small, produces no pressure effects, but is associated with hyperplasia of the adrenal cortex and Cushing's syndrome (see page 385).

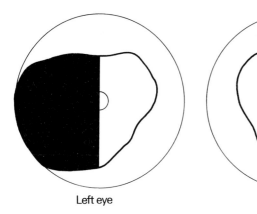

Left eye   Right eye

Fig. 10.8. Visual field chart in a patient with a pituitary tumour. Note the blindness in both temporal fields (bitemporal hemianopia), marked black on the chart.

Secondary tumours

Particular primary sites of origin are from carcinomas of the lung, breast and kidney. Small multiple deposits tend to be scattered through the brain, so that early features are personality change and confusion leading later to coma.

Special investigations

X-rays of the skull. Areas of calcification may be seen in 10% of tumours. The pineal gland is often calcified in adults and inspection of the films of the skull may show a shift of the pineal to one side, indicating a space-occupying lesion. Enlargement or erosion of the pituitary fossa suggests the presence of a pituitary tumour. The development of *computerised axial tomography* (C.A.T. scan), using a new technique of X-ray scanning and recording, has greatly improved the radiological diagnosis of intracranial masses.

X-ray of the chest must always be performed to exclude a primary bronchogenic carcinoma, which is the commonest source of brain metastases.

Brain scan with radioactive isotopes is extremely important as a simple and painless method of obtaining a positive localising diagnosis (Fig. 10.10).

Air studies. Air may be introduced into the ventricles either through a burr-hole (*ventriculography*) or via a lumbar or cisternal puncture (*air encaphalography*). Deformity or displacement of the ventricles may outline a space-occupying tumour.

Cerebral angiography. An intracranial tumour may be localised by injecting radio opaque dye into the carotid artery. An abnormal vascular pattern may be seen in the tumour or the vessels may be

Fig. 10.9. Acromegaly due to an eosinophil adenoma of the pituitary. Note the coarse enlarged features.

Fig. 10.10. Brain scan demonstrating a cerebral tumour, which shows as the relatively dense area.

Fig. 10.11. A large right-sided cerebral tumour demonstrated by angiography. Note that the anterior cerebral artery, which should be in the mid-line, is displaced over to the left by the tumour mass.

seen to be displaced by the growth from their normal positions (Fig. 10.11).

Aspiration biopsy of the tumour may be performed through a burr hole.

Electro-encephalography (EEG) may give useful localising information in tumours of the cerebrum.

Treatment

Slowly growing encapsulated intracranial tumours are capable of surgical removal and these include many meningiomas, acoustic neuromas and pituitary tumours. Of the gliomas, only the well differentiated tumours are amenable to surgical removal. Malignant primary growths have an extremely poor prognosis and are treated by palliative radiotherapy after the diagnosis has been established by a biopsy.

INTRACRANIAL VASCULAR LESIONS

Aneurysms

The vast majority of intracranial aneurysms are congenital in origin, although occasionally they may be due to atherosclerosis or trauma. These congenital aneurysms are saccular ('berry aneurysm') which arise on the circle of Willis, the anastomotic communication between the internal carotid arteries and the vertebral arteries at the base of the brain. About 20% are multiple and the sexes are equally affected (see Fig. 8.3).

Clinical features

The importance of these aneurysms is that they are the commonest cause of spontaneous subarachnoid haemorrhage, but when they rupture they may also produce intracerebral or subdural bleeding. Rupture may occur at any age, but especially after 40; increasing atheromatous changes in the arteries and hypertension are probably precipitating factors.

The haemorrhage usually presents as a sudden severe headache with vomiting. The patient may become unconscious and the blood in the subarachnoid space causes severe cerebral irritation resembling meningitis (meningism). There may be neck retraction and the patient resists attempts to flex the neck. Lumbar puncture confirms the presence of blood in the CSF. If the blood is allowed to settle it will be noticed that the supernatant fluid is yellow in colour (*xanthochromic*) and by this means we can differentiate between a true subarachnoid haemorrhage and a 'bloody tap', produced by pricking a small blood vessel during the diagnostic lumbar puncture.

Haemorrhage from a ruptured aneurysm is serious and no less than a quarter of the patients die without recovering consciousness. Half the patients will bleed again within six weeks of the initial haemorrhage and the mortality in such cases is high. After six weeks the likelihood of recurrent haemorrhage becomes less, but it is still present.

Treatment

While the patient is in coma there is nothing to be done except careful nursing—exactly like the outline of treatment described for the nursing care of the unconscious head injury (page 146). If the patient recovers from the initial haemorrhage then cerebral angiography is performed to locate the site of the aneurysm and this should be carried out as soon as possible, preferably before the peak incidence of recurrent haemorrhage, which is after about 2 weeks.

If an aneurysm is demonstrated (Fig. 10.12) treatment comprises either direct or indirect surgery. In the direct attack the aneurysm is exposed via a craniotomy and is obliterated, either by excision, or by applying a silver clip to its base or to its supplying vessels, or by inducing thrombosis by wrapping it in a detached piece of muscle. The indirect approach comprises ligation of the common carotid artery in those instances where the aneurysm is supplied by the internal carotid artery, since diminution of the blood flow through the aneurysm encourages its thrombosis. About one third of the angiograms are negative and probably indicate that thrombosis has taken place spontaneously in a small aneurysm. Such cases are treated conservatively and the prognosis is good.

Angiomas

Developmental angiomatous malformations may occur in any part of the central nervous system, but particularly over the surface of the cerebral hemisphere. They may produce epilepsy, headaches, slowly progressive paralysis or may leak and result in subarachnoid haemorrhage. This is less catastrophic than in rupture of an aneurysm but accounts for about 10% of all examples of spontaneous subarachnoid bleeding.

The exact diagnosis and localisation is made by cerebral angiography.

Fig. 10.12. A large cerebral aneurysm demonstrated by carotid angiography.

In some cases excision of the angioma is possible and this should be carried out particularly if marked symptoms are present, or if there has been preceding subarachnoid haemorrhage. In many cases, however, the angioma is too extensive or too deeply situated to make operation feasible.

HEAD INJURIES

One of the most serious responsibilities undertaken by a nurse is the care of a patient who has sustained a head injury. It is no exaggeration to say that his life depends upon her careful nursing and observation. Hippocrates, the father of medicine, wrote 'no head injury is so trivial that we can neglect it, nor so severe that there is no hope' and each year in this country patients die because what at first appears to be a trivial head injury is ignored, whereas others, rushed to theatre while being artificially ventilated or even undergoing cardiac massage, make a complete recovery. There is no mystique about head injuries and we hope to show, in this chapter, that their management is based on common sense.

The causes of coma

An everyday problem is the patient brought into Casualty unconscious. The following are the common causes to be considered:
1. Trauma to the brain.
2. Cerebral disease; for example, a stroke (the commonest), epilepsy, cerebral tumour, abscess or meningitis.
3. Drugs, especially the barbiturates and alcohol. For convenience, we can include carbon monoxide and coal gas poisoning in this group.
4. Diabetes—either hyperglycaemic or hypoglycaemic coma.
5. Uraemia—patients in advanced renal failure pass into coma.
6. Hepatic coma, the patient being deeply jaundiced and usually in the terminal stages of cirrhosis.
7. Profound toxaemia—for example in advanced peritonitis or septicaemia.
8. Hysteria.

The first four groups account for the great majority of emergency admissions. If there is any doubt about the cause of coma, blood should be taken for glucose, barbiturate and alcohol estimations.

It is usually easy enough to tell from witnesses that unconsciousness is due to trauma, but it is vitally important to remember that a drunk or an epileptic may have struck his head in falling so that his initial condition is complicated by a head injury. In contrast, a patient may have suffered a stroke, be seen to fall down and sustain what is, in fact, a trivial head injury which disguises the real cause of his coma being a serious intracerebral vascular accident.

The management of the unconscious head injury

This must be considered under three headings:
1. Nursing the unconscious patient.
2. Observation.
3. Indications for operative treatment.

The first two apply to every case but operative intervention is only needed in about 10% of head injuries. Although we consider these topics under separate headings, all three lines of management may be going on at one and the same time.

The nursing care of the unconscious patient

1. *The airway*

Without any doubt at all, the most important single factor in the care of the deeply unconscious patient, whatever the cause, is the maintenance of the airway. The patient in coma has lost his cough reflex and so cannot protect his respiratory passages from inhalation of vomit and blood; furthermore, the unconscious patient loses the ability we possess, even when asleep, of maintaining the tongue held forward so that it does not obstruct the laryngeal orifice. The patient must therefore be transported and nursed lying on one side with the body tilted head downwards ('the tonsil position'). This simple but absolutely vital manœuvre ensures that the tongue falls forwards and also that bronchial secretions or vomit drain from the mouth rather than being inhaled (Fig. 10.13). Suction may be required to remove excessive secretions or vomit from the pharynx. If the airway cannot be maintained satisfactorily by this technique, and this is particularly so when the presence of other injuries make it necessary for the patient to lie on his back (for example, associated fracture of the femur) then an endotracheal tube may be necessary (Fig. 10.14). If the patient remains unconscious, a tracheostomy using a cuffed tube may be required.

2. *Restlessness*

The unconscious head injury may be extremely restless. Morphia is contra-indicated since this will depress respiration, disguise the level of coma and will also produce constriction of the pupils, which masks a valuable physical sign. Phenobarbitone or paraldehyde may be required for severe restlessness or epileptic fits. Judicious restraint, cot-sides and padding may be required to protect the patient from injuring himself. A cause of restlessness may be a distended bladder and often if the retention is relieved by means of a catheter the patient will calm down considerably.

3. *Feeding*

Many head injuries were allowed to die in the past due to dehydration and starvation. If it is obvious that the patient is going to

Fig. 10.13. The 'tonsil position' for transportation of an unconscious patient. Note the 'head down, feet up' inclination.

Fig. 10.14. Maintenance of an airway by means of the passage of an endotracheal tube via a laryngoscope.

remain unconscious and unable to swallow after 12 hours then a naso-gastric tube should be passed so that adequate fluid, electrolytes and calories can be provided. It is, of course, essential to ensure that the tube is lying correctly in the stomach since, if coiled in the oesophagus, there is the risk of regurgitation and inhalation into the respiratory passages.

4. *Skin and general nursing care*

A deeply unconscious patient is liable to bed sores; careful nursing attention is required for their prevention. Eye toilet to prevent exposure keratitis, frequent mouth hygiene and full range passive movement to all limbs to prevent contractures are all part of the nurse's heavy responsibilities.

5. *Sphincters*

The unconscious patient is frequently incontinent; the resultant excoriation of the skin makes him still more liable to pressure sores. The use of Paul's tubing on the penis, or of an indwelling catheter in the female patient, will help in the nursing care. Faecal impaction is quite common if the bowels are neglected; the unconscious patient usually requires regular enemas to clear the bowel, but digital disimpaction may be necessary.

Observations

The observations which must be carried out on an unconscious head injury fall into two groups.

The first is the complete clinical examination of the patient to determine whether or not other injuries are present. Following most accidents, the patient can tell us which parts of his body have been injured, but this is obviously not the case when he is in coma! An injury which has been sufficient to render a patient unconscious, a severe car crash for example, is likely to have produced damage elsewhere—it is surprising how common such gross things as fracture of the femur or a serious chest injury are overlooked in these cases and it is essential for the head injury patient to be checked over from head to toe.

Secondly, our observations are concentrated on looking for signs of deterioration in the patient which, for practical purposes, indicate that intracranial bleeding is taking place.

Three things can happen to unconscious head injury patients while under observation:

1. The great majority become lighter and recover completely.
2. A small proportion remain in relatively deep coma as a result of severe cerebral trauma and this state of affairs may persist for weeks or even months.
3. Another small proportion of patients pass into progressively deeper coma. This may be caused either by intracranial bleeding, with clot pressing on the brain, or oedema of the damaged cerebral tissues or, at a later stage, intracranial infection. The last is now fortunately rare except in some cases of penetrating compound fractures of the skull.

Since it is extremely difficult to differentiate between the progressive coma produced by intracranial haemorrhage (which requires urgent surgical intervention) and cerebral oedema, for practical purposes one may state that a patient with a closed head injury who becomes more deeply unconscious after the accident requires immediate surgery.

The repeated observations that are ordered for the unconscious head injury should not be regarded as a routine chore but as an essential process to detect that minority of patients who are developing the features of cerebral compression.

The observations fall into three groups which are, in order of importance:

1. The conscious level
2. The reaction of the pupils
3. The pulse, respiration and blood pressure.

In the early hours following a head injury these observations must be repeated at ten or fifteen minute intervals and plotted on a chart.

Conscious level

Vague terms such as comatose, semi-comatose, unconscious or stuperose should be avoided—they mean nothing when compared one to the other and are useless when charting changes in conscious level. Instead, we use the patient's responses to stimuli and these are very much the reactions of a person recovering from a deep anaesthesia. As the patient becomes progressively lighter, we can chart the following levels:

1. No response at all to painful stimulation—the deepest level of unconsciousness.
2. Inco-ordinated response to pain—for example, the patient moves all four limbs following a pin prick.
3. Co-ordinated response to pain—the patient is now light enough to push away the examiner's hand when pricked or pinched.
4. Response to simple commands—for example he now puts out his tongue when ordered to do so.
5. The patient is now able to talk but is disorientated and does not know his name, his whereabouts, the day or the time. Gradually he passes from this state to full orientation.

Any shift from a higher to a lower level in this scheme is highly significant of deepening coma and is undoubtedly the most valuable of all the observations that we can make.

Pupils

If a cerebral hemisphere is pressed upon by an enlarging blood clot, the third cranial nerve on that side becomes stretched and put out of action. Its paralysis results in dilatation of the corresponding pupil, since the third nerve transmits the nerve supply to the pupillary constrictor muscle. The pupil is also unable to respond to light. An important sign of acute cerebral compression is dilatation and loss of light reaction of the pupil on the same side as the cerebral compression. As compression continues, the third nerve on the opposite side becomes compressed and the opposite pupil, in turn, dilates and becomes fixed to light. Bilateral fixed dilated pupils in a patient with a head injury indicates great cerebral compression and the prognosis is now extremely grave (Fig. 10.15).

A At first the pupil is dilated
on the affected side

B Later stage, both pupils are widely
dilated and do not respond to light

Fig. 10.15. The pupil changes in acute cerebral compression.

Pulse, respiration and blood pressure

With increasing cerebral compression, the pulse progressively slows, the respirations become stertorous and the blood pressure rises. These changes usually go hand in glove with increasing coma and pupil dilatation.

Special investigations of the unconscious patient

We have already mentioned that if there is any doubt about the traumatic nature of the coma, blood should be sent to the laboratory for sugar, alcohol and barbiturate levels, as well as testing a specimen of urine for sugar.

High quality X-rays of the skull are obtained for evidence of fracture but it should be noted that an extensive fracture at the base of the skull may not show up at all on X-rays which demonstrate, for the most part, lesions of the skull vault (Fig. 10.16).

If the patient shows progressive deterioration in the first few hours after head injury we have noted that the diagnosis lies between intra-cranial bleeding and cerebral oedema. In a neurological unit, the diagnosis may be greatly aided by a cerebral arteriogram which can demonstrate the site and size of any intracranial clot. Many centres are now able to carry out computerised axial tomography ('C.A.T. scan') which can accurately delineate the clot within a few minutes. If such facilities are not immediately available, the only safe procedure is rapid burr-hole exploration of the skull over the suspected by means of an external wound on the scalp or via the nasal or aural cavities.

Depressed fractures in adults are nearly always compound; it stands to reason that if the blow is severe enough to drive a fragment of the skull below its surrounds, it is also severe enough to tear through the overlying scalp. In children with their softer, more elastic bones, a 'pond' fracture may occur over which the skin remains intact and which rather resembles a dent in a table-tennis ball.

A compound fracture to the exterior is treated like any other compound fracture; the wound edges are narrowly excised, dead tissue, bone deprived of its periosteum and any pulped brain removed, the dura repaired if possible and the skin then sutured.

A special variety of compound fracture is where continuity to the exterior occurs through the nose or ear and is demonstrated by a discharge of cerebrospinal fluid through these orifices (C.S.F. rhinorrhoea or otorrhoea—the latter is far less common). In these instances a dural tear associated with a fracture of the skull base allows a ready pathway of infection along the nose or the ear to the meninges and brain. In such cases the patient is barrier nursed and placed on sulphadimidine, since the sulphonamides readily pass into the cerebrospinal fluid. If the leak persists then it may be necessary to repair the tear in the dura mater using a piece of fibrous deep fascia cut from the thigh.

Clinical accompaniments of skull fractures

Examination of the patient's head will often reveal features produced by the fracture of the skull itself or of injury to adjacent structures. There is frequently bruising, swelling and abrasions over the site of the blow and it is here that the fracture line is most likely to be placed (Fig. 10.17A) Fractures which involve the orbit are often accompanied by an orbital haematoma, in which the eyelids are swollen and bruised, the bruising being limited exactly to the orbital margin. The eyelids can be opened only with difficulty but then blood can be seen tracking beneath the conjunctiva. This is in contrast to the common 'black eye' due to a direct blow on the face, when bruising extends over the eyebrow and cheek and in which there is no blood beyond the conjunctiva. A haemorrhage may be seen, in these circumstances, in the conjunctiva itself, but this does not track posteriorly (Fig. 10.18).

Fractures of the base of the skull are frequently accompanied by bleeding from the nose or ear and we have already mentioned that occasionally cerebrospinal fluid or even pulped brain tissue may be seen to be escaping from either orifice.

(A) SUBCONJUNCTIVAL
    HAEMORRHAGE
    —NO POSTERIOR LIMIT

(B) CONJUNCTIVAL
    HAEMORRHAGE
    —POSTERIOR LIMIT SEEN

Fig. 10.18. The differential diagnosis between subconjunctival (A) and conjunctival haemorrhage (B).

Cranial nerves may be injured if the fracture line passes across the foramina from which they emerge from the skull. Fractures involving the anterior part of the skull frequently damage the first cranial (olfactory) nerve and loss of smell (anosmia) is quite common following frontal injuries. The optic nerve may be torn with resultant blindness. The 7th (facial) nerve and 8th (auditory) nerve may be injured producing facial palsy and deafness. Any of the other cranial nerves may be involved but such injuries are relatively rare.

INTRACRANIAL HAEMORRHAGE

Following injury, haemorrhage may take place within the skull in a number of compartments (Fig. 10.19).

The extradural space lies between the dura mater and the skull. These two structures are usually firmly adherent to each other but may be stripped apart by haemorrhage.

The subdural space, between the brain and the dura.

The subarachnoid space, between the arachnoid and the brain.

Rarely haemorrhage occurs into the substance of the brain (*intracerebral*) and this may rupture into the ventricular system.

Extradural haemorrhage

This is sometimes badly named middle meningeal haemorrhage— a term that should not be used. It may indeed arise from a tear of the middle meningeal artery or vein, but an extradural collection of blood may also develop from a laceration of one of the other blood vessels running over the meninges, from the torn sagittal venous sinus or simply from blood oozing out of the bone marrow or stripped dura mater on either side of a fracture.

CLINICAL FEATURES

The typical story is of a relatively minor head injury which produces temporary concussion. The patient recovers from this (the 'lucid

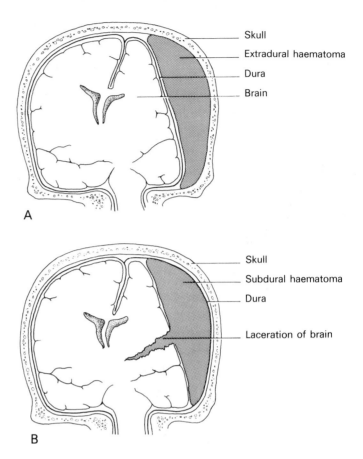

Fig. 10.19. Extradural haematoma (A) and subdural haematoma (B). The latter is associated with a severe brain laceration.

period') then, some hours later, develops headache and progresses to deeper and deeper coma due to cerebral compression produced by the extradural clot. Each year we read of tragedies in which someone has had too much to drink, falls down and hits his head, recovers enough to get home to bed and is found dead there in the morning, or the cricketer who is mildly concussed by a cricket ball, recovers enough to carry on with the game and dies that night. It is important to note, however, that this picture of recovery only accounts for about 50% of the cases. Often there is no lucid period and the patient progressively passes into deeper and deeper coma from the time of the initial injury.

The physical signs are those of rapidly increasing intracerebral pressure, which have already been discussed (page 149)—deepening coma, dilatation of the pupil on the affected side, a falling pulse rate, rise in blood pressure and stertorous respiration.

In addition, hemiplegia may develop on the side opposite to the lesion and occasionally Jacksonian fits occur. A boggy haematoma of the scalp usually overlies the site of the extradural haemorrhage; this is because some of the blood escapes through the fracture line into the subcutaneous tissues.

Skull X-rays may be very helpful; the haematoma is likely to be on the side of, and beneath, the fracture if one is present. In special neurosurgical centres, computerised axial tomography ('C.A.T. scan') or a carotid angiogram may accurately localise the position of the clot. Echo-encephalography has recently been introduced with great success to demonstrate shift of mid-line structures within the brain because of clot compression. This instrument works on the same principle as a depth-finder on a ship.

Treatment

An extradural haemorrhage is one of the few surgical emergencies where minutes really do matter both to prevent irreversible brain damage from taking place and to avert death as a result of compression of the respiratory centre in the medulla. The patient is taken immediately to the operating theatre, care being taken to maintain the airway, if necessary by an endotracheal tube and artificial ventilation. Under local anaesthetic a burr-hole is made over the suspected site of the clot by means of a drill (Fig. 10.20), the opening enlarged with nibbling forceps and the blood evacuated (Fig. 10.21). The source of bleeding on the dura is controlled either with silver Cushing clips, with diathermy or by under running the vessel with a

Fig. 10.20. A skull perforator with drill attachment.

Other complications which require mention include meningitis, hyperpyrexia, post-traumatic neurosis and epilepsy.

MENINGITIS

Infection of the meninges may complicate a fracture of the skull which is compound either directly to the exterior or via a dural tear into the nasal or aural cavities. Confirmation of the diagnosis of meningitis is made by lumbar puncture and bacteriological examination of the fluid.

Treatment is appropriate chemotherapy, both systemically and into the spinal theca by means of lumbar puncture.

Occasionally, the infection of a penetrating wound of the brain may result in cerebral abscess (see page 137).

HYPERPYREXIA

Severe injury to the brain stem may result in prolonged unconsciousness, decerebrate rigidity with the legs held rigidly extended and the arms flexed to the sides (Fig. 10.22), pin-point pupils and, very dangerously, hyperpyrexia with a temperature rising up to 105° or more. This latter results from injury to the heat regulating centre and, unlike most fevers, there is no accompanying sweating.

Treatment requires most vigorous nursing care. All blankets are removed and the naked patient is treated with tepid sponging. If this proves ineffective, then crushed ice placed in polythene bags is applied over the trunk. Chlorpromazine may be useful to stop shivering since the latter will prevent cooling.

POST-TRAUMATIC NEUROSIS

This is not uncommon after a head injury. Unless reassured and rapidly rehabilitated a patient may easily be left to imagine that his brain has been irrevocably damaged and that he will never lead a normal life again.

Some idea of the severity of the injury is given by the period of amnesia, both the retrograde amnesia up to the time of the accident and the post-traumatic amnesia following injury. If this period amounts to only minutes or a few hours, the ultimate prognosis is good. Amnesia of several days or even weeks means that the chance of ultimate return to full mental function is much less.

Fig. 10.22. Decerebrate rigidity
in severe brain stem injury.

PERSISTENT EPILEPSY

This may especially complicate penetrating compound wounds with
resultant scarring of the cerebral cortex. All such patients are given
phenobarbitone for at least six months following injury. Established
post-traumatic epilepsy is treated by means of anti-convulsant drugs
(phenobarbitone, epanutin etc.); alcohol should be forbidden.

Chapter 11. Oesophagus, stomach and duodenum

Introduction

The alimentary canal extends from the lips to the anus. The mouth and pharynx are considered elsewhere and the rest of the alimentary canal will be taken in anatomical order from the oesophagus down.

Oesophagus

Anatomy

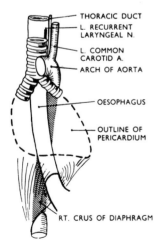

THORACIC DUCT
L. RECURRENT LARYNGEAL N.
L. COMMON CAROTID A.
ARCH OF AORTA
OESOPHAGUS
OUTLINE OF PERICARDIUM
RT. CRUS OF DIAPHRAGM

Fig. 11.1. The oesophagus and its anterior relations.

The oesophagus is a muscular tube which extends from the level of the cricoid cartilage, in the neck, to its junction with the stomach. In its entire length it is closely applied to the front of the bodies of the vertebrae. In the neck it is situated behind the trachea and it continues this relationship as it descends into the thorax in the posterior mediastinum (Fig. 11.1) until the trachea divides into the right and left main bronchi. It continues down behind the heart and pericardium, with the right and left vagus nerves closely applied to it, to enter the abdomen through the hiatus in the diaphragm. Just beneath the hiatus it enters the stomach at the cardia, the right vagus nerve becoming posterior and the left vagus nerve becoming anterior.

The oesophagus is lined by stratified squamous epithelium, which is both smooth and tough. At its upper end the muscle wall of the oesophagus is of the voluntary, striated kind, which allows the act of swallowing to be voluntarily initiated. This type of muscle gradually changes, until at the lower end the muscle is completely involuntary, resulting in the automatic nature of the peristaltic wave that forces food and fluid into the stomach, even if the subject stands on his head.

Symptoms of oesophageal disease

1. *Dysphagia*—this term is used either to describe difficulty in swallowing or pain on swallowing. It always indicates that full investigation should be undertaken. Generally, with a progressive disease such as a cancer, the dysphagia will first cause a 'sticking' of solid foods. As it progresses, however, it results in difficulty in swallowing liquids.

2. *Regurgitation*—this occurs when saliva, food, or a mixture of the two, pool within the oesophagus. It is distinguished from vomiting by the fact that it frequently occurs soon after a meal; the ejected contents are slimy and contain food residue unstained by bile, alkaline to litmus paper, and recognisable as having been eaten with the previous meal.

A special form of regurgitation occurs with a pharyngeal diverticulum. In this case the patient learns how to empty the diverticulum, or pouch, by external pressure on the neck, or by adopting a head-down position.

3. *Pain*—severe pain can arise from damage to the oesophageal lining or wall. Usually the pain is referred anteriorly to the neck, chest, or upper abdomen, according to the site of the injury. Occasionally, however, the pain is experienced in the back. Regurgitation of acid stomach contents produces inflammation in the oesophagus and this is experienced as a burning pain in the upper epigastrium or lower chest, a symptom commonly described as 'heartburn'.

4. *Chest complications.* A confusing and important symptom arises when dysphagia has progressed to the point when liquids cannot be swallowed. In this case saliva, constantly being produced, gradually fills up the oesophagus. During the daytime this will be regurgitated but, at night, when the patient is asleep, the saliva, together with other swallowed oesophageal contents, spills over into the trachea, resulting in an aspiration pnemonia. It is even possible for a young patient with achalasia of the cardia to present as an asthmatic. It is also quite common for newly born babies with oesophageal atresia to present as pneumonia for the same reason.

5. *Loss of Weight.* This results quite obviously from the fact that less food can be eaten and the total calorie intake falls below the level required to maintain the weight. Patients with long-standing severe

near its lower end. The history is usually all that is required to make the diagnosis and a chest X-ray confirms it (Fig. 11.3, see also Fig. 20.46).

Treatment comprises oesophagoscopy under a general anaesthetic, which allows forceps extraction of the foreign body.

Adults with foreign bodies stuck in the oesophagus fall into two categories. In the first the foreign body is sharp, often a fish bone or sometimes a rabbit bone which has become swallowed and which has imbedded itself in the mucosa preventing its further passage into the stomach.

Many such objects are not radio-opaque but the diagnosis may be confirmed by a barium swallow examination.

Extraction is through an oesophagoscope, which may require considerable dexterity when the object is large, sharp and irregular. Numerous cases are recorded in which the foreign body has not been extracted and has then worked its way through the wall of the oesophagus, resulting in a perforation and peri-oesophageal abscess or, worse still, penetration of the aorta with a massive and fatal haemorrhage.

The second category in adults is when swallowed material cannot negotiate the oesophagus because of a pre-existing abnormality such as a stricture from either a malignant growth or peptic oesophagitis.

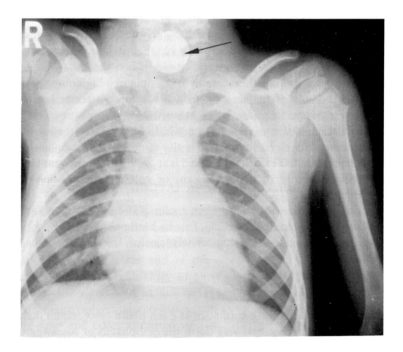

Fig. 11.3. X-ray of the chest of a child showing an opaque foreign body (an old-fashioned penny) lodged in the upper oesophagus.

Once again, these patients require full investigation by barium swallow and oesophagoscopy. Following this, treatment will be required to correct the basic abnormality of the oesophageal wall.

OESOPHAGEAL WEB

This is a narrowing of the upper end of the oesophagus which occurs in middle-aged women in association with iron-deficient anaemia and is given the name of the Plummer-Vinson or Patterson-Kelly syndrome. This syndrome may develop into a post-cricoid carcinoma, that is a carcinoma of the upper end of the oesophagus.

Treatment of this condition is aimed at the treatment of the iron deficiency by oral iron and requires frequent checks to detect possible development of a carcinoma.

OESOPHAGEAL (PHARYNGEAL) POUCH

See page 477.

ACHALASIA OF THE CARDIA

Achalasia of the cardia is a condition in which the normal peristaltic wave of the oesophagus, which occurs as food material is being swallowed, is not transmitted at the lower end of the oesophagus.

Clinical features

It is slightly more common in women than men, the onset tends to be insidious and patients may not even notice that they have had difficulty in swallowing for a considerable number of years. Generally the patients are underweight and aged between 35 and 50 years. As onset is so insidious, advanced malnutrition may occur. Sometimes the oesophagus becomes full of food and fluid debris, and when the patient becomes recumbent at night some of this material is aspirated into the lungs, so that he or she may present with pneumonia.

Special investigations

A chest X-ray may reveal a mediastinal mass produced by the grossly distended oesophagus.

A barium swallow clinches the diagnosis. The dilated, tortuous oesophagus is outlined, usually half full of retained food and fluid.

Fig. 11.4. Barium swallow in achalasia. Note the grossly dilated oesophagus above the narrow terminal segment (arrowed).

At its lower end it tapers into a short narrow segment that drains into the stomach (Fig. 11.4).

Oesophagoscopy is like going down a tunnel the bottom of which contains a puddle of food debris.

Treatment

Some patients may respond to regular dilatation of the lower end of the oesophagus or to one or more forcible stretches by means of a balloon introduced through an oesophagoscope. Most surgeons in this country prefer to carry out *Heller's Operation*, in which the thickened muscle wall of the lower end of the oesophagus (approached through a left thoracotomy), is split down to the mucosa. Most patients respond dramatically to this procedure (Fig. 11.5).

HIATUS HERNIA

In the normal person gastric juice cannot pass from the stomach up into the oesophagus because of a number of mechanisms, which include the physiological sphincter at the lower end of the oesophagus, the angle between the oesophagus and the stomach, the positive intra-abdominal pressure which tends to keep the oesophagus shut and the muscle fibres of the diaphragm which are wrapped around the lower end of the oesophagus, particularly from the right crus. In a considerable number of patients, especially females, with advancing years and increasing obesity, the oesophageal hiatus in the diaphragm becomes unusually wide, allowing the oesophago-gastric junction, sometimes together with part of the fundus of the stomach, to pass into the chest. The precise anatomical relationship between the oesophago-gastric junction and the hiatus allows hiatus herniae to be classified as follows (Fig. 11.6).
1. *Sliding hiatus hernia*—in this type the oesophago-gastric junction passes into the chest.
2. *Rolling hiatus hernia*—in which the oesophago-gastric junction remains in the abdomen but the fundus of the stomach passes into the chest.

Clinical features

The most common symptom to be associated with a hiatus hernia is produced by gastro-oesophageal reflux, resulting in a peptic oesophagitis. This is experienced as heartburn, a burning pain which is situated retrosternally and which is relieved by alkalis and an upright posture. Regurgitation of recently eaten food mixed with gastric juice commonly occurs when the patient bends forwards. Such common tasks as gardening and housework, which involves bending over, result in this reflux.

In the case of a rolling hiatus hernia it is quite possible for a significant portion of the stomach to enter the chest with the result that the stomach assumes an upside-down position (*a gastric volvulus*). In these patients acute symptoms may be precipitated by a heavy meal when the patient feels nausea and makes attempts at vomiting but without oesophageal regurgitation being able to occur. It is also common for these patients to have a competent oesophageal sphincter with no gastro-oesophageal reflux.

Complications

Continued peptic oesophagitis at the lower end of the oesophagus may result in *stricture formation* with progressive dysphagia. The inflamed mucosa may bleed, either acutely (haematemesis) or insidiously with the development of an iron-deficiency anaemia.

Special investigations

A Barium swallow and meal will delineate the hernia, although it may be necessary to tip the patient head-down in order to demon-

Fig. 11.5. Heller's operation. The muscle of the lower oesophagus is split down to the mucosa (compare Ramstedt's operation, Fig. 11.11).

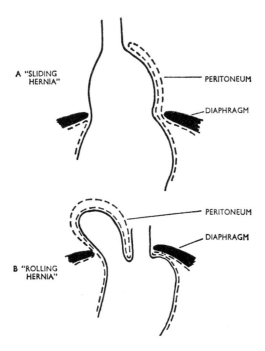

A "SLIDING HERNIA"

PERITONEUM

DIAPHRAGM

B "ROLLING HERNIA"

PERITONEUM

DIAPHRAGM

Fig. 11.6. (A) A sliding hiatus hernia. (B) A rolling hiatus hernia. In the first, the stomach and lower oesophagus slide into the chest through the enlarged oesophageal hiatus; in the second the stomach rolls upwards through the hiatus alongside the lower oesophagus.

strate this (Fig. 11.7). Reflux will be shown by barium regurgitating into the oesophagus from the stomach and any associated stricture will also be revealed.

Oesophagoscopy may be necessary, particularly when the radiologist cannot be certain whether a stricture in these circumstances is benign or due to a coexistent carcinoma, a not infrequent situation.

Treatment

1. *Conservative*

Very many of the patients who complain of the symptoms of a hiatus hernia are overweight and the first line of treatment in such subjects will therefore be aimed at weight reduction with consequent lowering of the intra-abdominal pressure. An upright posture will aid in the maintenance of gastro-oesophageal continence, thus minimising oesophagitis. To this end patients are advised to raise the head of the bed slightly and to avoid stooping and bending positions.

Fig. 11.7. Barium meal showing a sliding hiatus hernia. Note the large pouch of stomach above the diaphragm (arrowed).

The acid and peptic activity at the lower end of the oesophagus is then reduced to a minimum with non-absorbable alkalis, for example aluminium hydroxide or magnesium trisilicate.

These measures are successful in removing the symptoms due to a hiatus hernia in the majority of patients. It is even possible to arrest the progress and in a number of patients reverse the development of a peptic stricture. However there are some patients in whom these measures are not effective and who require surgery.

2. *Surgical treatment*

Numerous operations have been described for the repair of a hiatus hernia. The fact that so many procedures are available to the surgeon clearly indicates that none of them is entirely satisfactory. Allison has advocated the repair of the oesophageal ligaments using an approach through the chest. Belsey also uses an approach through the chest in which the oesophagus is firmly stitched to the underside of the diaphragm, the oesophago-gastric angle is restored and the diaphragmatic ligaments are repaired. Other surgeons employ an abdominal approach, pointing out that the virtue of this method is that an abdominal exploration can be carried out at the same time which permits the exclusion or treatment of other pathology producing similar symptoms, for example those associated with the presence of non-opaque gall stones. The hiatal procedure in this case comprises repair of the hiatus itself by means of several silk or nylon sutures through the crura of the diaphragm which may be combined with a Nissen fundoplication, carried out by wrapping the fundus of the stomach up around the lower end of the oesophagus.

A stricture of the oesophagus due to reflux may respond to conservative medical therapy or, if not too severe, may dilate up once the hiatus hernia is repaired and further reflux prevented. A severe stricture, however, may require dilatation via an oesophagoscope or surgical resection.

OESOPHAGEAL CARCINOMA

Pathology

The most common primary tumour of the oesophagus is the squamous cell carcinoma. It is more common in men than in women and in this country usually occurs in the age range from 50 to 70. There is a striking and curious racial and geographical distribution in that it is extremely common in the Bantu in Southern Africa. It is also common in Eastern races, particularly the Japanese. The most common site in the oesophagus to be affected is the lower one third. Rarely adenocarcinomas are found at the lower end of the oesophagus, arising either from islands of columnar epithelium which exist in the oesophagus near its junction with the stomach or from the epithelium of the stomach itself, the tumour then spreading up the oesophagus.

Non-epithelial tumours are also found, the most common of these is the leiomyoma which is the benign, or the leiomyosarcoma which is the malignant form of this smooth muscle tumour. Other tumours such as lymphosarcoma and secondary malignant tumours are rare.

Clinical features

The commonest symptom by far is difficulty in swallowing (*dysphagia*). At first this is for solids only but as the tumour grows the difficulty extends to liquids. Associated with this is a progressive loss of weight. There may be positive occult blood in the faeces, with anaemia. If dysphagia is complete there may be the symptoms and signs of aspiration pneumonia. It is common for patients who have progressed to this extent to complain of 'sialorrhoea' which is the production and expectoration of large volumes of saliva. Sometimes the tumour spreads to the cervical lymph nodes.

Special investigations

As with all oesophageal conditions, the diagnosis is by means of preliminary barium swallow followed by oesophagoscopy and biopsy (Fig. 11.8).

Fig. 11.8. Barium swallow in carcinoma of the oesophagus. This is demonstrated by the narrow stricture in the mid-oesophagus (arrowed).

Treatment

If the patient is dehydrated and cachectic on admission, it is first necessary to improve his nutritional state. Often if food debris is cleared from the oesophagus by gentle lavage or at oesophagoscopy, he will then be able to swallow liquids such as milk and Complan to which vitamins can be added. If not, a plastic nasogastric tube may be threaded through the malignant stricture. Only if these simple measures fail is a feeding gastrostomy required in order to prepare the patient for further treatment.

If investigation reveals the carcinoma to be limited and in the lower third of the oesophagus, resection of the tumour is carried out using a thoraco-abdominal approach, either as one continuous incision from the abdomen into the left chest or as two incisions, one in the midline of the abdomen and the second at the level of the right fifth rib. The tumour is completely excised and the upper end of the oesophagus is joined to the fundus of the stomach, which is mobilised and brought into the chest. This always results in division of the vagus nerves and a pyloroplasty has therefore to be added.

In tumours of the middle third of the oesophagus resection is again the procedure of choice although technically this is much more difficult as the line of the anastomosis between the oesophagus and the stomach comes to lie above the arch of the aorta or is fashioned in the neck.

Tumours of the upper third of the oesophagus and post-cricoid carcinomas are usually treated by radiotherapy.

A tumour that has extended into tissues around the oesophagus thus preventing resection can be palliated by passing a tube such as the Mousseau-Barbin or Celestin tube (see Fig. 5.8) through it, to enable the patient to swallow food until extension of the carcinoma produces the inevitable death of the patient.

After intubation all food must be sieved and has to be followed by a drink to remove food debris from the lumen of the tube; it is found an advantage to use some form of effervescent fluid such as lemonade or soda water.

Unfortunately the long-term results after resection of oesophageal carcinomas are not good and under 5% of patients are alive and free from tumour five years after the operation.

Stomach

Anatomy

The stomach (Fig. 11.9) is divided into a fundus, body, antrum and pylorus. The lines of division between these parts of the stomach are ill-defined but nevertheless serve as useful descriptive terms. There is an extremely important functional difference between the fundus and the body, on one hand, and the antrum on the other and this relates to the type of cells found in the mucosa. Acid is only secreted in the body and fundus of the stomach. No acid is secreted from the antrum and it is from here that mucosal cells termed 'G-cells' produce the hormone *gastrin*. It is not possible by external inspection to distinguish between the body and the antrum.

The whole of the gastrointestinal tract is lined by an inner circular and outer longitudinal coat of involuntary muscle, but in the case of the stomach these are arranged in loops which permit considerable distension of the organ as it fills with food, allowing it

Fig. 11.9. The stomach and its subdivisions.

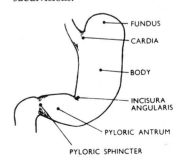

to fulfil its function as a reservoir. The muscle of the antrum is thicker than that in the body. The antrum undergoes vigorous, segmenting contraction with the result that food is broken down and converted to gastric chyme so that the process of digestion can continue rapidly in the intestine.

The pylorus is marked by a small vein which passes over its anterior surface, the 'pyloric vein of Mayo'. At operation the pylorus can be felt as a definite ring which will admit the tip of one finger. The precise function of the pylorus is still in some doubt. It does not seem to be concerned with the regulation of gastric emptying so much as in the prevention of duodeno-gastric reflux, although naturally if the pylorus is unable to expand sufficiently for any reason, such as scarring following duodenal ulceration, gastric emptying will be delayed.

The stomach is richly supplied with blood from the coeliac axis via the left and right gastric arteries and the left and right gastroepiploic arteries. The venous drainage follows the arteries and is to the portal vein; the ascending branch of the left gastric vein communicates with the azygos vein in the chest. These anastomotic channels in the lower oesophages and cardia become dilated in the condition of portal hypertension, a fact of considerable importance in the development of oesophageal varices. The lymphatic drainage tends to follow the venous drainage, there being lymph nodes along the lesser curve of the stomach with the lymphatics extending to the porta hepatis, and inferiorly along the greater curve of the stomach via the greater omentum to the transverse mesocolon and the superior border of the pancreas. The nerve supply is from the vagus nerves (Fig. 11.10) and from the sympathetic nerves travelling with the arteries.

Gastric secretion

The cells lining the fundus and body of the stomach produce a complicated secretion which contains hydrochloric acid with inorganic ions, principally chloride, sodium and potassium, together with enzymes concerned with digestion, particularly pepsin, but also amylase and lipase in small quantities. The acid is produced from cells which can be readily identified on histological section called parietal cells. Thus the secretion from the body of the stomach is of a highly acid nature and the pH falls to the region of 1.5. In contrast to this is the secretion of the antrum, which is almost neutral. Antral cells produce gastrin, which is a hormone. This enters the bloodstream and when it recirculates and reaches the parietal cells it stimulates them to produce hydrochloric acid (HCl).

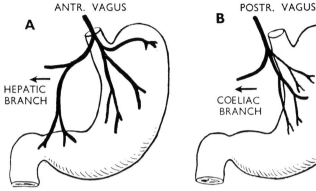

Fig. 11.10. The vagal supply to the stomach. (A) The anterior vagus; (B) the posterior vagus.

The stimuli to gastric juice production are:

1. *The psychic phase* of gastric secretion, that is the thought, sight or smell of food which results in the vagus nerve becoming active with consequent stimulation of both parietal cells and antral G-cells.

2. *Gastric phase of secretion*, which results from direct contact between the swallowed food and the stomach. Certain foods, particularly digested meat products, are powerful stimulators of the G-cells and result in the release of gastrin and an increased secretion of acid.

GASTRIC FUNCTION TESTS

The old term 'test meal' is misleading and should not be used. The amount of acid that the stomach can produce is measured by means of a gastric function test. In this the patient fasts for 12 hours overnight and a plastic tube is passed through either the nose or the mouth into the stomach. This is usually 45 cm from the incisors or 50 cm from the external nares. The juice is aspirated from the fasting stomach and usually only amounts to 25 ml, or so. The tube is then aspirated at a negative pressure of 5 cm of mercury for the next hour, the suction being broken every 10 minutes and 20 ml of air being blown down the tube to clear it of any plugs of mucus. This hour's secretion is termed the *basal hour* and is kept separate. The patient is now given an injection of Pentagastrin (which is a synthetic product composed of the terminal 5 peptides from the gastrin molecule, and is produced by I.C.I.) the dose being 0.02 micrograms/kg body weight administered intramuscularly. The secretion of the stomach is collected for the next 1 hour, as for the first hour, divided into separate 15 minute samples. The acid is measured by titration. The 'peak acid output' is calculated from the two highest 15 minute outputs in the hour expressed as milliequivalents

From the surgical point of view the drug and alcohol induced group is the most important since the acute erosions of the gastric mucosa that result are a common cause of gastric haemorrhage (see page 195).

TUMOURS OF THE STOMACH

The only common tumour to affect the stomach is the carcinoma which arises from its epithelium; other tumours are quite rare. These include the benign leiomyoma, the malignant leiomyosarcoma and lymphosarcoma, infiltration by Hodgkin's disease and rare invasion from adjacent tumours (pancreas or colon).

LEIOMYOMA

This arises from the muscle of the stomach wall, projects into the lumen of the stomach and becomes ulcerated at its apex, so that it may be an occasional cause of a brisk haematemesis. Rarely it undergoes malignant change to form a leiomyosarcoma.

LYMPHOSARCOMA

This rare tumour arises from lymphoid tissue in the wall of the stomach. It produces gross distortion and irregularity of the stomach and may fistulate into the colon. Spread takes place to the lymph nodes—first to those adjacent to the stomach and then widely to nodes in the neck, axillae and groins.

Treatment is by resection of the primary tumour, where possible, and radiotherapy to involved nodes.

CARCINOMA OF THE STOMACH

Pathology

This is an extremely common and important tumour. In this country it is headed in incidence only by cancer of the lung and large bowel in the male, and by carcinoma of the breast, uterus and large bowel in the female. Distribution is world-wide, although it is particularly frequent in some races, especially the Japanese. Any age may be involved, but it especially affects the age range 50—70. The incidence is raised in patients with pernicious anaemia and there is a definite link with subjects having blood group A, which suggests a genetic factor. Occasionally a gastric carcinoma arises in a previous chronic benign gastric ulcer.

About a quarter of stomach cancers arise in the pyloric region of the stomach. The remainder are distributed fairly evenly throughout the rest of the organ, or diffusely involve the whole of the stomach.

The tumour may take the form of a malignant ulcer with heaped overhanging edges (Fig. 11.16), or it may form a polypoid mass which proliferates into the stomach lumen, or it may widely infiltrate the submucous planes of the stomach which results in a thickened, contracted, organ with little if any superficial ulceration to which the title *'leather-bottle stomach'* is applied.

Spread of the tumour occurs locally through the wall of the stomach and adjacent organs (pancreas, abdominal wall, transverse colon) may be directly invaded. A gastro-colic fistula may develop.

Adjacent lymph nodes are commonly affected. Blood stream dissemination occurs via the portal vein to the liver and thence occasionally to the lungs and the skeleton. Seedlings of tumour may disseminate throughout the peritoneal cavity (transcoelomic spread) and this is characteristically accompanied by ascites.

Clinical features

Symptoms may be produced by the local effects of the tumour, by the secondaries, or by general features associated with malignant disease.

Local symptoms include epigastric pain, which may be indistinguishable from that produced by a chronic gastric ulcer. Vomiting is especially associated with a pyloric tumour producing gastric outlet obstruction and dysphagia (difficulty in swallowing) occurs in tumours at the cardio-oesophageal junction. Only occasionally does a carcinoma of the stomach present with either perforation or acute haemorrhage.

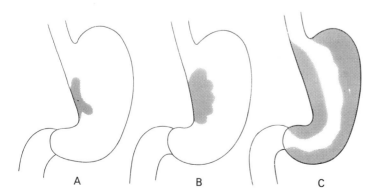

Fig. 11.16. The types of gastric cancer: (A) ulcer, (B) polypoid, (C) leather bottle stomach (linitis plastica).

Secondaries: the patient may first report with jaundice due to liver involvement or abdominal distention due to ascites.

General features: a frequent form of presentation are the general symptoms associated with malignant disease—anorexia, loss of weight and anaemia.

Clinical examination may reveal features which correspond to these three headings. There may be a mass to feel in the abdomen which is the tumour itself. An enlarged liver may be obvious, or the surgeon may detect ascites. Weight loss and anaemia may be present (see Fig. 5.7).

Special investigations

The barium meal is highly accurate; it may demonstrate an irregular stricture, a polypoid tumour, or an ulcer with raised edges (Fig. 11.17). Occasionally, however, the radiologist has considerable

Fig. 11.17. Barium meal demonstrating a polypoid carcinoma of the stomach—note the filling defect (arrowed) projecting inwards from the lesser curvature of the stomach.

difficulty in distinguishing between a benign and malignant stomach ulcer. If necessary *gastroscopy* can then be performed using the fibre-optic instrument. The ulcer can then be directly visualized and a biopsy taken for microscopic examination.

Treatment

The only possible chance of cure for this condition is surgical removal, and this depends on early diagnosis. A tumour at the pylorus or antrum can be removed by partial gastrectomy in which the distal two-thirds of the stomach is removed, the duodenum closed, and a loop of the first part of the jejunum joined to the stomach (Polya gastectomy). If the tumour occupies the body of the stomach or the cardia, it may be necessary to carry out total gastrectomy, close the duodenum and anastomose the jejunum to the divided oesophagus (the Roux-en-Y anastomosis). These procedures are illustrated in Fig. 11.18.

If the tumour cannot be resected because of local invasiveness it may be possible to carry out a gastro-enterostomy to relieve obstruction of the pylorus or intubation by means of a plastic tube (see Fig. 5.8) may relieve the dysphagia of an advanced carcinoma at the cardia. Irradiation and cytotoxic therapy are of only limited value.

Prognosis

This depends on how extensive the tumour is at the time of surgery and on its microscopic nature; the more undifferentiated or anaplastic the tumour, the worse the prognosis is likely to be. The overall outlook is poor; only 5% of all patients presenting to hospital survive for 5 years. However, 20% of patients who undergo radical curative surgery are alive at the end of a five-year period.

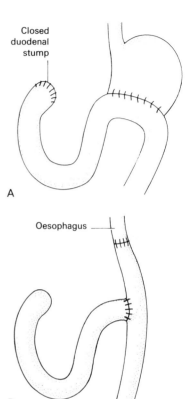

Fig. 11.18. Diagram of the Polya partial gastrectomy (A) and total gastrectomy (B). In the first, the duodenum has been closed and a loop of jejunum anastomosed to the gastric remnant. In the second, the duodenum has again been closed and Roux-loop of jejunum brought up and sutured to the oesophagus.

Duodenum

Anatomy

The duodenum commences immediately after the pylorus and travels in a C-shape to join the jejunum at the duodeno-jejunal junction (Fig. 11.19). Enclosed within the concave border of the 'C' is the head of the pancreas. The common bile duct runs behind the first part of the duodenum and then, after traversing the posterior aspect of the head of the pancreas, enters the medial wall of the

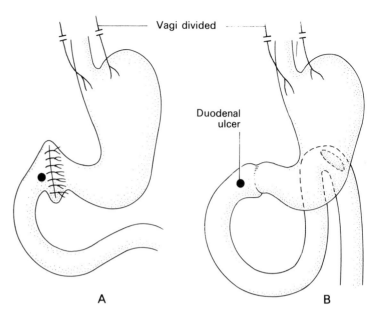

Fig. 11.21. Types of gastric drainage after vagotomy: (A) pyloroplasty and (B) gastro-jejunostomy.

of weakness associated with sweating and palpitations following meals. Satisfactory results can be anticipated in between 85 and 90% of patients.

Before submitting a patient with peptic ulcer to surgery he should be checked for four things:

1. The haemoglobin level; these patients have often been on a diet low in iron and may also have had occult bleeding.

2. The teeth; these often require dental treatment, since gross dental caries predisposes to postoperative parotitis and there is always the risk of dislodgement and inhalation of a loose and septic tooth during anaesthesia.

3. Vitamin C; peptic ulcer patients are often deficient in this vitamin because of their long use of a diet which lacks fruit and vegetables.

4. These patients are often heavy smokers with a chronic cough. Smoking is forbidden and intensive chest physiotherapy given in order to reduce the incidence and severity of postoperative pulmonary collapse.

PERFORATED PEPTIC ULCER

Pathology

Perforation complicates about 10% of all peptic ulcers. Of all perforations, 90% occur in duodenal ulcer, and 90% are in males, especially in the 25–50 year age group. Infants and the very elderly,

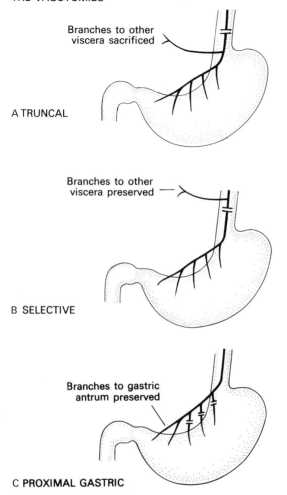

Fig. **11.22.** (A) Truncal, (B) selective and (C) proximal gastric vagotomy.

however, are not immune. There is a high incidence of perforation in patients with peptic ulcer who are on heavy cortisone therapy, and in these the perforation may be relatively silent. Gastric carcinomas occasionally perforate.

Clinical Features

A previous history of peptic ulceration is often obtained, although this may be forgotten by the patient in his agony. Typically there is a sudden severe generalised abdominal pain. Irritation of the lower aspect of the diaphragm by gastric contents may be indicated by radiation of the pain to one or both shoulders, usually the right.

The pain is aggravated by movement and the patient lies rigidly still. There is nausea but only occasionally vomiting.

Examination reveals a patient in severe pain, cold and sweating, with rapid shallow respiration. However, in the early hours, there is no clinical evidence of true shock; the pulse is steady and the blood pressure normal. In the early stages also the temperature is either normal or a little depressed. The abdomen is retracted and when touched is as rigid as a board. On auscultation bowel sounds are absent.

In the delayed case, after 12 hours or more, the features of late peritonitis with paralytic ileus become manifest; the abdomen becomes distended, effortless vomiting occurs and the patient is extremely toxic and in shock.

X-ray of the abdomen with the patient erect may show free gas below the diaphragm in about 70% of cases (Fig. 11.23).

Treatment

The stomach is emptied by means of a nasogastric tube to diminish further leakage through the perforation, and is an essential pre-anaesthetic measure. Morphia is given to relieve pain and an intra-

Fig. 11.23. A chest X-ray in a patient with perforated duodenal ulcer. Note that there is free air in the abdomen which is seen between the liver and the diaphragm on the right and between the fundus of the stomach and diaphragm on the left (arrowed).

venous drip commenced. Ampicillin is given to contend with the peritoneal infection. At operation the peritoneal cavity is sucked clear of all contaminating material and the perforation closed with three or four catgut sutures (Fig. 11.24). Provided undue delay has been avoided, prognosis is good but the mortality is high in patients who do not reach hospital until 12 hours or more from the perforation and this delay is particularly serious in elderly patients.

The late prognosis following perforation depends on whether or not the ulcer is chronic. If there is a previous history of ulceration, about 50% have further serious symptoms and usually come to later elective surgery. If the ulcer is acute with no previous history, this figure falls to 20%. A second subsequent perforation is not rare.

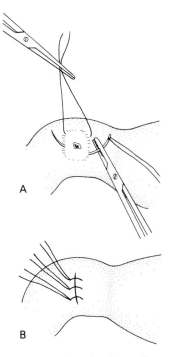

Fig. 11.24. Repair of a perforated duodenal ulcer by means of interrupted catgut sutures.

PYLORIC STENOSIS

By common usage, this term has come to include all conditions which result in obstruction to the outflow of the stomach, whether situated in the distal antrum, at the pylorus itself, or in the first part of the duodenum.

The common causes in the adult are scarring due to chronic duodenal ulcer, a benign peptic ulcer of the antrum, or a carcinoma of the pyloric end of the stomach.

Congenital pyloric stenosis in infants is considered on page 176.

Clinical features

The cardinal symptom of pyloric stenosis, whatever the cause, is vomiting. This is characteristically profuse, free from bile, and may contain food eaten one or two days previously. If the obstruction is due to a stenosing duodenal ulcer there is usually a history of peptic ulceration which has been present for some years. However, if obstruction is due to a carcinoma of the pyloric end of the stomach, the history is usually much shorter, often only weeks or months in duration.

If vomiting persists, the patient's nutrition suffers and he loses weight. There may be dehydration and weakness due to loss of fluid and electrolytes.

On examination the patient may appear dehydrated and wasted. The abdomen may reveal the characteristic succussion splash which is elicited by gently shaking the patient from side to side and listening for the noise produced by the fluid and air contents splashing within the dilated stomach. Sir James Walton, a surgeon at the London Hospital, described three stages of pyloric stenosis:

1. 'the stomach that you can hear'; this is the succussion splash.

2. 'the stomach that you can see'; when a patient with advanced pyloric stenosis is observed, it is possible to see waves of gastric peristalsis which pass from left to right in the epigastrium.

3. 'the stomach that you can feel'; in this very marked case the wall of the stomach is so hypertrophied that it can be palpated through the abdominal muscles.

Investigations

1. *Gastric aspiration* yields a morning resting juice of over 100 ml. It may, in fact, amount to a litre or more of foul-smelling gastric contents containing stale food residue.

2. *Barium meal* shows dilatation of the stomach with a narrow outlet and considerable delay in emptying (Fig. 11.25). It may be difficult or impossible for the radiologist to be certain whether or not the obstruction is due to a benign peptic ulcer of the distal stomach or duodenum, or due to a carcinoma.

3. *Biochemical investigations.* Prolonged vomiting results in loss of

Fig. 11.25. Barium meal in pyloric stenosis due to a duodenal ulcer. The stomach is grossly dilated due to obstruction at its outlet. Note that the greater curvature of the stomach is actually in the patient's pelvis!

water, hydrochloric acid and electrolytes. The loss of acid results in the condition of alkalosis so that the plasma bicarbonate is elevated. The serum chloride, sodium and potassium may be lowered. The blood urea may rise, partly as a result of dehydration and partly because of renal impairment secondary to the electrolyte disturbances.

Treatment

The treatment for established pyloric obstruction, whatever its cause, is invariably surgical. Before operation dehydration and electrolyte depletion are corrected by intravenous replacement of normal saline and of potassium. Daily gastric lavage is performed to remove the debris from the stomach and in addition this often restores function to the stomach and allows fluid absorption to take place by mouth. Vitamin C is given, since the patient with chronic duodenal ulcer is often deficient in ascorbic acid.

Surgical correction is carried out as soon as the patient's general condition is satisfactory, usually about 7 days after admission to hospital. If the obstruction is due to carcinoma of the stomach a partial gastrectomy of the Polya type is performed. A stenosing duodenal ulcer is best treated by vagotomy combined with gastrojejunostomy.

GASTRO-INTESTINAL HAEMORRHAGE

Gastro-intestinal haemorrhage may comprise *haematemesis* (the vomiting of blood), *melaena* (the passage of altered black, tarry, blood per rectum) or a combination of the two. In this country the commonest single cause of this entity is duodenal ulcer. It is a common condition which complicates about 10% of all patients with peptic ulcer, and is also dangerous, bearing with it a mortality rate of about 10%.

The management of patients presenting with gastro-intestinal haemorrhage is threefold:
1. The assessment and replacement of the blood loss.
2. An attempt to diagnose the source of the bleeding.
3. The treatment and control of the source of bleeding.

Blood loss

Before doing anything else, it may be necessary to initiate a blood transfusion in a patient who is obviously shocked with pallor, sweating, a pulse rate above 100, and a blood pressure which has a systolic below 100 mmHg. Every case is grouped on admission and blood made available by cross-matching even if this is not immediately required.

The source of bleeding

Bleeding may be from some local source or result from a general bleeding tendency, such as haemophilia or anticoagulant therapy.

It is useful to consider the possible local causes anatomically:

Oesophagus—oesophageal varices associated with portal hypertension or peptic oesophagitis associated with hiatus hernia.

Stomach—gastric ulcer, acute erosions (including those associated with aspirin, alcohol, butazolidine and cortisone), gastric tumours.

Duodenum—duodenal ulcer, and rarely erosion of the duodenum by a pancreatic tumour.

Intestine—tumours, Meckel's diverticulum.

About 85% of patients with acute gastro-intestinal haemorrhage in this country have either a peptic ulcer or an erosion of the stomach or duodenum. About 5% of patients have oesophageal varices, and the remainder are accounted for by the other causes listed above.

Diagnosis, as always, is made on history, examination, and special investigations.

There may be a typical story of peptic ulceration and perhaps the patient has had a positive barium meal previously. Careful enquiry must be made about ingestion of drugs which may produce acute gastric erosion. A story of alcoholism or previous virus hepatitis may suggest cirrhosis with the development of oesophageal varices and an alcoholic debauch may also have precipitated acute gastric erosion.

Clinical examination is usually negative, apart from those features suggesting blood loss, but the presence of jaundice, an enlarged liver and spleen suggest oesophageal varices, secondary to cirrhosis.

If the bleeding settles, it may be possible to investigate the patient by means of a barium meal together with gastroduodenoscopy, but if the patient is bleeding actively, these are extremely difficult because of clot in the stomach.

Treatment

In the first instance this is medical. The patient is admitted to hospital and put to bed. He is reassured and reassurance is supplemented with morphia if he is restless. If shocked, as assessed by pallor, rapid pulse, and a low blood pressure, a blood transfusion is commenced and a careful shock chart instituted in every case. As soon as active bleeding ceases, milk is allowed by mouth in the form of regular hourly or two-hourly drinks, and as soon as possible the patient is transferred to a semi-solid gastric diet. Aluminium hydroxide gel 10 ml is prescribed every two hours by day and during waking hours at night. Cimetidine, a powerful inhibitor of gastric acid secretion, can be given via the patient's intravenous drip. Since some of these patients have been shown to be deficient in vitamin C this should be given at the rate of 200 mg t.d.s. for five days and then continued at a dosage of 100 mg per day.

On this regime three out of four patients will settle down. In the remaining patients, bleeding either continues or recurs while under observation and it is in these that emergency surgery is obligatory. Unless operation is performed and the bleeding point controlled the patient will die of continued haemorrhage.

In such cases, the blood transfusion is continued and urgent preparation made for laparotomy. At operation the source of bleeding is found and controlled. This usually takes the form of a gastrectomy for a chronic gastric ulcer and either a gastrectomy or a vagotomy with pyloroplasty and undersewing of the bleeding ulcer for duodenal ulceration. In cases of acute erosion it may be possible to undersew the bleeding vessel after opening the stomach (gastrostomy).

In the patients who are treated medically and who settle down, careful assessment is made in the convalescent period. If the presence of a chronic duodenal or gastric is established, then surgery is usually advised as an elective procedure since once a chronic ulcer has bled subsequent haemorrhages are likely to occur.

The management of haemorrhage from oesophageal varices

This is considered on page 290.

Chapter 12. The intestine

The small intestine

Anatomy

The upper half of the small intestine is termed the jejunum and the lower half the ileum. There is no obvious junction between the two parts, and it is not possible to tell exactly where one ends and the other begins. However, at operation, the jejunum has a thicker wall and only one arterial arcade, whereas the ileum has a much thinner wall and a double arterial arcade (Fig. 12.1). The small intestine is richly supplied with blood vessels, the arterial source being derived exclusively from the superior mesenteric artery. If this vessel is occluded, the small intestine will inevitably undergo necrosis. The veins from the small intestine drain into the superior mesenteric vein which, after joining the splenic vein, becomes the portal vein. Thus all the blood from the small intestine passes directly through the liver.

The mucosa of the jejunum is thrown up into folds or *villi* which have the effect of producing a very large surface area of mucosa for the absorption of food material. When the surface of the mucosa is examined at operation it has a velvety appearance due to the villi, in addition to which the mucosa is folded on itself, producing a series of ridges which run around the wall of the intestine, the valvulae conniventes.

Physiology

As might be expected from the anatomical distinctions described above, the jejunum is responsible for the absorption of the majority

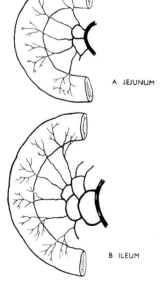

Fig. 12.1. The simple arterial arcades of the jejunum (A) compared with the complex arcades of the ileum (B).

A JEJUNUM

B ILEUM

of foodstuffs. The transmission of the contents however are quite rapid, and barium if ingested with a meal is seen to enter the ileum after only 30 to 60 minutes. In distinction to this, the ileum slows down the transit of its contents and this is the reason that patients who lose significant sections of the terminal ileum tend to develop the symptoms of intestinal hurry, which include diarrhoea. The ileum is responsible for the absorption of water and in addition has some special functions for the absorption of certain substances. The first of these is Vitamin B_{12}, bound to intrinsic factor, which is absorbed by the terminal 100 cm of ileum. The second is conjugated bile salts which have been secreted into the duodenum, have played their part in the digestion of fat and are then re-absorbed so that they can re-circulate in the so-called entero-hepatic circulation for the digestion of more fat.

MECKEL'S DIVERTICULUM

Pathology

Meckel's diverticulum is a pouch which is found on the ante-mesenteric border of the terminal ileum and is a remnant of the vitello-intestinal tract. This duct in the fetus communicates with the yolk sac and protrudes through the gap in the anterior abdominal wall which later becomes the umbilicus. Normally, the duct closes just prior to birth, but in some people the small blind remnant persists (Fig. 12.2). As an aid to memory the 'rule of 2's' has been formulated; and this is that Meckel's diverticulum occurs in 2% of the population, 2 feet from the ileo-caecal valve and is on average 2 inches long. Obviously this is merely a useful approximation. It occurs equally in both men and women.

Section of the Meckel's diverticulum reveals that there are all layers of the bowel wall present and the mucosa is generally similar to normal ileal mucosa. In a few cases, however, ectopic gastric mucosa is found which is capable of secreting hydrochloric acid.

Clinical features

The vast majority of Meckel's diverticula do not give rise to any symptoms, and either are never found or are incidental observations at autopsy. A few cases of Meckel's diverticulitis occur, however, when the diverticulum becomes inflamed in an exactly similar way to the appendix in appendicitis. The symptomatology is indistinguishable from that of appendicitis, being initially central abdominal pain, later shifting to the right iliac fossa, associated with anorexia and vomiting.

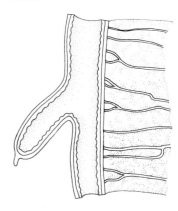

Fig. 12.2. A Meckel's diverticulum.

is uncontrolled sepsis or an abdominal mass. The initial dosage is high, e.g. prednisone 40–60 mg per day, rapidly reducing to a maintenance level 5–15 mg daily after two weeks or so.

One of the interesting recent developments, the evidence for which is now beginning to accumulate, is that when a remission in the disease is produced by steroids this may be maintained by the use of immuno-suppressive therapy. In this case Imuran is given in a dose varying between 50 and 100 mg per day controlled by initially frequent white cell counts, every third day or so, and then being continued in the long term. It must be realised that immuno-suppressive therapy is difficult to maintain and is attended by the significant dangers of uncontrolled infection and possibly, in the long term, the development of carcinoma of various tissues. It may be justified, however, by virtue of the fact that Crohn's disease is an extremely serious condition which may result in the death of the patient.

Surgery is frequently required for this condition when there is a persistent intestinal obstruction or fistula formation. In a patient who has not had previous surgery the affected portion of the intestine should be completely excised, a method of treatment obviously only applicable if a relatively short segment is involved. Discussion has existed in the past as to whether the diseased segment should be excised or bypassed, but it would seem that results of excision are better than those for simple bypass. Unfortunately, long term results of surgery are not entirely satisfactory because of recurrence of the disease and in a series of patients investigated in Leeds 10 years after primary surgery, 40% had required a second operation. In addition, the early post-operative mortality is high, being between 3 and 5%, this being due to a combination of infective complications and fluid and electrolyte imbalance. However, the long-term outlook is better after surgery than after medical treatment alone and proponents of this form of therapy point to the fact that following surgery over 70% of persons are in good general health compared with under 20% before surgery has been carried out.

VASCULAR DISEASE OF THE INTESTINE

Obstruction to either the artery or the vein which supplies a segment of intestine will result in gangrene. Arterial occlusion may occur either as a result of an embolus or thrombosis due to degenerative arterial disease. Venous thrombosis occurs, but is rarer, and the cause is more difficult to determine.

In a case of vascular gangrene of the intestine laparotomy is required with resection of the affected portion of the intestine and reconstitution by end-to-end-anastomosis. Occasionally embolectomy or removal of the thrombus may restore circulation to all or part of the infarcted intestine. The patients who develop this condition usually have generalised arterial degenerative disease which results in a poor general outlook from resection.

TUMOURS OF THE SMALL INTESTINE

One of the many mysteries of tumour formation is the rarity of growths from beyond the pylorus to the ileo-caecal valve, in spite of their great frequency in the stomach and large intestine.

The epithelium may give rise to a benign adenoma or malignant adenocarcinoma. It is also a site for the carcinoid tumour which is considered below. The walls of the small intestine may give rise to benign or malignant tumours of its plain muscle (leiomyoma and leiomyosarcoma respectively), and its lymphoid tissue may be the site of a lymphosarcoma. Secondary invasion may occur directly from adjacent stomach or colon or by metastases from, for example, the breast.

Tumours of the small intestine may present with intestinal bleeding, obstruction, intussusception or volvulus and treatment, where possible, is by resection.

THE CARCINOID SYNDROME

Carcinoid tumours occur most commonly in the appendix, but may be found anywhere in the alimentary tract, and occasionally in the lung. The tumour arises from cells which take up special silver stains and which occur in the crypts of the intestinal mucosa. The tumour is very slowly growing, and those of the appendix are relatively benign. However, those arising in the small intestine and large bowel spread eventually to the regional lymph nodes and the liver.

Where there is an extensive mass of tumour, symptoms are produced because of the serotonin (5-hydroxytryptamine or 5 HT) which is secreted by the carcinoid cells.

Clinical features

The carcinoid syndrome comprises any of the following features:
1. An abdominal mass or an enlarged liver produced by the tumour itself or by its secondaries.
2. Flushing with attacks of cyanosis.
3. Diarrhoea with noisy bowel sounds (borborygmi).
4. Bronchospasm.
5. Pulmonary stenosis.
   The diagnosis is confirmed by estimating the breakdown product

of 5 HT which is 5-hydroxyindole acetic acid (5-HIAA), which can be readily estimated and whose level is considerably raised in this syndrome.

Treatment

This comprises resection of the tumour in early cases. Local deposits in the liver are also occasionally amenable to surgical excision. Even if widespread deposits are present, the tumour is slowly growing and the patient may survive for many years.

SMALL INTESTINAL OBSTRUCTION

This may be divided into adynamic and dynamic.

ADYNAMIC OBSTRUCTION

This is due to the loss of propulsive power of the small intestine and is termed 'paralytic ileus'. This inevitably follows laparotomy and also occurs when any form of irritation to the peritoneum occurs, such as peritonitis. It is also encountered in patients with extensive retroperitoneal haemorrhage such as may occur in fractures of the lumbar spine.

Clinical features

In the post-operative case, the patient has no more pain than would be expected from his laparotomy wound. The abdomen is distended, generally rather tender, and silent on auscultation. There may be nausea or vomiting and no flatus is passed.

Treatment

The treatment of this condition is that of its underlying cause in many instances (see peritonitis below). However, one of the important effects of paralytic ileus is that the intestine is not only unable to move, but also unable to absorb fluid, which therefore pools within its dilated loops. In order to maintain the patient in satisfactory general condition, intravenous saline will be required, together with supplements of up to 80 mEq (or mmol) of potassium per 24 hours. A strict fluid chart is obligatory. A naso-gastric tube is passed in order to keep the stomach empty. This prevents vomiting and the possibility of aspiration of gastric contents.

If the ileus is very prolonged, that is for more than three or four days, intravenous feeding with amino acids, fructose and fat should be given in order to maintain nutrition.

DYNAMIC OBSTRUCTION

Dynamic obstruction occurs when there is some mechanical block along the length of the bowel.

Classification

Whenever one considers obstruction of a tube anywhere in the body this should be classified into:
1. Causes in the lumen
2. Causes in the wall
3. Causes outside the wall (Fig. 12.5)

Applying this classification to obstruction of the small intestine, we have:

1. *Causes within the lumen*—these are rather unusual, but may result from the presence of an inspissated mass of food, particularly fruit pith or vegetable material. Occasionally a gall stone enters the small intestine via a fistula between the gall bladder and the duodenum; if sufficiently large it may impact in the bowel producing a *gall stone ileus*.

2. *In the wall*—congenital atresia, Crohn's disease, tumours, etc.

3. *Outside the wall*—This is the commonest type of obstruction of the small intestine and may be due to a strangulated hernia, volvulus, intussusception or intraperitoneal adhesions or bands.

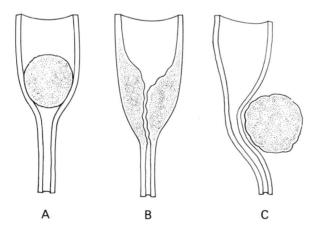

A   B   C

Fig. 12.5. Any tube in the body may be obstructed by causes in the lumen (A), causes in the wall (B) and causes outside the wall (C).

Pathology

Simple obstruction occurs when the bowel is occluded without damage to its blood supply; in *strangulation obstruction*, the blood supply of the involved intestine is cut off, and if unrelieved, gangrene of the involved segment will take place.

When the intestine is obstructed by a simple occlusion, the intestine above the obstruction becomes dilated, partly with gas (most of which is swallowed air) and partly by fluids secreted by the stomach, intestinal wall, liver and pancreas. There is increased peristalsis in an attempt to overcome the obstruction. As the bowel distends, the blood supply to the tensely distended gut wall becomes impaired and in extreme cases there may be mucosal ulceration and eventually perforation. Perforation may also occur from the pressure of a band or the edge of the hernia neck on the bowel wall producing local ischaemia.

In strangulation obstruction the situation is even more serious since the ischaemic bowel is unable to contain its bacteria and their toxins within its lumen so that a transudation of organisms into the peritoneal cavity rapidly takes place, with secondary peritonitis. Unrelieved strangulation is followed by gangrene of the ischaemic bowel with perforation (Fig. 12.6).

The lethal effects of intestinal obstruction result from fluid and electrolyte loss due to the copious vomiting and exudation into the bowel lumen, protein loss into the gut and toxaemia due to the migration of toxins and bacteria either through the intact but ischaemic bowel wall or through an actual perforation.

Clinical features

The cardinal symptoms of intestinal obstruction are four in number:
1. Colicky pain
2. Distension
3. Absolute constipation (for flatus as well as for faeces)
4. Vomiting

These features can easily be deduced from the pathology described above. The *colicky pain* results from the increased peristalsis in the obstructed gut, and is usually the first symptom. The *distension* results from progressive dilatation of the gut above the site of occlusion by gas and fluid. The *absolute constipation* is produced by the blockage of the bowel. However, a partial or chronic obstruction may be accompanied by the passage of small amounts of flatus and even in complete obstruction the patient may pass one or two normal stools as the lower bowel empties after the onset of the obstruction. *Vomiting* usually occurs early when the obstruction is high in the intestine,

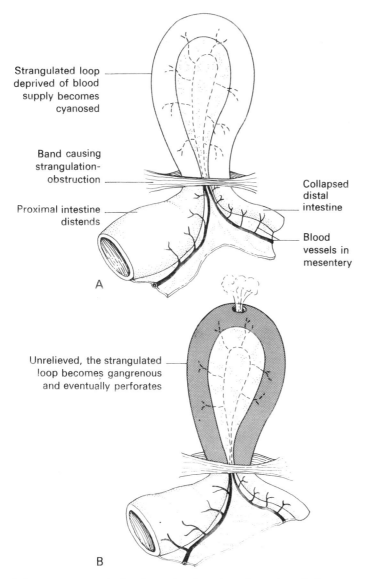

Strangulated loop
deprived of blood
supply becomes
cyanosed

Band causing
strangulation-
obstruction

Proximal intestine
distends

Collapsed
distal
intestine

Blood
vessels in
mesentery

A

Unrelieved, the strangulated
loop becomes gangrenous
and eventually perforates

B

Fig. 12.6. Unrelieved strangulation obstruction (A) results in gangrene of the affected segment and eventually perforation (B).

but is late or even entirely absent in chronic or large bowel obstruction. In the late stages the vomiting becomes faeculent due to bacterial decomposition of the stagnant contents of the gut.

On examination the patient may be obviously dehydrated, he is in pain and may be rolling about with colic. The pulse is usually elevated but the temperature frequently is normal. The abdomen is distended, visible peristalsis may be present and noisy bowel sounds are heard on listening to the abdomen. It is important to look carefully for two features; the presence of a strangulated external hernia, which will make the diagnosis easy, and the presence of an abdominal scar. Intestinal obstruction in the presence of this evidence of a previous operation immediately suggests either adhesions or a band as the cause.

Special investigations

Plain X-rays of the abdomen are valuable in the diagnosis of intestinal obstruction. Dilated loops of small intestine can be seen when the patient is in the supine position. When the patient is X-rayed in the standing position, the gas floats to the top of the fluid within the dilated loops and appears as multiple fluid levels (Fig. 12.7).

Treatment

All cases of dynamic intestinal obstruction require laparotomy. It is essential, before this is carried out, to resuscitate the patient. Blood is taken for estimation of haemoglobin, urea and electrolytes as well as for the grouping and cross-matching of blood. A nasogastric tube is passed so that the stomach can be maintained empty. An intravenous drip of saline is commenced to replace the losses the patient has

Fig. 12.7. X-rays of the abdomen in a case of intestinal obstruction due to post-operative adhesions. (A) supine position; the dilated loops of small intestine are visualised. (B) in the standing position multiple fluid levels are seen.

A

B

suffered by virtue of vomiting and loss of fluid into the dilated intestine and to maintain the patient during the time fluids cannot be absorbed normally through the small bowel. It is an important rule that the only person who can give an analgesic to the patient is the surgeon who makes the decision whether to operate or not. If analgesics are given too early in the process of diagnosis and treatment there is the danger that all pain will be removed and the true diagnosis will be missed with resulting delay in effective treatment.

When the patient is fully resuscitated, rehydrated and has a normal blood pressure (the pulse rate usually takes some time before it falls to normal levels) and is passing urine, then and only then is laparotomy performed. At laparotomy the small intestine will be found to be dilated proximal to the obstruction, that distal to the obstruction is collapsed. If the obstruction is of long standing, the wall of the proximal intestine will be oedematous and soft. The dilated proximal intestine is decompressed by means of a long sucker (a Savage decompressor) and the obstructing agent is removed, or if this is not possible, for example in some cases of secondary carcinoma, it is bypassed. If the intestine is strangulated, the necrotic section of the intestine is resected and continuity is restored by end-to-end anastomosis.

There are some cases in which it is not possible to tell whether the intestine is necrotic or not. In this situation the segment in question is wrapped in warm, moist packs and is left for 10 minutes or so. Its viability or otherwise is then assessed on the basis of pulsation of the vessels in the mesentery, colour of intestinal wall and the presence of intestinal movement. If in doubt, and a massive length of small intestine is involved, it is quite permissible to return the intestine to the peritoneal cavity and to re-inspect it at a second laparotomy 24 hours later. Fortunately this circumstance is extremely rare.

Post-operatively a long continued paralytic ileus is the rule. During this period fluid will be lost into the paralysed intestine, via the urine and by insensible losses through the skin and in expired air, which are often increased by virtue of post-operative pyrexia. It is extremely important, therefore, to keep up with the additional fluid losses and there is a tendency for patients to be dehydrated after operation because too rigid a policy of fluid restriction is adopted. It is likely that in the first 24 hours after operation an adult male patient will require between 5 and 6 litres of fluid to maintain his normal fluid balance and provide additional water for urinary output in excess of one litre. In the second post-operative day less fluid volume is required, in the region of 3 to 5 litres, depending upon circumstances.

When the paralytic ileus recovers, fluid within the lumen of the intestine is absorbed and excreted in the urine and this is found to result in a diuresis. It is interesting that when this diuresis occurs, and the paralytic ileus recovers with the passage of flatus, patients seem to have turned a corner in the process of recovery, their comfort and well-being are then rapidly improved.

OBSTRUCTION OF THE SMALL INTESTINE IN CHILDREN

A number of important conditions produce obstruction of the small intestine in infants and children. These include congenital intestinal atresia, volvulus neonatorum, meconium ileus and intussusception. Neonatal obstruction of the large bowel due to Hirschsprung's disease and ano-rectal atresias are dealt with in the section on rectum.

Continuous vomiting in the newborn may be due to intracranial injury, infection, or intestinal obstruction. If the vomit contains bile, this indicates, almost without exception, that intestinal obstruction is present. In addition to vomiting there may be constipation, abdominal distention and visible peristalsis.

A plain X-ray of the abdomen is invaluable in demonstrating the distended loops of intestine with fluid levels.

CONGENITAL ATRESIA

This may be a septum across the small intestine which may be complete or partial, or a complete gap (Fig. 12.8); multiple segments may be involved.

Treatment

This comprises resection of the stricture and end-to-end anastomosis, but the operation is difficult and the mortality high.

VOLVULUS NEONATORUM

Occasionally the normally wide attachment of the small bowel mesentery to the posterior abdominal wall is defective and this allows torsion, or volvulus, of the whole of the small intestine together with the right side of the large bowel (Fig. 12.9). Untreated, the whole of this segment of intestine becomes gangrenous. There may in addition be a congenital band which passes from the large bowel across the duodenum (Ladd's band) and which may produce secondary obstruction of the duodenum.

A

B

C

Fig. 12.8. Varieties of congenital atresia of the small intestine.

Treatment

Comprises untwisting the volvulus, dividing the transduodenal band and attaching the abnormally mobile ascending colon to the lateral abdominal wall.

MECONIUM ILEUS

This is a manifestation of mucoviscidosis, which is a generalised defect of mucus secretion of the intestine, the bronchial tree and the pancreas (*fibrocystic pancreatic disease*). Because of the loss of intestinal mucus and a blockage of pancreatic ducts with loss of tryptic digestion, the lower ileum of the new born babe is blocked with sticky, thick meconium (Fig. 12.10). The x-rays of the abdomen

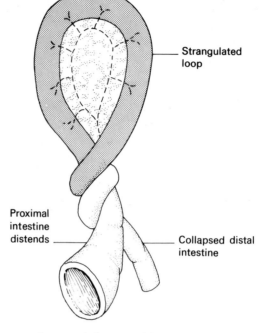

Strangulated loop

Proximal intestine distends

Collapsed distal intestine

Fig. 12.9. Volvulus neonatorum—diagram to show the torsion of the intestine on its mesentery.

are characteristic. In addition to the distended coils of bowel, a typical mottled 'ground glass' appearance of meconium can be seen within the abdominal cavity.

Treatment

The inspissated meconium may require removal by lavage through a small incision in the intestine. Occasionally the impacted segment of small intestine may show areas of gangrene from pressure necrosis and requires resection. Post-operatively the infant is given pancreatic extract by mouth to replace the deficient trypsin.

Prognosis is poor, and because of lack of mucus secretion in the bronchi, recurrent chest infection is almost inevitable.

INTUSSUSCEPTION

Intussusception is the invagination of one portion of the gut into the lumen of the immediately adjoining bowel (Fig. 12.11).

Aetiology

95% of cases occur in infants or young children where there is usually no obvious cause. The mesenteric lymph nodes in these cases are

Fig. 12.10. Meconium ileus. (A) This segment of small intestine was so impacted with meconium that it required resection. (B) The sticky meconium from the bowel lumen.

usually enlarged and it has been suggested that the lymphoid tissue in the bowel wall becomes swollen due to a virus infection. In adults and in some children a polyp, a tumour, or an inverted Meckel's diverticulum may form the apex of the intussusception.

The inner layer of the intussusception has its blood supply cut off by the direct pressure of the outer layer, as well as by stretching of its supplying mesentery so that, if left untreated, gangrene is inevitable.

Most cases affect the ileo-caecal region so that the small intestine protrudes into the ascending colon.

Clinical features in infants

Usually previously healthy children are affected aged between 3 and 12 months; boys twice as often as girls.

The history is of spasms of abdominal colic typified by screaming and pallor. There is vomiting and a mixture of blood and slime ('red currant jelly') is passed per rectum. A sausage-shaped mass may be felt on abdominal palpation.

Fig. 12.11. Diagram of an intussusception.

Treatment

In most centres operative treatment is employed. The intussusception is reduced at laparotomy or, if gangrene has already taken place in a late case, resection or short circuit may be necessary.

It is sometimes possible to reduce the intussusception by running barium into the rectum in the X-ray department. The pressure of the head of the barium reduces the intussusception and X-rays are taken to confirm that this has taken place.

The appendix

Anatomy

The appendix arises from the caecum about one inch below the ileo-caecal valve. It is a diverticulum that varies in length from about $1\frac{1}{2}$ to 9 inches. Its position is extremely variable, more so than any other organ. Most commonly it lies behind the caecum, but it may hang down into the pelvis or pass in front or behind the terminal ileum (Fig. 12.12). The mesentery of the appendix carries the blood supply to this organ along the appendicular artery, a branch of the ileo-colic artery (Fig. 12.13). This represents the entire vascular supply of the appendix and if any of its branches are thrombosed secondary to acute infection of the appendix, then gangrene and subsequent perforation are inevitable.

ACUTE APPENDICITIS

This is the commonest abdominal emergency, and it is estimated to affect 1 in 6 of the British population. However, it is only found in civilised communities or in primitive peoples who have been unwise enough to change to Western diet.

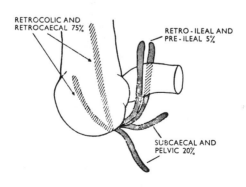

RETROCOLIC AND
RETROCAECAL 75%

RETRO - ILEAL AND
PRE - ILEAL 5%

SUBCAECAL AND
PELVIC 20%

Fig. 12.12. The positions in which the appendix may lie, together with their approximate incidence.

Acute appendicitis usually occurs when the appendix is obstructed. This may be due to a pellet of faecal material (faecolith), a kink from inflammatory adhesions, or enlargement of the lymph collections in its wall secondary to a catarrhal inflammation of its mucosa. Since the appendix of the infant is wide-mouthed and well drained, and since the lumen of the appendix is almost obliterated in old age, appendicitis in the two extremes of life is relatively rare. The obstructed appendix acts as a closed loop; bacteria proliferate in its lumen and invade the appendix wall, which is damaged by pressure necrosis. Thrombosis of its supplying blood vessels then results in gangrene and perforation (Fig. 12.14).

The acutely inflamed appendix may resolve, but, if so, a further attack can usually be expected, so that it is not uncommon for a patient to admit to one or more previous milder episodes of pain. More often the inflamed appendix undergoes gangrene and then perforates, either with a general peritonitis, or with the formation of a localised appendix abscess.

Fig. 12.13. The blood supply of the appendix.

Clinical features

A typical attack of acute appendicitis commences as a central abdominal colic which shifts after approximately 6 hours to the right

Fig. 12.14. A perforated gangrenous appendix removed at operation.

lower abdomen. The central abdominal pain is visceral in origin; the shift of pain is due to involvement of the sensitive peritoneum lining the abdominal wall which is irritated by the inflammatory process. Nausea and vomiting are usually present, so that Murphy described as a diagnostic sequence: central abdominal pain, followed by vomiting, followed by a shift of the pain to the right iliac fossa.

With perforation of the appendix there may be a temporary remission of pain, but this is followed by a more severe and generalised pain with profuse vomiting as general peritonitis develops.

On examination, the temperature and pulse are usually raised. The patient is flushed and is in obvious pain. The tongue is coated and the breath is foul. Examination of the abdomen reveals localised tenderness in the region of the inflamed appendix. There is usually guarding of the abdominal muscles over this site.

In late cases with generalised peritonitis the abdomen becomes diffusely tender and rigid, bowel sounds are absent, and the patient is obviously very ill.

Special investigations are of little value in making the diagnosis though they may have been needed to exclude other possibilities. The white cell count is usually raised with a polymorph leucocytosis. X-rays of the abdomen have no truly diagnostic features.

Differential diagnosis

Although the diagnosis of appendicitis is frequently quite straightforward, it may be a great mimic of other diseases, and these should be considered systematically:

1. *Other intra-abdominal conditions.* These include perforated peptic ulcer, acute cholecystitis, acute intestinal obstruction, gastroenteritis, acute Crohn's disease and acute diverticulitis of the colon.
2. *Urinary tract.* Renal colic and acute pyelonephritis. The urine must be tested for blood and pus cells in every case of acute abdominal pain.
3. *The chest.* Basal pneumonia and pleurisy may give referred abdominal pain, which may be surprisingly difficult to differentiate, especially in children.
4. *Central nervous system.* The pain which precedes the eruption of herpes zoster (shingles) affecting the 11th and 12th thoracic segments and the irritation of these posterior nerve roots in spinal disease may give referred pain to the lower abdomen.
5. *Gynaecological causes.* The commonest pitfalls are acute salpingitis, ruptured ovarian cyst and ruptured ectopic pregnancy. It is useful to consider that 'every lady is pregnant until proved otherwise'!

Treatment

Treatment of acute appendicitis is appendicectomy unless an appendix mass has formed without evidence of general peritonitis (see below) or in those rare circumstances where operation would be difficult or impossible, for example in a small boat at sea, or in a mountain hut in a blizzard. Here reliance must be placed on the hope that the attack will resolve or that a local abscess will form rather than on one's surgical skill using a razor blade and a bent spoon.

If at operation the appendix is found to have become gangrenous, or perforated with general peritonitis, then, in addition to removing the appendix, antibiotic therapy is commenced and here ampicillin is the first drug of choice. If there is considerable local infection a drain is inserted in the wound.

THE APPENDIX MASS

It is not rare for a patient to present with a history of several days of abdominal pain, by which time a localised mass has developed in the right iliac fossa. In these circumstances the inflamed appendix has become walled off by adhesions to adjacent organs and immediate surgery in such circumstances may simply spread the infection through the peritoneal cavity.

Treatment

At first this should be conservative. The mass is outlined on the skin with a marking pencil (Fig. 12.15). The patient is put to bed on a fluid diet and his general condition, together with temperature and

Fig. 12.15. The outline of an appendix abscess marked on the skin.

pulse are carefully observed. Antibiotics are *not* prescribed since these may simply produce a chronic inflammatory mass, which is honeycombed with abscess cavities, a condition that has received the nickname 'antibioticoma'. On this treatment 3 out of 4 cases resolve, the temperature settles and the mass subsides. In the remainder, the mass enlarges and the temperature persists. Under these circumstances the abscess requires surgical drainage.

After the mass has resolved (whether under conservative treatment or following drainage) then appendicectomy is carried out after an interval of 2 or 3 months when the inflammatory condition has settled completely. Unless appendicectomy is performed, there is a considerable risk of a further attack of acute appendicitis.

PERITONITIS

Perforation of the acutely inflamed appendix is the commonest cause of peritonitis in this country. This is a convenient point, therefore, to consider this subject in detail.

Aetiology

Peritonitis can be defined as inflammation of the peritoneal cavity. Bacteria may enter this space by four portals:
1. *From the exterior*—a penetrating wound of the abdominal wall, or by infection introduced at laparotomy.
2. *From intra-abdominal viscera*—either from perforation (for example perforated duodenal ulcer, perforated appendicitis, or rupture of the intestine from trauma), gangrene of a viscus (e.g. acute cholecystitis or infarction of the intestine), or post-operative leakage of an intestinal anastomosis.
3. *Via the bloodstream*—as part of a septicaemia, a rare source of infection today.
4. *Via the female genital tract*—following acute salpingitis or puerperal infection (inflammation of the genital canal during childbirth). Approximately 40% of all cases of peritonitis are due to acute appendicitis, 20% result from post-operative complications, and 20% are due to perforated peptic ulcers.

Clinical features

Peritonitis inevitably follows some precipitating lesion which itself may have definite clinical features. For example, the onset may be an attack of acute appendicitis, or a perforated duodenal ulcer, or abdominal trauma, each with its appropriate symptoms and signs.

In the early hours, peritonitis is characterized by a generalised severe pain. The patient wishes to lie still because any movement aggravates his agony. Irritation of the lower aspect of the diaphragm may be accompanied by pain which is referred to the shoulder tip. Vomiting is frequent. The temperature is usually elevated and the pulse rises progressively. Examination at this time shows a seriously ill patient with localised or generalised tenderness of the abdomen, depending on the extent of the peritonitis. The abdominal wall is held rigidly and rebound tenderness is present. The abdomen is silent on stethoscopic examination.

In advanced cases, the abdomen becomes distended, signs of free fluid are present, the patient becomes increasingly toxic with a rapid, feeble pulse. Vomiting becomes faeculant and the patient is obviously shocked with moist, cold and cyanosed skin.

Treatment

Specific causes of peritonitis may require specific therapy. These are dealt with in their appropriate sections. The general principles of treatment are as follows:

1. *Relieve pain* by means of morphia.

2. *Gastric aspiration* by means of a naso-gastric tube; this reduces the risk of inhalation of vomit and prevents further abdominal distention by removing swallowed air.

3. *Fluid and electrolyte replacement* by intravenous therapy. Blood may be required in the presence of shock.

4. *Antibiotic therapy.* Ampicillin or a combination of gentamicin and metronidazole (Flagyl) are commonly employed but therapy is guided where possible by checking the sensitivity of the responsible organisms.

5. *Surgery* is indicated if the source of infection can be removed or closed. For example, a perforated peptic uler is sutured, a gangrenous perforated appendix removed and ruptured gut resected or repaired.

Conservative treatment is indicated where the infection has been localised (e.g. an appendix mass), or where the primary focus is irremovable as in pancreatitis, or post-partum infection, where the patient is moribund, or where there is a lack of surgical facilities, as on board ship. Here reliance must be placed on intravenous therapy, gastric aspiration, and antibiotics.

Any localised collection of pus requires drainage and later surgery may be required for the evacuation of residual abcesses. Following peritonitis, pus may collect in the subphrenic spaces or in the pelvis.

Pus may collect between the diaphragm and the liver or immediately below the liver on either the right or left side; indeed rarely they are bilateral.

About one third follow perforated appendicitis, one third from perforations of peptic ulcer, and a sixth from abdominal operations.

Clinical features

Subphrenic infection usually follows a general peritonitis after 10 days to 3 weeks, although if antibiotics have been given, an abscess may be disguised and may only become obvious weeks or even months after the original episode. Often there are no localizing symptoms, but the patient merely presents with a swinging pyrexia, malaise, nausea, loss of weight and anaemia. There may, however, be localising features of pain in the upper abdomen, the lower chest, or referred to the shoulder, and there may be swelling or tenderness in the upper abdomen or lower chest.

Special investigations

The white cell count is raised to the region of 15,000 to 20,000, with a relative increase in polymorphs.

Screening of the chest is the vital investigation which reveals an abnormality in nearly all cases. The signs are elevation of the diaphragm on the affected side, diminished or absent mobility of the diaphragm, a pleural effusion, and/or collapse of the lung base on the affected side, and gas together with a fluid level below the diaphragm (Fig. 12.16).

Treatment

If there is no gas and free fluid on X-ray, an early case may respond to antibiotic therapy, but if there is clinical or X-ray evidence of a localised abscess or if resolution fails to occur on antibiotic therapy, then surgical drainage is indicated.

PELVIC ABSCESS

A pelvic abscess may follow any general peritonitis, but it is particularly common after acute appendicits (75%), or after gynaecological infections. In the male the abscess lies between the bladder and the

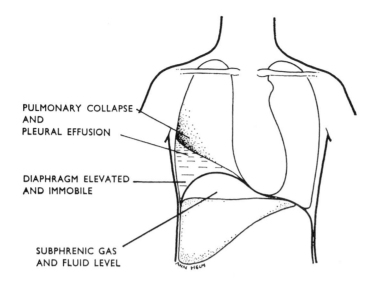

PULMONARY COLLAPSE
AND
PLEURAL EFFUSION

DIAPHRAGM ELEVATED
AND IMMOBILE

SUBPHRENIC GAS
AND FLUID LEVEL

Fig. 12.16. Diagram of the X-ray appearances of a right subphrenic abscess. The diaphragm is raised (and fixed on screening), a fluid level is present beneath it and there is a pleural effusion with compression and collapse of the lung base.

rectum, in the female between the uterus and posterior fornix of the vagina anteriorly, and the rectum posteriorly (pouch of Douglas).

Left untreated the abscess may burst into the rectum or vagina, or may discharge onto the abdominal wall, particularly if there has been a previous abdominal laparotomy incision at the time of the original episode of peritonitis. Occasionally the abscess may rupture into the peritoneal cavity.

Clinical features

1. General—swinging pyrexia, toxaemia, weight loss with leuco-cytosis.
2. Local—diarrhoea, mucous discharge per rectum, the presence of a mass felt on rectal or vaginal examination, which is occasionally large enough to be palpated abdominally.

Treatment

An early pelvic cellulitis may respond rapidly to a short course of chemotherapy, but there is the risk that the prolonged antibiotic treatment of an unresolved infection may produce a chronic inflammatory mass studded with small abscess cavities in the pelvis. It is safer, therefore, where there is an established pelvic abscess, to withhold chemotherapy and await pointing into the vagina or rectum through which surgical drainage can be carried out. Very often even this is not required since firm pressure by the finger in the rectum may be followed by rupture of the abscess through the rectal wall.

The colon

Anatomy

The colon is a bulky muscular tube which extends from the caecum in the right iliac fossa via the ascending colon, the hepatic flexure, the transverse colon, the splenic flexure, the descending colon and the pelvic (sigmoid) colon to terminate in the rectum, which commences opposite the centre of the third piece of the sacrum and which empties to the exterior via the anal canal (Fig. 12.17).

The junction between the ileum and caecum is protected by the ileocaecal valve. This is a thickening of the circular muscle of the terminal ileum which exerts some regulation of the emptying of ileal contents, and prevents reflux from the caecum. Just beneath the ileocaecal junction is attached the appendix.

The characteristic appearance of the colon is due to two main features in the arrangement of the muscle coat. The first of these is the regular pouching of the colon into 'haustra' and the second is the condensation of the outer longitudinal muscle into three separate bands known as the *taenia coli*.

Fig. 12.17. The colon and its blood supply.

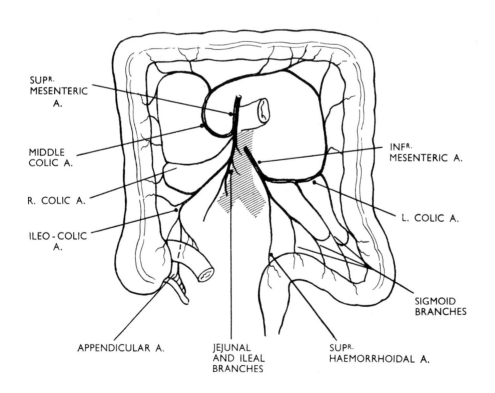

SUPR. MESENTERIC A.

MIDDLE COLIC A.

R. COLIC A.

ILEO-COLIC A.

INFR. MESENTERIC A.

L. COLIC A.

SIGMOID BRANCHES

APPENDICULAR A.

JEJUNAL AND ILEAL BRANCHES

SUPR. HAEMORRHOIDAL A.

The taenia coli become a continuous coat over the surface of the appendix and distally over the rectum. The ascending colon and the descending colon are retroperitoneal in situation; the transverse colon however is an intra-peritoneal structure, its blood supply being carried to it along the transverse mesocolon. Hanging from the under surface of the transverse colon is the fatty sheet, the greater omentum, which, above the colon, becomes attached to the greater curve of the stomach. The pelvic colon is also intra-peritoneal and also has a mesocolon.

The blood supply of the caecum, the right side of the colon and the transverse colon is derived from the superior mesenteric artery via the ileo-colic, right colic and middle colic branches. The descending and pelvic colon, together with the upper part of the rectum, are supplied with blood from the inferior mesenteric artery, which arises from the front of the aorta just above its bifurcation. The venous drainage of the colon passes to the portal vein. The lymphatic drainage follows the venous drainage and lymph nodes are found at the edge of the colonic wall and alongside the aorta.

As with the whole of the intestine, the nerve supply is both from the sympathetic and parasympathetic nervous systems. The sympathetic nerves are carried to the wall of the intestine both from the retro-peritoneal plexuses and with blood vessels. The parasympathetic supply is derived for the right side of the colon and half of the transverse colon from the vagus nerve and for the left side of the colon from the parasympathetic sacral outflow.

Considering the function of the colon, its wall is surprisingly thin. This has the effect that it is extremely distensible. The mucosa appears on inspection to be pale pink in colour with a shiny, smooth surface. When viewing the normal mucosa through a sigmoidoscope it is possible to distinguish individual blood vessels running beneath its surface.

The colon acts as a reservoir. Water is reabsorbed so that liquid ileal contents are converted into solid faeces.

Contraction of the colon and a desire to defaecate result when the wall becomes distended or with the gastro-colic reflex which follows taking a meal.

Apart from these normal causes of colonic contraction, certain drugs, including Senokot, castor oil and phenolphthalein, have a similar action.

ULCERATIVE COLITIS

Ulcerative colitis is a disease of the colon and rectum of unknown cause. Among many suggestions as to its aetiology are psychosomatic factors, an allergy or auto-immune disease.

Pathology

Females are more commonly affected than males. Although the disease may occur at any age, the peak incidence is between 20 and 40 years. In the majority of cases the condition affects the rectum first, but later spreads to involve the whole of the colon. Initially there is oedema and reddening of the mucosa. This is followed by bleeding from the inflamed mucosa when it is touched ('contact bleeding'), then ulceration (Fig. 12.18.). Eventually the wall of the colon becomes oedematous and fibrotic so that it is rigid with loss of its normal haustrations.

Clinical features

The patient complains of profuse diarrhoea, which contains blood, mucus and pus. There may be accompanying cramp-like abdominal pains. There may be an acute onset of fulminating disease accompanied by fever, toxaemia, severe bleeding and the risk of perforation. More often attacks are less severe and intermittent, or the patient may pass into a stage of chronic active disease.

Investigations

Sigmoidoscopy reveals oedema of the mucosa with contact bleeding in the early mild cases, proceeding to granularity of the mucosa and then frank ulceration, with pus and blood in the bowel lumen. Biopsy will give confirming histological evidence of the diagnosis.

Fig. 12.18. Ulcerative colitis. The specimen removed at operation has been opened to demonstrate the diffuse ulceration of the mucosa.

A barium enema shows ragged ulceration and in the chronic case the fibrosis and loss of haustration produces the typical appearances of the 'drainpipe' colon (Fig. 12.19.).

Stool examination reveals pus and blood but no specific organism can be grown.

Differential diagnosis must be made from other causes of diarrhoea especially those due to specific infecting organisms producing amoebic or bacillary dysentery. This is particularly true in patients who are, or have been, domiciled overseas. Carcinoma of the colon and Crohn's disease of the large bowel are also important differential diagnoses.

Complications

These may be either local or general.

Local complications are perforation of the colon, haemorrhage, which may either be acute or chronic with progressive anaemia, stricture formation, peri-anal infection, fistula-in-ano, and malignant change. Patients with ulcerative colitis, particularly those with long-standing disease, are at far greater risk of developing carcinoma of the large bowel than normal individuals.

General complications are toxaemia, loss of weight, anaemia, arthritis, iritis, ulceration of the legs and abscesses of the skin, which may break down into ulcers (pyoderma gangrenosa).

Fig. 12.19. Barium enema in advanced ulcerative colitis to show the typical 'drain pipe' appearance of colon and fine ulceration of the mucosa.

Treatment

Initially this is medical in the uncomplicated case, but surgery is required when medical treatment fails or if complications supervene.

1. *Medical treatment*

A high protein diet is prescribed with vitamin supplements and iron. Blood transfusion is given if the patient is severely anaemic. If there has been severe depletion of fluids and electrolytes due to profuse diarrhoea, this must be corrected by an intravenous drip. In many cases the acute attack may be brought under control by a combination of steroids given systemically and also as retention enemas. Sulphasalazine (salazopyrine), which is a sulphonomide/salicilate compound, is also of value. Diarrhoea may be controlled with codeine or isogel.

2. *Surgical treatment*

Surgery is required in a fulminating attack of colitis which does not rapidly respond to conservative measures, particularly where there is any suspicion that the bowel may have perforated. Local complications, including severe haemorrhage, stricture, or any question of malignant change, or the development of any general complications also make surgery obligatory. Operation is also advised where the patient is in chronic ill health due to repeated episodes of the disease or continued colitis.

The only certain cure for ulcerative colitis in our present state of ignorance about its aetiology is total excision of the colon, rectum and anal canal, with permanent ileostomy. In some patients it is possible to resect the colon and then to anastomose the ileum to the rectum (colectomy with ileo-rectal anastomosis). This has the clear advantage of preservation of the rectum and anus, although, because of the loss of most of the reservoir capacity of the large bowel, the patient usually experiences frequency of defaecation in the region of 3–7 bowel actions daily. The surgery is also technically more difficult with a greater number of post-operative complications. With the rectum left in place there is also the risk of later development of a carcinoma in the stump.

At present the choice of operation depends on a careful assessment of the individual patient; the presence of gross disease of the rectum obviously makes its preservation hazardous, but a patient may well wish to take any risk in order to preserve the anal sphincter. If an ileostomy is necessary, the patient must be reassured that a full and active life can be lead, thanks to the development of modern adhesive ileostomy appliances (Fig. 12.20). It is useful to introduce him pre-operatively to a patient who has already well adapted to the ileostomy life.

ISCHAEMIC COLITIS

This condition has been recognised quite recently and results from a defective blood supply to the region of the splenic flexure of the colon. It is at this point that an anastomosis occurs between the arterial supply of the colon from the superior mesenteric and inferior mesenteric arteries (see Fig. 12.17). The lesion is found in old people with generalised atherosclerosis.

Gross ischaemia may result in frank gangrene of the bowel, but more often there is mucosal ulceration and fibrotic narrowing of the affected segment.

The diagnosis is confirmed by barium enema X-ray which reveals a short segment of irregularity with narrowing in the splenic flexure region.

The majority of patients recover without permanent damage to the colon, but stricture formation may require resection and, of course, gangrene of the bowel precipitates emergency surgery.

A   B

Fig. 12.20. An adhesive ileostomy appliance, (A) without and (B) with bag.

Pathology

A diverticulum is a small pouch of mucosa pouting through the muscular wall of the colon, rather like the inner tube of a bicycle tyre bursting through the outer casing. Diverticula are found most commonly in the pelvic colon and become increasingly rare in passing from the left to the right side of the large intestine. They are unusual before the age of 40, but in the elderly they are found in about 30% of all post mortems. Sex distribution is roughly equal. Although the exact cause of diverticula is not known, they are associated with hypertrophy of the muscle of the colon wall, which undergoes contraction and produces out-pouchings at the sites of potential weakness in the muscle wall, which correspond to the points of entry of the supplying vessels to the bowel. (Fig. 12.21). Although colonic diverticula are so common in Western civilised communities they are extremely rare among primitive peoples, and it may be that the modern refined low roughage diet may be responsible for the muscle thickening which is the primary lesion in this condition.

Complications

The majority of patients with diverticula of the colon are symptomless, and this condition is termed *'diverticulosis'*. Some patients have symptoms produced by the thickening of the colonic wall (Fig. 12.22) and this is termed *chronic diverticular disease*. A diverti-

Fig. 12.21. The relationship of diverticula of the colon to the penetrating blood vessels. (A) normal colon, (B) colon with diverticula.

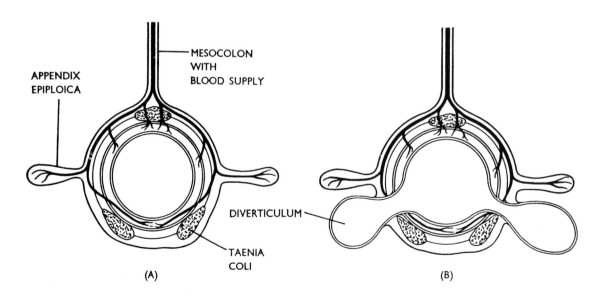

APPENDIX
EPIPLOICA

MESOCOLON
WITH
BLOOD SUPPLY

DIVERTICULUM

TAENIA
COLI

(A)   (B)

which is specific for Bacteroides fragilis, the common anaerobic organism in faeces.

The operation that is carried out is a hemicolectomy; for a caecal carcinoma this is a right hemicolectomy, for a transverse colon carcinoma a transverse hemi-colectomy, and for a carcinoma of the descending colon or pelvic colon a left hemicolectomy (Fig. 12.28).

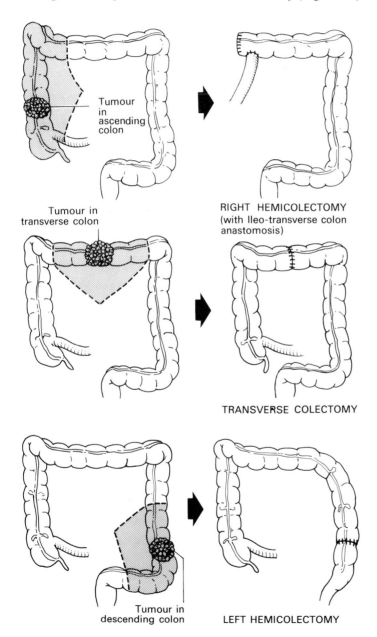

Tumour in ascending colon

RIGHT HEMICOLECTOMY (with Ileo-transverse colon anastomosis)

Tumour in transverse colon

TRANSVERSE COLECTOMY

Tumour in descending colon

LEFT HEMICOLECTOMY

Fig. 12.28. The types of partial colectomy.

An end-to-end anastomosis is performed and if there is any technical difficulty in performing this anastomosis or if the suture line encroaches on the rectum, a protecting side colostomy is performed proximal to the anastomosis.

If the patient has any degree of obstruction due to the carcinoma it is essential to perform a preliminary colostomy. This allows the colon to deflate to its normal dimension and the faecal residue held up by the carcinoma to be evacuated. The second stage of the procedure then involves the hemicolectomy. The third and final stage is the closure of the colostomy.

If there is any evidence of spread of the disease beyond the confines of the resected specimen of colon, cytotoxic agents such as 5-Fluorouracil administered at weekly intervals intravenously have been found to be of use in checking the continuing growth of the carcinoma.

COLOSTOMY

A colostomy is an artificial opening between the colon and the skin of the abdominal wall. When it is fashioned in the operating theatre the mucosa of the colon is stitched to the cut edge of the skin in the opening in the abdominal wall that has been made to receive it. Flatus and faeces are then discharged through this opening on to the surface of the abdomen, where they are collected into a plastic or rubber bag.

There are a number of different types of colostomy which are carried out for a variety of different reasons (Fig. 12.29).

1. *Terminal colostomy.* This is formed when the divided end of the colon is brought out to the surface of the left iliac fossa following abdominoperineal excision of the rectum. This is obviously a permanent state of affairs.

2. *Side colostomy* is formed when the anterior wall of the colon is sutured to the abdominal wall, a small side hole being made in the colon. This is used in two main situations. The first of these is when the distal colon is obstructed, for example by a carcinoma. Relief of the obstruction in this way will prevent further dilation of the proximal intestine and relieve pain and vomiting. The second indication is to 'protect' an anastomosis in order to ensure that it is not placed under any pressure and that if a leak does occur it remains small and localised. For example, when anterior resection of the rectum is carried out the descending colon is joined to the rectum quite low down in the pelvis. This anastomosis is not only technically quite

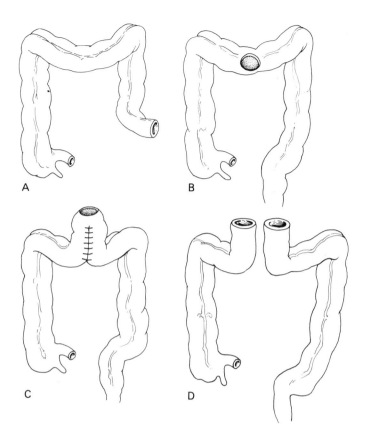

A

B

C

D

Fig. 12.29. The types of colostomy. (A) terminal, (B) side, (C) loop, (D) defunctioning.

difficult but also has a reputation for leaking as it has been estimated that this will occur in up to one-third of these cases.

3. *Loop colostomy* is performed when a loop of the colon, usually the transverse colon, is exteriorised and passed over a glass rod. This is used for similar cases to the side colostomy but suffers the disadvantage of being bulky and relatively difficult to manage. However, it is easy to carry out and almost completely defunctions the distal bowel, at least for the first few days after operation. The glass rod is withdrawn after 5 to 7 days and the exteriorised colon falls back into the abdomen with the exception of the muco-cutaneous junction. The end result of this manoeuvre is a side colostomy.

4. *Defunctioning colostomy*, (Devine Colostomy) It is sometimes necessary to ensure that *no* faeces pass into the distal colon. In this case the colon is transected, and the two ends, proximal and distal, are brought out through separate openings in the abdominal wall.

5. *Double-barrelled colostomy*, (Paul-Mikulicz Operation) This is an

old fashioned procedure for the removal of an obstructing carcinoma of the pelvic colon. The loop of the pelvic colon, with the tumour at its apex, is exteriorised from the abdomen and after the peritoneal cavity has been closed and the colon fixed to the surface of the skin, the loop with its contained carcinoma is excised. The two ends of the colon then discharge on to the surface of the skin, rather like the barrels of a double-barrelled shotgun. This operation is no longer performed for cancer because the excision of the carcinoma is inadequate as it does not include the regional lymph nodes. It is still used in cases of gangrene or perforation of the transverse or pelvic colon, for example gunshot wounds, and in gangrenous volvulus of the pelvic colon.

Colostomy care

Broadly speaking the care of a colostomy falls into one of two categories. The first of these employs the 'wash-out' technique. Each morning the patient washes out the colon with water, using a special syringe and nozzle, until no more faecal material can be obtained. Providing that the diet has been well controlled the colon will not discharge any more of its contents for the rest of that day and the stoma merely requires a small dry dressing held in place by a suitable pad and plastic tape or a belt. The second method is to allow the colon to assume a normal rhythm in which it will usually discharge faeces once, twice or three times per day. In this case a suitable receptacle in the form of a disposable plastic bag has to be applied to the surface of the abdominal wall. These plastic bags may be held in place by a belt and a ring protected by plastic foam. An example of this type of appliance is the Schacht device, which is useful for a temporary colostomy fashioned for the relief of obstruction which will be closed a week or two after its formation (Fig. 12.30). A more appropriate appliance for longer-term use is a flange which is stuck to the surface of the skin by adhesive. In this case the disposable plastic bags are attached to the flange either by more adhesive or by being slipped over a specially designed ring. An example of this type of apparatus is the Translet appliance (Fig. 12.31).

There must be almost as many different detailed methods of colostomy care as there are patients with colostomies. One of the first things to convey to a patient faced with this enormous alteration in the pattern of his or her life is to emphasise that near normal activity can be carried out. There need be no interruption in the social, recreational, sexual or domestic life of the patient. The patients can swim, meet their friends, marry and have children in

Fig. 12.30. The Schacht colostomy appliance.

spite of what may be initially regarded as a totally disastrous alteration of anatomy.

It is probably wrong to advocate one method of colostomy care to the exclusion of all others. Many intelligent patients prefer to wash-out their colostomies each morning and thereby to be free of the difficulties of bag changing during working hours. For less intelligent patients the wash-out method can have some dangers because if the nozzle of the syringe is introduced into the colostomy in the wrong direction or with too much force it is possible to pump a large volume of 'wash-out' water through a tear in the wall of the colon into the peritoneal cavity. For these patients therefore, some sort of adhesive flange is more appropriate.

Diet is found to be extremely important. Increase in roughage will often produce colostomy diarrhoea which, as may be imagined, is

Fig. 12.31. The Translet colostomy appliance.

much more difficult to cope with than in the normal person. Onions and certain other pungent foods may result in an unpleasant odour which is difficult to control. Most patients learn very quickly how to regulate their diet so as to avoid these complications.

The rectum and anal canal

Anatomy

The rectum is continuous with the pelvic (sigmoid) colon opposite the middle of the third piece of the sacrum and is 5 inches long (Fig. 12.32). It is supplied with blood from 3 haemorrhoidal arteries, the upper one being derived from the inferior mesenteric artery, the middle and lower ones from the internal iliac arteries.

The veins follow the arteries and the submucosa of the rectum is therefore a point of junction between the portal and systemic venous systems. The nerve supply is from the lumbar sympathetic and the sacral part of the parasympathetic outflow. The sensations that the rectum is capable of initiating are those of distension together with the ability to distinguish between flatus and faeces. Pain may also be experienced but this is deep seated and ill localised—a visceral type of pain.

The *anal canal* is $1\frac{1}{2}$ inches long and terminates at the anal orifice. Its lower half is lined by a squamous epithelium, unlike the columnar mucosa that lines the rest of the intestine. This lower part of the anal

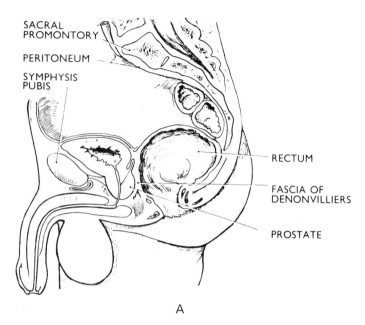

SACRAL
PROMONTORY

PERITONEUM

SYMPHYSIS
PUBIS

RECTUM

FASCIA OF
DENONVILLIERS

PROSTATE

A

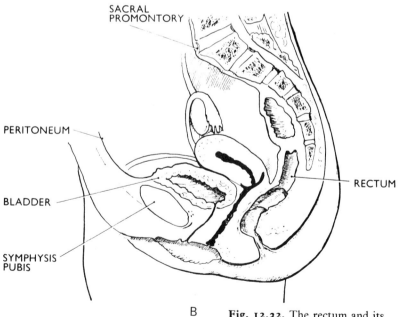

SACRAL
PROMONTORY

PERITONEUM

BLADDER

SYMPHYSIS
PUBIS

RECTUM

B

Fig. 12.32. The rectum and its
related viscera (A) in the male
and (B) in the female.

canal receives innervation from the inferior haemorrhoidal nerve which subserves normal cutaneous sensation; the lower canal is therefore extremely sensitive to the prick of a needle, whereas injection of a haemorrhoid, by inserting a hypodermic needle into the mucosa of the upper part of the anal canal, is almost painless.

ANO-RECTAL ATRESIA

The anal canal is formed in the embryo by a junction between the distal extremity of the hind gut and an invagination of the epithelium between the buttocks termed the proctodaeum. This accounts for the upper part of the canal becoming lined with an intestinal mucosa and the lower part being covered with squamous epithelium. If the septum between the two structures fails to break down then the condition of atresia results (Fig. 12.33). Any degree of severity of this condition may occur, from imperforate anus, made up of a thin septum, to complete absence of the anal canal and rectum. About half the infants with atresia have an associated fistula, which in the female passes into the vagina and in the male into the bladder or urethra.

Clinical features

The anus may be entirely absent or represented by a dimple or by a blind canal. Of course the infant is unable to pass any meconium, although this escapes either through the vagina or through the urethra if there is an associated fistula.

The extent of the defect is judged by x-raying the child, held

Fig. 12.33. Atresia of the anal canal.

Imperforate anus   Rectum distended with meconium

upside down, with a metal marker at the site of the anus. The distance between the gas bubble in the lower bowel and the marker can then be measured.

Treatment

If the septum is thin it can be divided with suture of the edges of the defect of the skin. However, if there is an extensive gap between the blind end and the anal verge, a colostomy is made and a later attempt at a reconstructive operation is carried out when the child is about 2 years of age. If a vaginal fistula is present then surgery is not urgent, since the bowel decompresses through the vagina and elective surgery can be performed when the girl is older.

HIRSCHSPRUNG'S DISEASE

Pathology

This condition, which also receives the term congenital megacolon, is produced by faulty development of the parasympathetic nerve supply of the lower bowel. It is characterised by the absence of nerve cells in the rectum; this aganglionic segment sometimes extends into the lower colon and rarely affects the whole of the large bowel. The involved segment is spastic and the colon proximal to this becomes grossly distended (Fig. 12.34).

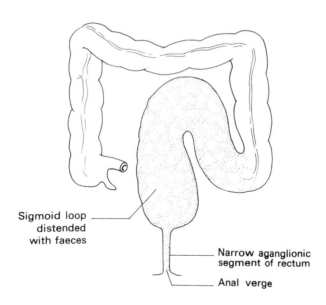

Sigmoid loop distended with faeces

Narrow aganglionic segment of rectum

Anal verge

Fig. 12.34. Hirschsprung's disease.

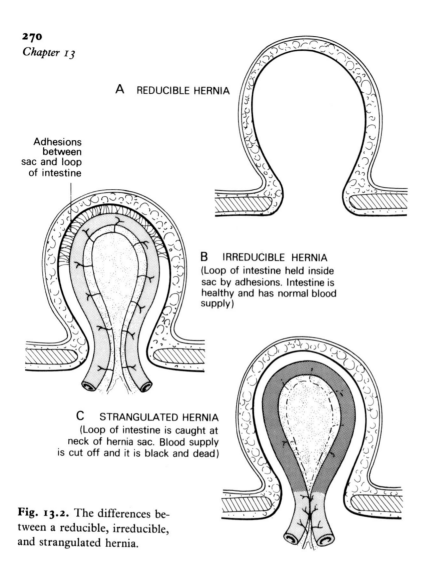

A   REDUCIBLE HERNIA

Adhesions
between
sac and loop
of intestine

B   IRREDUCIBLE HERNIA
(Loop of intestine held inside
sac by adhesions. Intestine is
healthy and has normal blood
supply)

C   STRANGULATED HERNIA
(Loop of intestine is caught at
neck of hernia sac. Blood supply
is cut off and it is black and dead)

Fig. 13.2. The differences between a reducible, irreducible,
and strangulated hernia.

and absolute constipation. Examination will show a tender, tense
hernia which cannot be reduced. The overlying skin becomes inflamed and oedematous and there are the signs of intestinal obstruction, with abdominal distension, tenderness and noisy bowel sounds.
The features of obstruction are absent and pain is less marked when
omentum rather than intestine is contained within the sac.

The three common types of hernia to strangulate are indirect
inguinal, femoral and umbilical. Direct inguinal hernia, incisional
and ventral hernias do so only rarely.

INGUINAL HERNIA

It has been estimated that 5% of the population of Great Britain have an inguinal hernia and that its repair accounts for about 10% of general surgical operations. 60% are right sided, 20% are left sided and 20% bilateral. Inguinal hernia comprises about 80% of all external hernias in the general population and the proportion of male to female is approximately 10 to 1. This is explained quite simply by the fact that the spermatic cord in the male, by its very size, produces a far greater weakness of the inguinal canal than the corresponding narrow round ligament in the female.

Anatomy (Fig. 13.4)

The inguinal canal is the oblique passage, $1\frac{1}{2}''$ long, which is taken through the lower abdominal wall by the testis and spermatic cord in the male and by the round ligament in the female. It lies immediately above the groin and passes downwards and medially from the internal inguinal ring to the external inguinal ring. The internal ring represents the point at which the spermatic cord (or round ligament) pushes through the inner aspect of the anterior abdominal wall and the external ring is the defect in the external oblique fascia through which it emerges.

An inguinal hernia may be classified as *indirect* when it enters the internal inguinal ring, traverses the canal and, if large enough, emerges through the external ring and descends into the scrotum

A Wide necked hernia

B Narrow necked hernia

Fig. 13.3. A hernia with a wide neck (A) is at less risk of strangulation than one whose neck is narrow (B).

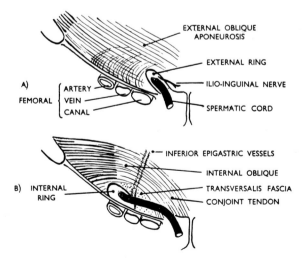

A) FEMORAL { ARTERY / VEIN / CANAL

EXTERNAL OBLIQUE APONEUROSIS
EXTERNAL RING
ILIO-INGUINAL NERVE
SPERMATIC CORD

B) INTERNAL RING

INFERIOR EPIGASTRIC VESSELS
INTERNAL OBLIQUE
TRANSVERSALIS FASCIA
CONJOINT TENDON

Fig. 13.4. The anatomy of the inguinal canal: (A) with the external oblique aponeurosis in place, (B) with the aponeurosis of the external oblique removed.

Fig. 13.5. An enormous indirect inguinal hernia which has descended into the scrotum and is irreducible.

(Fig. 13.5), or *direct* when it pushes through the posterior wall of the inguinal canal.

Indirect hernias may be *congenital*, due to the persistence of the *processus vaginalis*, which is the projection of peritoneum along which the testis descends into the scrotum in fetal life. These congenital hernias present at or soon after birth or arise in adolescence. The *acquired* variety may occur at any age in adult life and here the sac is formed by an evagination of the abdominal peritoneum. Some authorities maintain that indirect hernias at all ages represent congenitally formed sacs. The *direct hernia*, in contrast, is always acquired and therefore is usually seen in middle-aged or elderly patients. The difference between an indirect and a direct hernia is not just in the realms of exotic anatomy; a direct hernia has a large orifice and strangulation is consequently rare. In contrast, the internal inguinal ring is frequently narrow, so that the indirect hernia has a distinct tendency to strangulate.

Treatment

The treatment of inguinal hernia in infants and children comprises *herniotomy*, which is simple removal of the peritoneal sac. There is no optimum time for operating on the infant's hernia and surgery should be carried out as soon as possible after diagnosis has been made, since strangulation is not at all uncommon. In adults, surgery is usually advised; this comprises excision of the sac together with repair of the weakened inguinal canal and narrowing of the internal inguinal ring. A large variety of operations are employed, but particularly popular in this country is the nylon darn repair in which monofilament nylon is used to reinforce the posterior wall of the inguinal canal (Fig. 13.6).

A truss should only be prescribed for patients who are in very poor general health but even in such cases a painful hernia which threatens strangulation is much better repaired as an elective procedure, if necessary under a local anaesthetic, rather than as an emergency when strangulation has supervened.

If *strangulation* occurs, then, of course, emergency surgery is obligatory. A naso-gastric tube is passed, intravenous replacement of fluid and electrolytes commenced and the patient prepared as rapidly as possible for operation. The sac is opened and the constriction (which is usually at the neck of the hernia or at the external ring) is divided. It is now essential to assess the viability of the contents of the sac. If this is solely omentum, this can be excised if there is any doubt at all concerning viability. In the case of stran-

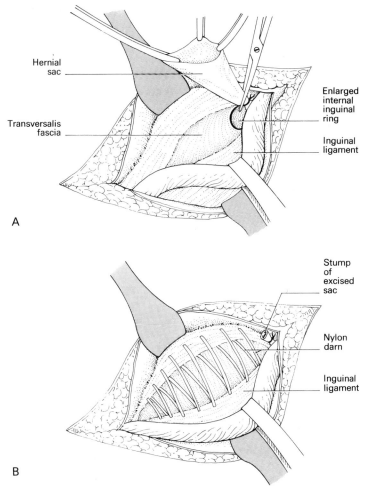

Hernial sac

Transversalis fascia

Enlarged internal inguinal ring

Inguinal ligament

A

Stump of excised sac

Nylon darn

Inguinal ligament

B

Fig. 13.6. Nylon darn repair of an inguinal hernia. The sac is transfixed and excised (A), followed by repair of the posterior wall of the inguinal canal (B). The spermatic cord is retracted by the sling.

gulated intestine, it is quite easy to identify perfectly healthy gut, which rapidly regains its normal colour, has a glistening covering peritoneum and has normal pulsation in its mesentery. Obviously non-viable intestine is green or black, oedematous, has lost its normal sheen and may be covered with fibrin flakes. The vessels in the mesentery supplying it are pulseless. If there is any doubt, the strangulated loop is wrapped in a warm saline pack and observed again after five or ten minutes. If there is still any doubt at all it is safer to resect the affected loop than to risk returning it into the peritoneal cavity where it may subsequently necrose completely and perforate. The healthy bowel is then reduced, the sac excised and a nylon darn repair is carried out.

Anatomy (Fig. 13.7)

A femoral hernia traverses the femoral canal. This is a gap that just admits the tip of the little finger and which lies at the medial extremity of the fascial tube, termed the femoral sheath, which contains the femoral artery and vein. The canal lies immediately medial to the femoral vein and presumably exists to allow considerable distension of the vein on exercise of the leg. It is filled by a plug of fat and contains a small lymph node. The neck of the canal is narrow and has a particularly sharp rigid medial border; for this reason irreducibility and strangulation are extremely common in hernias at this site.

Clinical features

Femoral hernias occur more commonly in females than in males because of the wider female pelvis which renders the canal larger in women than in men. The hernia is never due to a congenital sac

Fig. 13.7. The anatomy of the femoral canal.

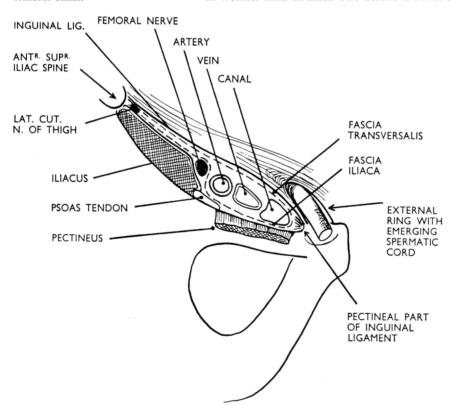

INGUINAL LIG. FEMORAL NERVE

ARTERY

ANT^{R.} SUPR.
ILIAC SPINE

VEIN

CANAL

LAT. CUT.
N. OF THIGH

FASCIA
TRANSVERSALIS

FASCIA
ILIACA

ILIACUS

PSOAS TENDON

EXTERNAL
RING WITH
EMERGING
SPERMATIC
CORD

PECTINEUS

PECTINEAL PART
OF INGUINAL
LIGAMENT

Fig. 13.8. An irreducible left femoral hernia in an elderly female.

but is invariably acquired. Cases rarely occur in children but are usually seen in the middle-aged and elderly (Fig. 13.8). The patient presents because of the lump in the groin. If strangulation occurs, the lump becomes tense and tender, and if bowel is incorporated in the contents of the hernia, features of intestinal obstruction supervene. It is surprising how often an old lady is unaware of the fact that she has a femoral hernia and she may present with intestinal obstruction without having noticed the irreducible lump in the groin; this must always be looked for specifically in such cases.

An interesting variety of strangulated femoral hernia is the *Richter's hernia*; here only a part of the wall of the small intestine is caught up and strangulated by the femoral ring. Because the lumen of the bowel is not completely encroached upon, symptoms of intestinal obstruction do not occur, although the knuckle of bowel may become completely necrotic and even perforate into the hernial sac (Fig. 13.9).

Treatment

All femoral hernias should be repaired because of this great danger of strangulation; the sac is excised and the femoral canal closed by sutures. If the patient presents with a strangulated hernia, treatment is carried out just as described above in the case of strangulated inguinal hernia.

UMBILICAL HERNIA

Congenital umbilical hernia

Normally at birth there is complete closure of the umbilical scar; if this is defective, the baby presents with a reducible bulge at the

Fig. 13.9. A Richter's hernia. Note that only a part of the wall of the gut is involved.

umbilicus. This is especially common in black children. The vast majority close spontaneously during the first year of life, but should the hernia persist after the child is two years old, then surgical repair should be carried out. The parents of a newborn infant with an umbilical hernia should be reassured that most disappear over the next few months without treatment. Strapping the hernia with adhesive is not required and may only give the baby a sensitivity rash, but from time to time it is necessary to carry out this procedure or provide a rubber truss simply to allay parental anxiety.

Exomphalos

This is a rare condition in which the baby is born with the intestine prolapsed through a translucent sac which protrudes through a defective anterior abdominal wall. Untreated this may rupture with fatal peritonitis.

Treatment comprises immediate surgical repair.

Acquired umbilical hernia

This is a common rupture which is found especially in obese multiparous women (Fig. 13.10). It occurs above or just below the umbil-

Fig. 13.10. A large umbilical hernia.

icus and is more accurately termed a para-umbilical hernia. The neck is narrow, and, like a femoral hernia, it is particularly liable to become irreducible or strangulated.

Treatment comprises excision of the sac and repair of the defect by overlapping the edges of the rectus sheath (Mayo operation, Fig. 13.11).

Fig. 13.11. Mayo repair of an umbilical hernia, using interrupted nylon sutures to overlap the rectus sheath.

EPIGASTRIC AND VENTRAL HERNIAS

An epigastric hernia is a small protrusion in the mid line of the upper abdomen which occurs through a defect in the linea alba, the dense fascial septum which passes from the xiphoid to the pubis, and which is especially wide in the upper abdomen.

The defect is small and usually only contains some extra peritoneal fat, but it is often surprisingly uncomfortable. Occasionally

Fig. 13.12. An incisional hernia. Note the transverse scar of a laparotomy performed many years previously.

a long gap occurs in the linea alba, producing a more extensive mid-line bulge which is termed a *ventral hernia*.

Treatment comprises suture of the defect.

INCISIONAL HERNIA

An incisional hernia occurs through a defect in the scar of a previous abdominal operation (Fig. 13.12). There is usually a wide neck and strangulation is consequently rare.

Treatment. If the general condition of the patient is good, the hernia is repaired by resuturing the layers of the abdominal wall. If operation is considered inadvisable, an abdominal belt is prescribed.

Chapter 14. Liver, gall bladder, spleen and pancreas

ANATOMY OF THE LIVER AND BILIARY TRACT

The liver, which is the largest single organ in the body, is situated in the upper abdomen, closely applied to the under surface of the diaphragm. It is divided into a right and left lobe by its peritoneal attachments and by the structures which enter the porta hepatis. It is enclosed by a capsule (Glisson's capsule) and outside this by peritoneum. It is suspended from the diaphragm by folds of peritoneum known as 'peritoneal ligaments', that which runs antero-posteriorly being termed the *falciform ligament* and at right-angles to this there are left and right triangular ligaments suspending the right and left lobes (Fig. 14.1).

The liver is supplied by blood from two distinct sources. The first of these is the *hepatic artery* derived from the coeliac axis and the second is the *portal vein*, which drains blood from the spleen, the stomach and the small and large intestine. Blood drains from the liver via *hepatic veins*, two or three in number, which are short and wide and pass straight into the inferior vena cava. The bile is drained from the liver by the bile ducts. There is a *left* and *right hepatic duct* draining the respective lobes of the liver which join at the porta hepatis to form the *common hepatic duct*. This passes out of the liver to the right of the hepatic artery and in front of the portal vein and is joined after two to five centimetres by the *cystic duct*. At this point the bile duct is called the *common bile duct* which is naturally divided into three parts. The first of these parts is superior to the duodenum, the second part runs behind the first part of the duodenum and the third part runs behind the head of the pancreas terminating at the

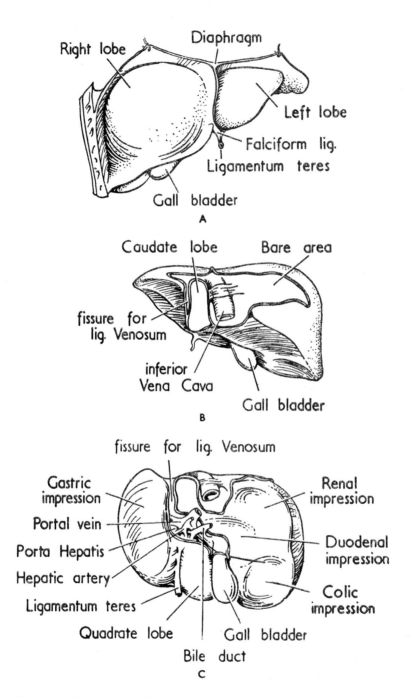

Fig. 14.1. The anatomy of the liver.

A. anterior, B, posterior and C, inferior view.

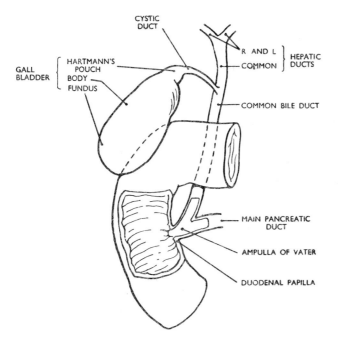

Fig. 14.2. The gall bladder and its duct system.

ampulla of Vater, where the bile duct enters the medial aspect of the second part of the duodenum (Fig. 14.2).

The gall bladder is a thin-walled sac which in life appears a bluish colour. Its duct, the cystic duct, joins the common hepatic duct.

The microscopic anatomy of the liver comprises a series of lobules, each having a central vein, which drains ultimately into the hepatic vein. The lobule is surrounded and separated from other lobules by the portal tracts, each of which contains terminal radicles of the hepatic artery and portal vein together with the fine commencing radicles of the bile ducts, the bile canaliculi. Thus blood filters from the hepatic artery and portal vein at the periphery of the hepatic lobule to the central vein through the hepatic capillaries, and the products of hepatic cell metabolism pass to the periphery of the lobule and enter the bile canaliculi. The capillaries along which the blood passes within the lobule are richly supplied with phagocytic cells which are capable of removing particulate matter, such as bacteria, from the blood stream. This arrangement of a dual blood supply ensures first that a ready supply of highly oxygenated blood is available to the hepatic cell which has a high metabolic rate, second that there is an intimate contact between the liver cell and the substances which have just been absorbed from the intestine and which are being carried into the body via the portal blood stream.

Physiology

The liver is responsible for a number of functions:

1. *Secretion of bile*

Bile contains water, inorganic ions (including sodium, bicarbonate, potassium and chloride and calcium) together with cholesterol, conjugated bile salts, bile pigments from which the characteristic greenish colour derives, certain lipoproteins and enzymes such as alkaline phosphatase.

In addition to this list, some breakdown products of, for example, hormones and drugs must be added.

2. *Storage*

The liver stores a considerable quantity of carbohydrate in the form of glycogen which is available for conversion to glucose should a source of energy be required. In addition, vitamin B_{12} and vitamin K are stored in the liver.

3. *Protein synthesis*

The liver is responsible for the synthesis of albumen and in conditions of impaired liver function the plasma albumen will be reduced. Vitamin K is converted in the liver to prothrombin, one of the factors concerned with the coagulation of blood.

4. *Protein breakdown*

Proteins which have no further function within the body are broken down to urea, which is excreted by the kidney.

5. *Detoxification*

Substances such as the oestrogenic hormones are rendered inactive by being combined (conjugated) with molecules such as taurine and glycine before being excreted.

JAUNDICE

Jaundice occurs when the level of bilirubin in the blood is such that the tissues, particularly the whites of the eyes, look yellow. The normal range of bilirubin is from 0.2 to 0.5 mg/100 ml of blood (3 to 8 μmol/litre) and in most people yellowness of the sclerae will become evident when the level rises to 2 mg/100 ml of blood (35 μmol/litre). There are three main groups of causes of jaundice:

1. *Pre-hepatic*

This is due to an increased production of bilirubin.

2. *Hepatic*

This type is usually due to damage to the liver cells by infection by toxic substances, by tumours or, in rare cases, it may be due to an hereditary abnormality of enzyme systems within the liver cell.

3. *Post-hepatic*

283
*Liver, gall bladder,
spleen and pancreas*

It is the post-hepatic jaundice with which surgeons are involved because in this case there is obstruction to either the common hepatic or the common bile duct preventing the passage of bile into the intestine. Post-hepatic jaundice can be further subclassified into the three groups of causes obstructing any tube in the body—causes in the lumen, in the wall and outside the wall.

(a) *Obstruction within the lumen of the bile duct*, for example gall stones, the commonest of all causes of post-hepatic or obstructive jaundice or, very rarely, parasites which include ascaris lumbricoides.

(b) *Obstruction due to an abnormality of the wall of the duct*, for example by accidental surgical division, congenital obliteration of the bile duct or carcinoma of the bile duct.

(c) *Compression of the bile duct or invasion of it from outside*, for example by carcinoma of the head of the pancreas, tumours in the lymph nodes in the porta hepatis, or acute and chronic pancreatitis.

It is important that surgeons should be aware of all types of jaundice so that the post-hepatic, obstructive jaundice can be distinguished from the other types of jaundice.

General features of obstructive jaundice

The major and minor bile ducts become dilated and if the liver is examined under the microscope plugs of bile may be seen in the bile canaliculi. Apart from this the architecture of the liver is usually normal, although long-standing obstruction may result in hepatic enlargement and the development of biliary cirrhosis due to scar tissue deposition. If infection of the static bile occurs, the process of hepatic cell damage is greatly accelerated; this condition is known as *cholangitis*.

The serum bilirubin rises and may reach extremely high levels. The patient appears yellow, later becoming a deep orange yellow, occasionally with a green tinge as the jaundice progresses. Since bilirubin is bound to protein, the superficial parts of the body with a high protein content appear to be more yellow than other parts and this is the explanation of the obvious yellow colour of the sclerae which persists for some time even after the relief of the obstruction. The urine is dark and contains an excess of bilirubin which will result in a positive reaction when tested with a labstix. If the urine is shaken it will be abnormally frothy. Flowers of sulphur sprinkled on the surface of urine in a jar will sink to the bottom whereas in the normal urine they remain floating on the surface. If

Careful pre-operative preparation is essential. As has been mentioned previously, these patients do not absorb fat and therefore they do not absorb fat soluble vitamins. One of these is vitamin K and failure to absorb it will ultimately result in lowered plasma prothrombin levels with the result that the patient has a blood coagulation defect. This is readily corrected by giving injections of vitamin K (for example Konakion) 10 mg intramuscularly per day. Before surgery is embarked upon, the prothrombin level must be checked and found to be normal. Another problem that exists in these patients is the sensitivity of the kidney to reduced blood flow. Whereas in a normal patient the kidney is quite able to function in spite of considerable operative trauma, the kidneys of a patient with obstructive jaundice are affected by short-lived and mild episodes of hypotension which result in renal tubular necrosis, the so-called *hepato—renal syndrome*. To protect the patient against this complication it is necessary to ensure that an active diuresis is occurring before, during and for 48 hours after the operation. To this end the patient is catheterised and an intravenous infusion of 10% mannitol is started. Mannitol is a sugar which is excreted unchanged in the urine and therefore carries water with it by virtue of its osmotic pressure. If the kidneys have already failed, however, it will act as a plasma expander and if too much is infused the patient will go into congestive cardiac failure. For this reason a preliminary test dose of 100 ml is infused on the night prior to operation and the urinary output is checked and should rise in the hour after the infusion to a level of 1 ml per minute. Providing this condition is fulfilled, the 10% mannitol infusion is commenced an hour prior to the operation at the rate of one litre per 24 hours and is continued throughout the operation and for 48 hours post-operatively.

The extra-hepatic biliary apparatus can be approached either through an upper right paramedian incision or a right subcostal (Kocher) incision (Fig. 14.5). The surgery from this point depends upon the precise cause of the obstructive jaundice. In general terms

Fig. 14.5. The incision used in biliary surgery (A) upper right paramedian, (B) right subcostal Kocher incision.

A   B

the obstruction may either be removed, as is the case with gall stones which are extracted through an incision made in the dilated common bile duct, or the obstruction may be bypassed when, for example it is due to advanced irremovable carcinoma of the head of the pancreas. In this latter case bypass may be achieved by anastomosing the gall bladder to a loop of jejunum (Fig. 14.6).

Whenever the common bile duct is opened, a T-tube is inserted into it at the end of the procedure. The reason for this is that oedema at the site of the operation may result in a temporary block to the passage of bile from the liver to the intestine. A T-tube within the common bile duct allows free drainage to the exterior and thereby prevents leakage through the sutures in the duct into the peritoneal cavity. It should be remembered that the bile is normally sterile and that the connection between the T-tube and the bile-collecting apparatus should not be broken except under sterile conditions.

Since it is undesirable for large quantities of bile to be lost from the patient the T-tube is clamped for progressively longer periods starting on the fifth post-operative day. This not only ensures that bile has to pass into the intestine, but also serves as a test of patency of the bile duct. On the fifth post-operative day the tube is clamped for one hour and providing there is no abdominal pain, the next day it is clamped on two occasions for two hours. Again, as long as there is no reaction on the seventh it is clamped on three occasions for three hours and on subsequent days it is permanently clamped. On approximately the tenth day the

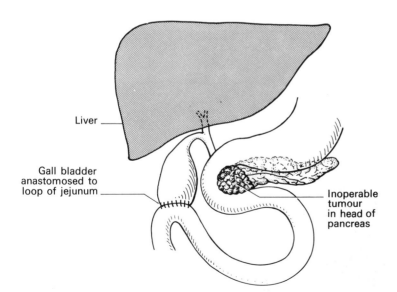

Liver

Gall bladder anastomosed to loop of jejunum

Inoperable tumour in head of pancreas

Fig. 14.6. Cholecyst-jejuno-stomy to bypass an inoperable carcinoma of the pancreas which is producing obstructive jaundice.

patency of the bile duct is checked by means of cholangiography. Radio-opaque dye is injected down the T-tube and X-rays are taken of the abdomen at the same time (Fig. 14.7). Providing there is no residual obstruction to the common bile duct, the T-tube, which is made of soft latex rubber, can be removed by simple traction. The small puncture wound in the abdominal wall will leak bile from between a half and one and a half hours only. In addition to the drainage of the common bile duct, a corrugated plastic drain is inserted to the region of the operation via a stab incision well to the lateral side of the main operative incision. Providing only small quantities of bile and haemoserous fluid are draining, this drain is shortened on the second post-operative day and removed on the third post-operative day.

ENLARGEMENTS OF THE LIVER

The main groups of causes of enlargement of the liver are:
(a) Polycystic disease, a rare congenital condition.
(b) Inflammatory—infective hepatitis, homologous serum hepatitis, leptospirosis and actinomycosis.

Fig. 14.7. A normal T-tube cholangiogram. The bile ducts are of normal size, no stones are visualised and the dye is seen to enter the duodenum. The arrow points to the T-tube outlined by the contrast material.

(c) Parasites—amoebic hepatitis and hydatid disease.

(d) Neoplasm—primary carcinoma of the liver and secondary carcinoma.

(e) Cirrhosis—portal, biliary, cardiac and haemochromatosis.

(f) The reticuloses—Hodgkin's disease, lymphosarcoma and leukaemia.

(g) Blood diseases—polycythaemia.

(h) Metabolic—amyloid, glycogen storage disease.

TRAUMA TO THE LIVER

Bleeding from this source may be massive and complicate the picture in multiple injuries if the patient is shocked and the peritoneal cavity contains blood.

If an isolated part of the liver is damaged, for example the left lobe, the most effective method of treatment is to remove it. If there are, however, general lacerations this will not be possible and haemorrhage will be controlled either by packing or by large gently placed sutures holding the fragile tissues loosely together. Partial hepatectomy is occasionally necessary where trauma is extensive.

CIRRHOSIS

Aetiology

This condition is characterised by a progressive infiltration of the liver by fibrous tissue with destruction of hepatic cells. There are a number of causes which include:

(a) *Portal*—this occurs in alcoholics, as a result of nutritional deficiency particularly protein deficiency, and following severe hepatitis. However it frequently may occur in the absence of any of these conditions and be idiopathic.

(b) *Biliary*—due to long-standing and unrelieved extra-hepatic bile duct obstruction or primary, of unknown cause, found in women between the ages of 40 and 50 (Hanot's cirrhosis).

(c) *Cardiac*—due to congestive cardiac failure.

(d) Cirrhosis may also occur in *haemochromatosis* due to the deposition of iron.

Clinical features

As the condition progresses from whatever cause more and more hepatic cells are destroyed. Eventually this will lead to hepatic failure. The time span from the commencement to the hepatic failure is usually of the order of several years and other effects of the condition therefore become obvious before death from liver failure occurs. One of these effects is an increase of the pressure of the blood in the portal vein—*portal hypertension*. There is also an increased incidence of chronic duodenal ulcer.

Apart from acute haemorrhage, the clinical picture of a patient with cirrhosis is one of steadily deteriorating liver function and on examination the liver is often palpable together with the spleen which also becomes enlarged. The skin of these patients occasionally contains large deposits of melanin which gives them an overall brown appearance. Also in the skin may be seen small angiomas— spider naevi—generally on the upper trunk, arms and face. If there is considerable loss of hepatic function an erythema of the thenar and hypothenar eminences may be seen. This is known as 'liver palm.'

If a patient is in incipient liver failure, the most common symptom is a loss of cerebral function with disorientation and inability to perform fine movements of the hands.

Portal hypertension

The pressure of the blood in the portal vein in a normal person is between 5 and 10 cm of water, this may rise to as high as 30 cm of water in patients with cirrhosis. The reason for the increased pressure is an intra-hepatic block to the flow of blood from the portal vein to the inferior vena cava. The reduced blood flow has two main effects, the first of which is an accelerated rate of damage to the liver and the second is the development of a collateral venous circulation. There are several potential sites at which portal blood can drain into the systemic veins. These are around the oesophagus and stomach, along the normally obliterated umbilical vein, in the region of the rectal venous plexus, and from veins associated with the ascending and descending colon. These collateral veins become greatly dilated and engorged with blood and those in the region of the oesophagus bulge into the lumen of the oesophagus, resulting in *oesophageal varices*. Bleeding from oesophageal varices is one of the causes of haematemesis and a not infrequent cause of death in these patients.

Treatment

1. *Conservative*

When a patient presents with bleeding from oesophageal varices, emergency treatment consists of blood replacement and, if necessary, the passing of a Sengstaken tube (Fig. 14.8) which has an arrangement of two balloons so that one balloon retains the tube in the

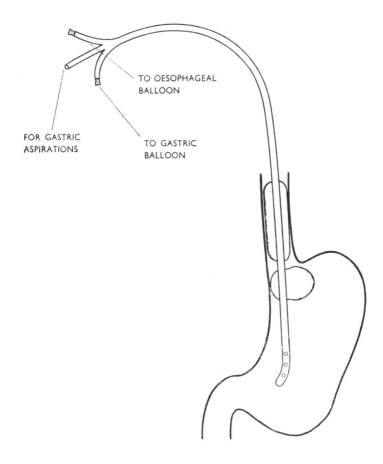

TO OESOPHAGEAL
BALLOON

FOR GASTRIC
ASPIRATIONS

TO GASTRIC
BALLOON

Fig. 14.8. The Sengstaken tube. Balloons in the oesophagus and in the cardia of the stomach compress the bleeding varices. The gastric tube can be used either for aspirating the stomach or for feeding purposes.

stomach while a second balloon presses against the oesophageal varices in the oesophagus and so occludes them. The lumen of the tube protrudes into the stomach and thus allows evacuation of any clot or secretion. Unfortunately, the tube can only be left in place for approximately 24 hours, otherwise oesophageal damage will occur. Other methods of treatment include giving intravenous Vasopressin which reduces the flow of blood into the splanchnic circulation.

In a patient with even a minor degree of liver failure an acute haemorrhage will tend to worsen the condition because blood, when it is passed into the bowel, will be digested and the products of digestion overload the liver's ability to deal with them. In this case the method of treatment is to evacuate the large bowel, where the incompletely digested products of the blood are fermenting, by means of an enema and to administer an oral non-absorbed antibiotic such as neomycin 1g 6 hourly.

2. Surgical

Emergency operations sometimes have to be carried out on these patients and the procedures which are required are either an oesophageal transection, in which the bleeding veins are ligated via a thoracotomy, or a high gastric transection which achieves the same object. Both these operations are attended by a significant mortality (10%) and morbidity and further, the results tend not to be permanent. In some centres, surgeons inject the varices with sclerosing fluid via an oesophagoscope very much like injecting piles.

The most permanent operative procedure, although one which is difficult and dangerous to perform when the patient is actually bleeding or soon after a major haemorrhage, is the diversion of portal blood to the systemic circulation, for example by means of a porto-caval anastomosis. In this procedure the side of the portal vein is joined to the side of the inferior vena cava in the region of the foramen of Winslow (Fig. 14.9).

GALL STONES

Initially at least gall stones form in the gall bladder. There are three main types (Fig. 14.10):
1. Cholesterol stones.
2. Pigment stones.
3. Mixed cholesterol, pigment and calcium phosphate stones.

Methods of formation

Cholesterol, which is a lipid, is excreted in the bile. Bile is an aqueous solution and in the normal person there exists a physico-chemical

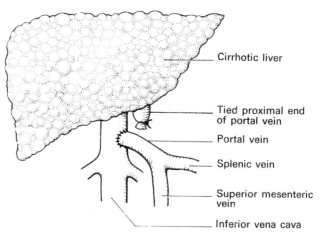

Fig. 14.9. An end-to-side porto-caval anastomosis between the portal vein and the side of the inferior vena cava. This decompresses the high pressure within the portal system.

Cirrhotic liver

Tied proximal end of portal vein

Portal vein

Splenic vein

Superior mesenteric vein

Inferior vena cava

MIXED

FACETED
MAY BE IN 'GENERATIONS'

CUT SURFACE—
CONCENTRIC RINGS

CHOLESTEROL

'SOLITAIRE'
OR CLUSTERS OF 'MULBERRIES'

CUT SURFACE—
RADIATING CRYSTALS

PIGMENT

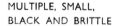

MULTIPLE, SMALL,
BLACK AND BRITTLE

CUT SURFACE —
AMORPHOUS

Fig. 14.10. The varieties of gall stones.

mechanism whereby the cholesterol is dissolved by means of Nature's detergents—the bile salts, together with phospho-lipids. If anything occurs to disturb the normal relationship between these three substances, cholesterol is deposited in a crystalline form. The gall bladder is responsible for concentrating the bile by absorbing water and it is therefore in this situation that the cholesterol concentration rises and precipitation of crystals is most likely to occur. Once crystals of cholesterol have been deposited more cholesterol attaches to the nucleus and a stone is formed.

In conditions in which there is an increased production of bilirubin, for example, any of the haemolytic jaundices such as hereditary spherocytosis (acholuric jaundice) the concentration of the pigment in the bile rises and pigment stones are formed in much the same way as are cholesterol stones.

Fig. 14.12. Normal cholecystogram (A) before (B) after a fatty meal. The fat has made the gall bladder contract, thus emptying its contents into the duodenum.

Fig. 14.13. Cholecystogram demonstrating multiple stones within the gall bladder. These appear as filling defects outlined by the radio-opaque dye within the gall bladder.

The mainstay of diagnosis is the *cholecystogram* in which the patient swallows tablets which contain an iodine compound which is excreted in the bile. Providing the patient is not jaundiced the dye passes with the bile into the gall bladder where it is concentrated and when x-rays are taken an outline of the gall bladder will be seen (Fig. 14.12). In approximately 40% of these investigations it is also possible to see the outline of the major extra-hepatic ducts as well. Stones may be seen within the gall bladder or bile ducts as filling defects (Fig. 14.13) and the diameter of the bile duct can often be judged. If significant obstruction has occurred, the common bile duct will be wider than the upper limit of normal which is 10 millimetres. Once the gall bladder has been visualised it is possible to give the patient a meal containing fat when a normal gall bladder will contract. If the contrast within the gall bladder is of inadequate concentration, an intravenous cholangiogram can be carried out in which a large quantity of dye is injected intravenously. This should not be done in the jaundiced patient as renal and more hepatic damage may result.

Treatment

Patients with acute cholecystitis are treated at first expectantly. They are put to bed and if vomiting has been severe and they are dehydrated an intravenous infusion is set up to correct and maintain their fluid and electrolyte balance. Antibiotics are given, the one of choice being ampicillin, 500 mg orally 6 hourly. Pulse rate and temperature are measured at hourly intervals and the abdomen is frequently examined to ensure that the inflammatory process which is occurring in the gall bladder is not spreading to the rest of the peritoneum. The danger with cholecystitis is that part of the wall of the gall bladder may necrose with release of infected bile into the peritoneal cavity and the development of generalised peritonitis. This occurrence is rare, but if in spite of bed rest and the treatment mentioned above the pulse rate and temperature do not rapidly settle, operation will be required.

If the attack of cholecystitis has been present for some days it may not be possible to carry out an emergency cholecystectomy and external drainage of the gall bladder with removal of the stones from the gall bladder will have to be performed—*cholecystostomy*. This can be a life-saving operation and may be performed even on the aged and infirm who are weakened by their cholecystitis. A small incision is made in the abdomen over the inflamed gall bladder, the gall bladder is opened and the stones within it removed and pus and bile is sucked out. The opening in the gall bladder is then sutured to the parietal peritoneum around a tube drain which protrudes through the abdominal wall. Since the major cause of the inflammation has been removed the patient's condition will rapidly improve.

It will be necessary when the inflammation has completely settled for the gall bladder to be removed. This usually will be three months after the acute attack of cholecystitis. Should the patient follow the more usual course and the attack of acute cholecystitis subsides over the period of 24 to 48 hours, cholecystectomy will be required three months later. These patients' gall bladders never return to normal and since the complications of stones in the gall bladder, that is obstructive jaundice, are so severe, cholecystectomy should be insisted on in every case. Indeed if gall stones are discovered by accident in a patient with only few symptoms, cholecystectomy is the safest course.

Cholecystectomy is performed through a right upper paramedian or right Kocher incision. Before the gall bladder is removed an

Fig. 14.14. Operative cholangiogram. There is a stone at the lower end of the common bile duct (arrowed) although dye can be seen entering the duodenum. (A) The stone was removed via an incision in the common bile duct which was then drained by means of a T-tube (B).

A

B

operative cholangiogram is performed. In this a tube is placed in the cystic duct and radio-opaque dye injected down it (Fig. 14.14). If stones are shown in the common bile duct, these are removed and the duct drained by means of a T-tube (see page 287).

The spleen

Anatomy

The spleen (Fig. 14.15) is situated in the upper left abdomen. Blood is supplied to the hilum by the splenic artery, which is one of the major vessels coming from the coeliac axis. A smaller but important

SURFACE RELATED TO STOMACH ACROSS LESSER SAC

SPLENIC FLEXURE

TAIL OF PANCREAS AND SPLENIC A.

L. KIDNEY

Fig. 14.15. The spleen and its immediate relations.

Fig. 14.16. The portal venous system.

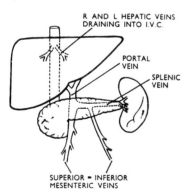

R AND L HEPATIC VEINS DRAINING INTO I.V.C.

PORTAL VEIN

SPLENIC VEIN

SUPERIOR ▪ INFERIOR MESENTERIC VEINS

supply is derived from the short gastric arteries from the fundus of the stomach. The splenic vein passes to the right along the superior border of the pancreas to join the superior mesenteric vein, the confluence becoming the portal vein (Fig. 14.16), which then passes to the hilum of the liver. Blood from the splenic artery becomes diffused within the splenic tissue, which has the structure of a sponge. There are numerous macrophage cells lining the sinuses within the spleen and these are capable of ingesting red cells, particularly at the end of their life. The spleen is thus the organ which is principally responsible for controlling the length of life of the red cell which, in the normal, is 120 days.

The spleen has to enlarge by about $2\frac{1}{2}$ times before it can be palpable. One of the characteristic features of a palpable spleen is that it moves from beneath the left costal margin in the direction of the right iliac fossa on deep inspiration as it is pushed down by the descending dome of the diaphragm.

299
Liver, gall bladder,
spleen and pancreas

Conditions for which splenectomy is required

1. Ruptured spleen—immediate

A not uncommon injury in road traffic accidents or other cases of abdominal trauma is rupture of the spleen. When this occurs the only safe treatment is rapid splenectomy otherwise the patient runs considerable risk of death from haemorrhage. When a patient has fracture of the left 10th, 11th or 12th ribs, those caring for him should be suspicious of splenic rupture. A blood transfusion is set up and the patient transferred to the operating theatre.

The operation is carried out via a left subcostal or upper midline incision through which the spleen can readily be lifted forward into the light which permits separate ligation of the splenic artery and the vein.

2. Ruptured spleen—delayed

One of the difficulties of this subject is that the spleen may not actually rupture although there has been disruption of the splenic pulp to such an extent that an extensive haematoma forms beneath the splenic capsule. This haematoma increases in size in much the same way as a subdural haematoma increases in size, and a full-scale rupture of splenic tissue occurs some time from 2nd to 10th day after the original trauma.

Very rarely spontaneous rupture of the spleen occurs in the complete absence of a history of abdominal trauma. This may follow an area of infarction of the splenic tissue, but is always sudden and calamitous. Usually the only diagnosis is one of massive intraperitoneal haemorrhage and immediate laparotomy has then to be carried out with subsequent removal of the spleen.

3. Haematological disorders

Several conditions may require splenectomy to remove the main source of erythrocyte destruction in those conditions where cells are unusually fragile. Notable amongst these are acholuric jaundice, primary thrombocytopenic purpura, acquired haemolytic anaemia, thalassemia and sickle cell anaemia. Occasionally splenectomy is also required for aplastic and myelosclerotic anaemia when the red cell destruction component of the blood picture is greatest.

4. Tropical diseases

Splenectomy may be indicated when the spleen becomes hugely enlarged in chronic malaria, Kala azar or schistosomiasis.

5. Neoplastic disease

Hodgkin's disease may require splenectomy for two distinct reasons. First, the spleen may be involved by Hodgkin's tissue and second splenectomy appears to exert a desirable influence on the regression of Hodgkin's disease. A third advantage is that when splenectomy is performed the abdominal cavity can be diligently searched for signs of disease, thus permitting accurate staging and allowing appropriate treatment to be carried out. Thus in a patient with Hodgkin's disease in the glands of the neck, the treatment of stage I, that is when the disease is localised to one group of glands, is different to the treatment of stage III when there is disease not only in the glands of the neck but also within the abdominal cavity. In the former case the glands will be completely excised or irradiated and in the latter case radiotherapy combined with cytotoxic drugs will be employed.

The pancreas

Anatomy

The pancreas is the best example of a mixed exocrine and endocrine gland. It is situated behind the peritoneum of the posterior abdominal wall and is a posterior relation of the stomach (Fig. 14.17). It is composed of the *head*, which fills the 'C'-shaped curve of the first, second and third parts of the duodenum. This is joined by a poorly defined *neck* to the *body* which extends across the posterior part of the abdomen, crossing in front of first the inferior vena cava and then the aorta at the level of the second lumbar vertebra. To the left of the vertebral column the body becomes the *tail* which

Fig. 14.17. The pancreas and its relations.

extends to the hilum of the spleen. An important posterior relationship of the head of the pancreas is the infraduodenal portion of the common bile duct, which runs in a groove before entering the medial aspect of the second part of the duodenum. In one third of patients the common bile duct is joined at its termination by the main pancreatic duct (the duct of Wirsung). Emerging from beneath the inferior border of the neck of the pancreas are the superior mesenteric vessels as they pass to the whole of the small intestine and to the ascending and transverse colon. Running along the superior border of the pancreas is the splenic artery and vein and these are both associated with a large number of lymph nodes. The superior mesenteric vein, which drains blood from the whole of the small intestine, passes upward behind the pancreas where it is joined by the splenic vein to become the portal vein.

The external appearance of the pancreas is of a lobular structure which reflects the microscopic anatomy. The lobules drain the exocrine secretion into a main duct which runs the whole length of the gland and which enters the duodenum just below the common bile duct at the ampulla of Vater (Fig. 14.18). There is in addition a smaller accessory duct which drains the superior part of the head of the pancreas (the duct of Santorini).

Microscopic examination of the gland reveals large clumps of cells that are quite distinct, these are the *'islets' of Langerhans*. They contain cells of several different types, the first of which are alpha cells which secrete glucagon. The second type of cell is the beta cell and these produce insulin. In certain disease processes other cells make their appearance, notably G-cells in the primary islet cell tumours responsible for the Zollinger-Ellison syndrome.

Physiology

1. *Exocrine pancreas*

The exocrine pancreas secretes a juice which passes into the second part of the duodenum and which is essential for normal digestion of carbohydrates, fats and proteins. The juice contains amylase, which hydrolyses polysaccharides, such as starch and glycogen, down to the disaccharide stage, lipase which acts on emulsified fat in the presence of bile salts resulting in the release of fatty acids and glycerol, and a group of proteolytic enzymes, including trypsin and chymotrypsin, which are responsible for breaking proteins down to their constituent molecules. As well as these enzymes, pancreatic juice is also rich in bicarbonate, and contains calcium, sodium, chloride and potassium.

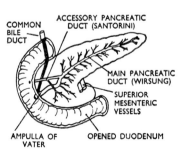

Fig. 14.18. The duodenum and pancreas dissected to show the pancreatic ducts and their orifices.

The stimulus to secretion is threefold. Firstly, there is a rich nerve supply derived from the vagus and sympathetic nerves which, when activated by food, results in a secretion of high bicarbonate content. Secondly, gastric chyme entering the duodenum causes the secretion of the hormone *secretin* which recirculates in the blood and stimulates the exocrine pancreas to produce juice also of high bicarbonate content. Thirdly, the duodenal chyme also results in the release of a second hormone, *pancreozymin*, which results in the secretion of a juice rich in enzymes.

2. *Endocrine pancreas*

Insulin is elaborated in the beta cells and secreted into the blood stream in response to variation in the level of the blood glucose. It is responsible for maintaining the blood glucose within closely defined limits. For example, following a meal, glucose tends to rise as it is absorbed from the intestine and this results in secretion of insulin which facilitates the inclusion of glucose into cells and its utilisation in the metabolic processes. This has the secondary result that the blood glucose level falls. In diabetes mellitus insufficient insulin is secreted in response to hyperglycaemia. This has the effect that the blood sugar rises and continues to rise, and metabolic pathways dependent on glucose become starved of their basic requirements.

The alpha cells secrete *glucagon* which has the opposite effect on blood glucose to insulin. That is, it results in an increase in blood glucose levels, but the mechanism of this increase is ill understood. Although it is produced in purified form so that it can be injected into patients, at the present time it has very little clinical application.

Two main groups of diseases affect the pancreas—inflammation (pancreatitis) and tumours.

PANCREATITIS

Pathology

This condition exists in one of three forms:
1. *Acute pancreatitis*, which may vary from mild to fulminating, with total destruction of all pancreatic tissue.
2. *Relapsing pancreatitis*.
3. *Chronic pancreatitis*.

In the condition of acute pancreatitis there is an inflammatory reaction throughout the whole gland. There are a number of conditions which may precipitate this and they are as follows:

1. *Infections*—for example mumps.
2. *Mechanical*—by the impaction of a gall stone at the lower end of the common bile duct, producing obstruction of the pancreatic duct.
3. *Metabolic*—for example, alcoholism, hyperparathyroidism.
4. *Vascular*—polyarteritis nodosa.
5. *Toxic*—alcohol poisoning.
6. *Traumatic*—due to external trauma, injuring the pancreas, for example a road traffic accident or gunshot wound.
7. Other causes—for example, pregnancy and Hodgkin's disease.

It must be admitted, however, that no aetiological factor can be determined in the majority of cases.

Clinical features

These depend on the extent of the inflammatory change within the gland. There may be upper abdominal pain, which characteristically radiates through to the centre of the midback. At first the abdominal pain is localised but as the process extends and the typical blood-stained exudate spreads into the general peritoneal cavity (this has been described as being like prune juice), so the pain becomes more generalised. Eventually the patient gives the appearance of someone suffering from peritonitis and this disease is an example of a chemical cause of this condition.

If the attack is a relatively minor one there may be some elevation of the pulse, the other vital signs being stable. As the severity of the attack increases, the pulse rate rises and eventually the blood pressure falls. The periphery of the patient becomes pale and he becomes shocked. This is partly due to the loss of fluid into the tissues around the pancreas, into the peritoneal cavity and into the intestine. Another factor, however, is the release of vaso-active substances from the inflamed pancreas itself which produce a shock-like state.

Special investigations

Serum Amylase The characteristic finding is an elevation of serum amylase, generally above 1,000 Somogyi units; this is because amylase is released into the peritoneal cavity from the inflamed pancreas and is absorbed into the bloodstream. The problem here is that the elevation may be transient, occurring only at the beginning of the attack, or in the case of haemorrhagic pancreatitis in which the pancreas is destroyed, the amylase will not rise at all, due to the destruction of the cells normally producing it.

In severe attacks the *serum calcium* is depressed, and this has been used as an index of prognosis. The more the calcium falls the worse the outlook for survival of the patient.

The urea and electrolytes are commonly normal unless the patient has been shocked or vomiting for a significant length of time, in which case the urea may become raised, sodium and chloride being low.

X-ray of the abdomen may show separation of loops of intestine by intraperitoneal fluid. A 'sentinel loop' of jejunum may be seen, this is due to the jejunum adjacent to the pancreas becoming paralysed because of the inflammatory process producing a localised area of paralytic ileus. Similarly, a colon cut off sign may be seen in which the transverse colon becomes distended with gas for the same reason.

Treatment

1. *Acute pancreatitis*

There is no effective specific remedy for pancreatitis. Therefore the treatment is supportive, aimed at relieving the pain and maintaining a satisfactory circulation. The patient is put to bed and given pethidine 100 mg 4 hourly, by intramuscular injection. Small quantities of water are allowed to be drunk for comfort and a fine nasogastric tube is passed to keep the stomach empty by aspiration, at first every hour and later every four hours. In every case intravenous fluid therapy will be required. From this point the vigour of the supportive measures depend upon the degree of inflammation in the pancreas. In severe haemorrhagic pancreatitis the patient may well be shocked, in which case fluid replacement should be controlled by means of a central venous pressure catheter and kept to a positive value (between +3 and +8 cm of water) with the use of plasma expanders such as plasma itself if necessary.

Trasylol inhibits the activity of proteolytic enzymes and since these are liberated by the process of acute pancreatitis, this drug has been suggested as being useful in acute pancreatitis. Unfortunately, although they have been extensively employed there is no evidence that they are effective. Antibiotics are valueless and should not be given. Similarly, steroids exert no beneficial effect. Occasionally, if the calcium level in the blood has dropped to an extremely low level it will be necessary to give intravenous calcium gluconate, 10 mg very slowly, to relieve the symptoms of tetany.

2. *Chronic relapsing pancreatitis*

In this condition there are episodes of acute pancreatitis interspersed with an entirely asymptomatic period or with a low background 'grumbling' pain. When they occur, the acute episodes of pancreatitis should be treated as above.

3. *Chronic pancreatitis*

This can exist in an entirely asymptomatic form in which a chance X-ray of the abdomen reveals extensive calcification throughout the whole pancreas. More commonly, however, it is associated with severe persistent abdominal pain. This condition has been said to result in some patients becoming drug addicts or alcoholics. However, the situation is usually that the chronic pancreatitis is initiated and maintained by the consumption of alcohol.

It is essential to exclude other disease within the abdominal cavity, particularly in the biliary tract, and if gall stones are demonstrated on cholecystography they should be removed surgically. The great lack in the investigation of the pancreas is an efficient test which shows the duct system. The pancreatic duct can now be demonstrated by catheterisation via a flexible gastroduodenoscope. (endoscopic retrograde cannulation of the pancreas, abbreviated to E.R.C.P.). This is an extremely useful technique but unfortunately cannot be successfully achieved in every case in which it is attempted. The only other method of demonstrating the main pancreatic duct is by operative pancreatography when at laparotomy a tube is inserted after the duodenum has been opened opposite the ampulla of Vater. This is clearly a major undertaking, but if by any of these means a localised constriction in the main pancreatic duct can be demonstrated, this should be relieved by surgery.

Many other surgical procedures have been described for pancreatitis but the sad fact remains that most of them are not effective. The pain in this condition can be so severe that some surgeons have advocated total removal of the pancreas. This obviously should only be reserved for the very severe degrees of this condition, as the quality of life without the pancreas is considerably impaired due to the 'brittle' diabetes and digestive abnormality.

CARCINOMA OF THE PANCREAS

Pathology

This is a fairly common malignant tumour and may be situated anywhere throughout the gland. As the greatest portion of pancreatic tissue is situated in the head, this is where the tumours are most commonly found, although a quarter occur in the body and 15% in the tail of the gland. Men are affected twice as commonly as are women and the peak age incidence is from 55 to 65.

In cut surface appearance the tumour is hard, white and infiltrates the normal pancreatic tissue and its surrounding structures (Fig. 14.19). Microscopically the tumours may be of duct origin or arise from the secreting cells of the termination of the ducts or rarely, may be associated with cystic spaces, the so-called cystadenocarcinoma.

Spread is by local infiltration, which may result in obstruction to the lower end of the common bile duct (producing jaundice) and of the common pancreatic duct, involvement of the medial wall of the duodenum with ulceration of the mucosa and eventually obstruction of the third part of the duodenum.

Clinical features

Unfortunately it is extremely difficult to diagnose an early carcinoma of the pancreas, with the result that this is one of the malignant tumours that tends to present by virtue of local or distant spread. Pain is a common feature and is usually experienced in the back, is ill-localised and of a deep seated type. Obstructive jaundice in the absence of a history suggestive of gall stones is common and is often associated with distension of the gall bladder, which can be palpated beneath the lower edge of the right lobe of the liver (Courvosier's law—see Fig. 14.3).

Special investigations

Barium Meal   If infiltration of the medial wall of the second part of the duodenum has occurred this can be seen as irregularity on

Dilated common bile duct

Tumour of head of pancreas

Duodenum

Fig. 14.19. Carcinoma of the head of the pancreas removed at a Whipple's operation together with the duodenum. (The specimen is viewed from the posterior aspect—note the dilated common bile duct.)

barium meal examination. As the head of the pancreas is expanded by the tumour the alteration in shape will also be detected on barium meal. A classic but rather unusual sign is the inverted '3' sign produced by bulging of the head of the pancreas around the ampulla of Vater.

Endoscopy The tumour may be seen and a biopsy can be obtained through the fibre-optic gastroduodenoscope if the lesion is involving the ampulla of Vater or ulcerating into the duodenum.

Treatment

Treatment can be divided into two types:

1. *Curative treatment*

If the tumour is small and has not infiltrated the neck of the gland to the left of the portal vein, it is possible to remove the head of the pancreas, the neck and part of the body together with the duodenum and part of the stomach (Fig. 14.20) in a pancreaticoduodenectomy (Whipple's operation). Unfortunately, the long-term results from this operation are not good, the five-year survival being only of the order of 5%.

2. *Palliative*

So often this condition presents with obstructive jaundice and since this leads to rapid liver function deterioration and is associated with very severe itching, its relief is important. This may be secured by performing *cholecystjejunostomy*, draining the gall bladder into a loop of jejunum (Fig. 14.6).

If no other palliation is possible, cytotoxic agents such as 5-Fluorouracil may be employed.

ISLET CELL TUMOURS

INSULINOMA

This is a tumour of the beta cells of the islet tissue which may be either benign of malignant. If considerably dedifferentiated the production of insulin is unlikely. Usually the tumour is benign and inappropriate secretion of insulin does occur. Presentation consequently is by hyperinsulinism which, in extreme cases, produces profound coma but more commonly the patient appears to undergo bouts of severe mental change, which includes antisocial manic behaviour, when in reality they are merely hypoglycaemic. In the

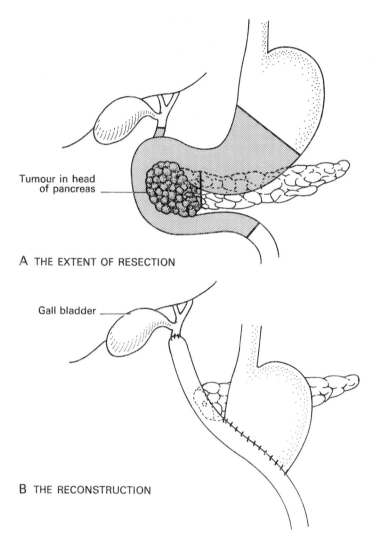

Tumour in head of pancreas

A THE EXTENT OF RESECTION

Gall bladder

B THE RECONSTRUCTION

Fig. 14.20. Whipple's operation, pancreaticoduodenectomy.

past, before this syndrome was widely recognised, these unfortunate patients found their way into mental hospitals where commonly they died from long continued bouts of hypoglycaemia. Diagnosis is made on the basis of a prolonged sugar tolerance test which demonstrates hypoglycaemia precipitated by fasting.

Treatment

Treatment is excision of the tumour. Unfortunately this is not always easy as the tumours may be quite small and difficult to find and within the substance of the pancreas.

ZOLLINGER-ELLISON SYNDROME

309
*Liver, gall bladder,
spleen and pancreas*

This extremely rare syndrome was first described in 1955 and consists of:

1. Fulminating duodenal ulcer diathesis, the ulcerative process usually extending into the upper jejunum.
2. Considerable gastric hyper-secretion of acid.
3. A tumour of the islet cells of the pancreas, which has the extraordinary property of producing the hormone gastrin.

Two-thirds of these tumours are malignant and of these two-thirds have metastases by the time the patient presents for treatment. The tumours may be distributed anywhere in the pancreatic tissue and occasionally exist in an unusual situation, for example the hilum of the spleen, the duodenum or the stomach. The syndrome is more common in males than in females in the ratio of 3 : 2 and the peak age incidence is in the 3rd, 4th and 5th decades. Adenomas of other endocrine glands occur in one patient out of four, including the pituitary, adrenal, parathyroid and in a combination of these glands.

Special investigations

Diagnosis is confirmed either by estimation of the hormone gastrin in the blood, when truly enormously high levels are found, or by the demonstration of a fasting gastric acid secretion which is at least 60% of the secretion that results from the injection of a maximum dose of pentagastrin.

Treatment

The treatment of choice is total gastrectomy. If subtotal pancreatectomy is attempted there is considerable danger that a small unheeded tumour may be left behind and this could be quite sufficient to produce disastrous recurrent ulceration. Total pancreatectomy leaves the patient with the problem of diabetes of a type which is very difficult to control, together with a considerable digestive defect and the quality of life following total pancreatectomy is not as good as that following total gastrectomy. Even though two-thirds of the Zollinger-Ellison tumours are malignant they appear to be very slow-growing and even when metastases have been found at operation, patients have lived for many years.

Good results have recently been reported using medical treatment with Cimetidine—a potent inhibitor of acid secretion.

Generally these are small and may be associated with cysts occurring in the kidney and the liver. They are due to obstruction to one or more of the ducts. No treatment is required and they do not give rise to symptoms.

In this condition the lesser sac of the peritoneal cavity becomes filled with fluid. The reason for this is that the opening into the lesser sac, the foramen of Winslow, becomes blocked because of an attack of pancreatitis. The inflammatory exudate which accumulates in the lesser sac from the anterior surface of the pancreas cannot find its way into the general peritoneal cavity and at the same time there must be a change in the permeability of the peritoneum lining the lesser sac, presumably due to the inflammatory processes.

Clinical features

The patient presents usually with central upper abdominal pain which may radiate through to the back. There may be a history of preceding pancreatitis and there may be a primary history of one of the precipitating causes of this, for example alcoholism. On examination a deep-seated mass is felt in the epigastrium, above the level of the umbilicus. It is usually difficult to define the borders of this mass accurately, impossible to get above it, and the mass may extend to diameters of 20 cm.

Special investigations

Plain x-ray of the abdomen will often reveal the edges of the cyst and there may be associated calcification within the pancreas. Barium meal demonstrates the stomach to be stretched over the front of the cyst and there may be distortion of the second part of the duodenum by the previously occurring pancreatitis (Fig. 14.21).

Treatment

Treatment is by making a wide anastomosis between the wall of the cyst and the posterior aspect of the stomach (Fig. 14.22). When this is done it might be supposed that the contents of the stomach leak into the cyst with disastrous results. This does not happen, however; fluid from the cyst drains into the stomach and if a barium meal is

311
*Liver, gall bladder,
spleen and pancreas*

Fig. 14.21. Barium meal in a
patient with a pseudocyst of the
pancreas. Note the way that the
barium within the stomach is
stretched over the cyst.

repeated after a few months in many cases it is found that there is
no evidence either of the stoma or of the cyst, the latter having collapsed and become permanently closed.

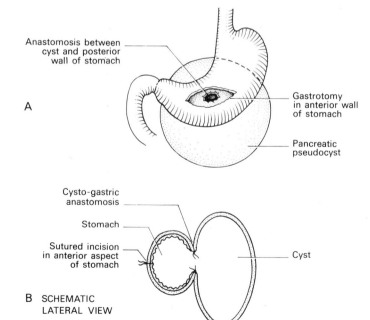

A

Anastomosis between
cyst and posterior
wall of stomach

Gastrotomy
in anterior wall
of stomach

Pancreatic
pseudocyst

Cysto-gastric
anastomosis

Stomach

Sutured incision
in anterior aspect
of stomach

Cyst

B SCHEMATIC
LATERAL VIEW

Fig. 14.22. Drainage of a pancreatic pseudocyst into the posterior aspect of the stomach.

Chapter 15. The urinary tract

The kidney and ureter

Anatomy

The kidneys lie retroperitoneally on the posterior abdominal wall. The right kidney is half an inch lower than the left, presumably because of its downward displacement by the bulk of the liver.

Each kidney lies against the diaphragm and the muscles of the posterior abdominal wall. Anteriorly the right kidney is related to the liver, duodenum (which may be accidentally injured in performing a right nephrectomy) and the hepatic flexure of the colon. In front of the left kidney lie the stomach, the pancreas, the spleen and the descending colon. On each side the adrenal sits as a cap on the kidney's upper pole (Fig. 15.1). The medial aspect of the kidney presents a deep vertical slit, the *hilum*, which transmits the renal

Fig. 15.1. The anterior relations of the kidneys.

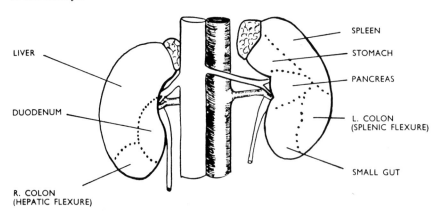

LIVER

DUODENUM

R. COLON
(HEPATIC FLEXURE)

SPLEEN

STOMACH

PANCREAS

L. COLON
(SPLENIC FLEXURE)

SMALL GUT

3. *Anuria*—due either to impaction of stones into the ureter on each side or blockage of the ureter in a remaining solitary kidney, the other kidney having either been previously removed or destroyed by disease. Very occasionally reflex anuria may result from a stone blocking one ureter with 'shut-down' of the normal opposite kidney.

4. *Retention of urine*—an unusual complication due to a stone becoming impacted in the urethra.

Treatment of stone in the urinary tract

Kidney

A small stone lodged in the kidney substance and not producing symptoms can be left alone although the patient must be kept under periodic X-ray survey. Large stones must be removed either by an incision through the substance of the kidney (*nephrolithotomy*) or, if at all possible, through the pelvis of the kidney (*pyelolithotomy*) since obviously this latter procedure can be effected with less damage to kidney tissue. If there is an associated hydronephrosis, removal of the stone alone is rarely sufficient and, indeed, may be followed in only a few months by recurrence of the calculus. It may be necessary to remove the lower pole of the kidney (*partial nephrectomy*) in order to ensure adequate drainage or to carry out a plastic operation on the pelvi-ureteric junction. Where the kidney is grossly and irreparably damaged, *nephrectomy* should be performed.

The ureter

Acute ureteric colic is treated by repeated injections of pethidine to relieve severe pain, together with a high fluid intake. The great majority of small stones within the ureter pass spontaneously. The smaller the calculus and lower down the ureter that the stone is situated, the more likely it is to pass, but stones up to the size and shape of a date stone, particularly if they are smooth, can be passed spontaneously.

If pain continues and X-rays show that the stone is not advancing, it may be possible to dilate the ureter via a ureteric catheter passed through a cystoscope, or it may be possible to fish out the stone by means of a number of ingenious snares and baskets which can be passed along catheters into the ureter under X-ray control in the operating theatre (Fig. 15.20). If these procedures fail then the stone must be removed surgically (*ureterolithotomy*).

Acute calculous anuria, due to blockage of both ureters by stone (or of the only remaining ureter where one kidney has lare?dy been destroyed by calculi, or removed surgically), is treated by

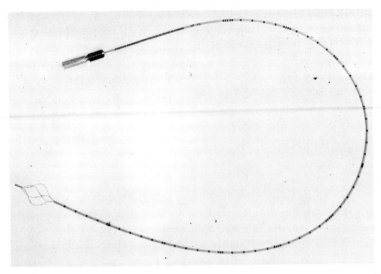

Fig. 15.20. A Dormia basket, which can be threaded through a cystoscope into the ureter for removal of a small ureteric calculus.

catheterising the ureters. If the ureteric catheter cannot be passed beyond the obstruction, the impacted stone must be removed at operation. If the patient is severely uraemic his general condition must first be improved, either by haemodialysis or peritoneal dialysis.

Bladder

If the stone is small it may pass spontaneously, but if not it may be removed either by means of crushing with a *lithotrite* (Fig. 15.21) or more commonly by open cystotomy through a suprapubic incision. At this operation, any underlying cause, such as a large obstructing prostate, must be dealt with or the stone will simply recur.

In every case of stone in the urinary tract an attempt is made to determine any predisposing factor and to eliminate this; thus renal infection is dealt with and any obstructive lesion within the urinary tract may require surgical correction. A small percentage of recurrent and bilateral stones are found to be due to a parathyroid tumour (see page 380) removal of which will prevent further recurrences. In every case the patient should be instructed to drink liberal amounts of fluid of any sort, in order to encourage the production of a copious, dilute urine.

Fig. 15.21. A lithotrite used for crushing a bladder stone.

Renal tumours are divided into those arising from the kidney itself and those derived from the renal pelvis. The latter grow from the transitional cell epithelium which lines the pelvis of the kidney as well as the ureter, the bladder and prostatic part of the urethra ('the uro-epithelium') so that tumours arising anywhere along this pathway are pathologically identical.

The two principal tumours of the kidney are the *nephroblastoma*, which usually occurs in children under four, and the *adenocarcinoma*, which usually occurs over the age of forty. Benign tumours and secondary tumours of the kidney are rare.

Tumours of the renal pelvis are the benign papilloma and malignant carcinoma.

NEPHROBLASTOMA

This is the commonest name for a cancer which is also termed Wilm's tumour, embryoma or adenomyosarcoma.

It is an extremely rapidly growing tumour which usually arises in children, although occasionally it affects adolescents. The tumour originates in the embryonic renal tissue and is made up of both epithelial and connective tissue elements. It is rapidly growing, soon invades surrounding tissues and the regional lymph nodes, and then spreads via the blood stream to the lungs and liver.

Clinical features

Rapid growth produces a large mass in the loin. Rather surprisingly, the renal pelvis is only involved late in the disease and therefore haematuria is relatively uncommon.

Treatment

If possible nephrectomy is performed and this is usually followed by radiotherapy. Occasionally a massive tumour may be shrunk down sufficiently by pre-operative irradiation to allow subsequent removal. In advanced cases cytotoxic agents may be employed.

ADENOCARCINOMA

This tumour is also termed the *Grawitz tumour*, after the German professor of pathology who first described it, or a *Hypernephroma*, an old term which dates back to the days when it was thought to arise from suprarenal tissue above the kidney.

Pathology

This tumour is the commonest of all renal growths. Men are more often affected than women and the patients are usually 40 years of age or over. The tumour appears as a large, vascular golden-yellow mass and is usually situated in one or other pole of the kidney (Fig. 15.22).

The tumour spreads directly through the renal substance and then invades the fatty capsule around the kidney. It disseminates by the lymphatics to the lymph nodes adjacent to the aorta and also tends to grow along the renal vein into the inferior vena cava; it then spreads by the blood stream to the lung, bones, brain and elsewhere.

Clinical features

About 40% of the patients present with haematuria; another 40% notice a mass in the abdomen or aching pain in the loin. The remaining 20% of patients manifest either with secondary deposits, for example a pathological fracture (Fig. 15.23), or else with the general features of malignant disease—anaemia, loss of weight and anorexia.

Investigations

The urine nearly always contains blood, which may be detected macroscopically or require microscopic examination. *The intravenous pyelogram* shows distortion of the kidney by the tumour

Fig. 15.22. A renal carcinoma (hypernephroma). The kidney has been bisected to show the massive tumour which occupies the upper half of the organ. Note that the kidney has been removed with a considerable amount of peri-renal fat.

artery, renal vein and the pelvis of the ureter. Within the kidney, the pelvis of the ureter divides into two or three major *calyces*, each of which divides into a number of minor calyces and each of these, in turn, is indented by a papilla of renal tissue onto which the collecting tubules of the kidney discharge urine.

The renal artery is derived directly from the aorta and is a massive vessel; indeed about 1/5th of the total circulation is passing through the kidneys at any one time.

The ureter is 10 inches long and runs as a muscular tube from the renal pelvis to the bladder. It passes first down the posterior abdominal wall, then on the lateral wall of the pelvis in front of the internal iliac artery. It has a thick muscular wall which is seen in the operating theatre to undergo typical worm-like writhing movements and it is this that enables the surgeon to identify it during pelvic and retroperitoneal operations.

EMBRYOLOGY AND CONGENITAL ANOMALIES

The ureter develops from the *metanephric duct*, a bud which pushes out from the cloaca, the common tube which is later to split up into bladder and rectum. On top of this metanephric duct develops a cap of tissue called the *metanephros*. The duct will form the ureter, the renal pelvis and the calyces; the metanephros will give rise to the kidney tissue itself. The kidney originally develops in the pelvis of the embryo then migrates headwards to reach the posterior abdominal wall. As it migrates, it acquires successively a fresh blood supply from higher and higher along the aorta.

This complex developmental process explains the high frequency with which congenital anomalies of the kidney, ureter and renal blood supply are found. Among the more important of these are (Fig. 15.2):

1. *Pelvic kidney*—due to failure of migration of the developing kidney upwards into the abdomen.
2. *Horse-shoe kidney*—produced by fusion of the two metanephric masses across the midline.
3. *Double ureter and/or kidneys*—due to reduplication of the metanephric bud.
4. *Congenital absence*—in one in every 2,400 births there is complete failure of the development of one kidney.
5. *Aberrant renal arteries*—it is not uncommon for there to be one or more additional arteries passing to the lower pole of the kidney; they represent persistence of aortic branches which pass to the kidney in its lower embryonic position.
6. *Polycystic disease* of the kidney results from failure of fusion of

Fig. 15.2. Common renal abnormalities. A, polycystic kidney; B, horseshoe kidney; C, pelvic kidney and double ureter; D, aberrant renal arteries and hydronephrosis.

the metanephros with its ducts—the result is multiple cyst formation throughout the renal substance, nearly always affecting both kidneys. Eventually the patient may die of renal failure or of hypertension.

It is important to note that polycystic disease, double kidneys and ureters and congenitally misplaced kidneys are all associated with an increased likelihood of infection when compared with kidneys that are anatomically normal. A child with recurrent episodes of urinary infection thus requires investigation to see whether some congenital urological abnormality may be present.

Renal physiology

The kidney functions to maintain water and electrolyte balance and has an important part to play in the regulation of the pH (acid/base relationship) of the blood, as well as acting as the excretory organ for many waste products of the body's metabolism and of foreign toxic substances.

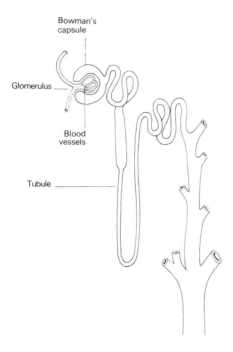

Bowman's
capsule

Glomerulus

Blood
vessels

Tubule

Fig. 15.3. Diagram of a nephron, comprising a Bowman's capsule and a tubule.

Each kidney is made up of approximately one million functioning units termed *nephrons* (Fig. 15.3) each comprising a glomerulus and a tubule. The *glomerulus* itself is made up of the expanded and thinned blind end of the renal tubule (termed Bowman's capsule) which is invaginated by a clump of capillaries.

The glomerulus acts as a simple filter through which the enormous amount of 180 litres of protein-free fluid is filtered from the blood-stream daily. This contains water, electrolytes and water-soluble substances such as glucose and urea. This filter is activated by the blood pressure—if the blood pressure falls then filtration slows or ceases.

In the *tubules* the greater part of this water is reabsorbed. Indeed since we produce approximately 1.5 litres of urine daily it means that 178 litres of glomerular filtrate is pumped back into the blood stream every 24 hours. The tubules select those substances which the body requires—all the glucose, for example, is completely reabsorbed in normal people—and lets pass those substances that are in excess and require elimination. In addition to this many toxic substances and poisonous chemicals, for example barbiturates, are cleared in this way.

Absorption is a property of the whole extent of the tubule, but the distal part is also capable of excreting substances into the urine, particularly hydrogen and potassium ions, and thus the distal duct plays an important part in maintaining the pH of the blood. It should be noticed that the tubules' power of absorption is limited so that, for example, if the blood glucose level is raised in diabetes mellitus not all the glucose can be absorbed by the tubules and this will then appear in the urine (glycosuria).

Water reabsorption is controlled by the anti-diuretic hormone of the posterior pituitary and sodium and chloride absorption is under the influence of aldosterone, one of the important hormones secreted by the adrenal cortex.

ANURIA

Having considered the normal physiology of the kidney we must now turn to the causes and treatment of failure of urine production of the kidney (*anuria*) or the only marginally less serious situation when the urine production falls to a level insufficient to maintain the body in health (*oliguria*).

The causes of this situation fall into three groups:

1. *Pre-renal*—here the kidneys themselves are initially healthy but if the blood pressure falls below the level necessary to maintain filtration through the glomeruli (usually below 80 mm of mercury), then renal function is impaired.

2. *Renal*—bilateral renal disease may be so severe that little or no urine can be produced. Examples are damage from certain poisons such as mercury, advanced chronic renal disease, transfusion reaction or tubular necrosis (see below).

3. *Post-renal*—complete bilateral obstruction of the renal drainage system, particularly by calculi or, fortunately rarely, by surgical injury.

ACUTE TUBULAR NECROSIS

The commonest cause of oliguria and anuria in modern surgical practice is acute tubular necrosis. This results from damage to the renal tubules as a result of ischaemia which may follow severe haemorrhage or result from the hypotension of severe toxaemia or burns. The damaged tubules become swollen, with blockage of their lumen, and suppression of urinary excretion takes place. Note that a patient who has a severe haemorrhage and becomes shocked may at first fail to produce urine because there is insufficient blood pressure to maintain filtration. However, if this state of affairs persists for several hours, there may then be the much more serious changes of tubular necrosis in the ischaemic kidneys and the anuria now becomes renal in origin.

There is always a good reason for the patient to become anuric—this may follow a serious accident, burns or heavy blood loss during operation which would suggest a pre-renal anuria which may proceed to acute tubular necrosis. The patient may be known to be suffering from severe chronic renal disease and the anuria is the end-stage of this condition. Anuria following hysterectomy indicates operative ligation of the ureters, or severe attacks of colicky pain preceding the anuria suggests calculous obstruction.

The patient fails to pass urine but, unlike retention of urine, the bladder is empty on clinical examination. If necessary this diagnosis is clinched by passing a catheter under full sterile precautions, when only a few drops of urine are obtained. At first the patient appears reasonably well, but then, within a few days, he becomes drowsy and thirsty with a dry brown tongue, develops anorexia, hiccups and effortless vomiting, and then lapses into coma. The progression of the condition can be monitored by estimation of the blood urea since the kidneys are now unable to excrete this product of protein break-down. It is not the urea itself which is particularly dangerous to the patient, but the retention of unexcreted electrolytes (particularly potassium, which, in high concentration, is toxic to the heart), the accumulation of non-excreted water which produces cerebral and pulmonary oedema, and the development of acidosis due to protein break-down.

Treatment

This will depend on the aetiology of the renal shutdown.

Pre-renal anuria requires replacement of blood volume, either by blood transfusion in haemorrhagic shock, plasma or plasma substitutes in severe burns, or saline in fluid depletion from vomiting or diarrhoea.

Post-renal anuria calls for surgical relief of the obstruction, for example, by catheterisation of the ureters blocked by stone (see page 337).

Tubular necrosis is the commonest variety of renal anuria. This is a reversible lesion and the aim of treatment is to keep the patient alive until the cells of the renal tubules recover. It is important not to overload the patient with water and electrolytes which cannot be excreted by the damaged kidneys, and to reduce protein metabolism as much as possible in order to limit the formation of protein break-down products, such as urea and potassium. The following regime is therefore instituted:

Fluid balance

The daily allowance of water is cut down to a basic 1 litre in 24 hours; this replaces the water lost in sweat and the water vapour excreted in the breath. To this ration must be added any additional fluid loss which occurs in vomiting, diarrhoea, a bowel fistula, or any other causes.

It may be necessary to give sodium bicarbonate to treat acidosis, but unless there are special circumstances such as this, the patient should not receive any electrolytes during the period of anuria.

Calorie replacement

If the patient is starved, he will simply utilise tissue protein and add to the toxic breakdown products already accumulating in the tissues. To reduce this as much as possible, the patient should be given Dextrose in 40% solution in his daily water ration. Since a gram of sugar produces four calories, one litre of 40% solution provides 1600 calories daily. This may be given in some cases orally or by naso-gastric tube, but more often the concentrated solution can only be tolerated by a nauseated patient if administered as an intravenous drip. Since the concentrated sugar solution will produce thrombosis in peripheral veins, it must be given by means of a caval drip via a fine catheter threaded into the inferior or superior vena cava via either the long saphenous vein or an arm vein.

Dialysis

In some cases this treatment alone will suffice, particularly if the patient's general condition is good at the onset of the anuria and the period of tubular necrosis only lasts for a few days. However, if the patient's general condition deteriorates, the blood urea continues to rise and if the serum potassium reaches a dangerous level of about 7 mEq/litre, it becomes necessary to maintain the patient by *haemodialysis* using the artificial kidney, which may be needed 2 or 3 times a week, or by *peritoneal dialysis*.

Haemodialysis. The principle of the artificial kidney is to pass the patient's blood through a coil of cellophane (a semi-permeable membrane), which is immersed in a bath of water to which electrolytes and sugar are added. Unwanted soluble substances in the patient's plasma (in particular, urea and potassium) pass from high concentration in the blood stream across the membrane into the bath fluid (Fig. 15.4). During dialysis coagulation of the blood within the

WASHING FLUID

BLOOD FROM ARTERY

PUMP

VEIN

CELLOPHANE
DIALYSER

WASTE

Fig. 15.4. Diagram of the circuit used in haemodialysis.

machine is prevented by heparinisation. Cannulae are placed in a suitable peripheral artery and vein and these can be used repeatedly by connecting the cannulae together, when not in use, by a plastic tube which maintains circulation and thus prevents clotting (the Scribner shunt Fig. 15.5). Another technique, recently introduced, is to anastomose a peripheral artery to its adjacent vein. Both vessels become distended in this artificial arteriovenous fistula and it is relatively easy to place large bore needles into these vessels under local anaesthesia whenever haemodialysis is required. This method is used when repeated dialyses are required in the treatment of chronic renal failure.

Peritoneal dialysis. The principle of this method is to use the peritoneal cavity as the semipermeable dialysing membrane. A plastic catheter is inserted into the peritoneal cavity and repeated lavage is carried out using an electrolyte-sugar solution similar to that employed in the bath of the artificial kidney (Fig. 15.6). The technique is relatively simple but strict precautions are required because of the risk of peritoneal infection.

Fig. 15.5. The Scribner shunt. This enables repeated dialyses to be performed, the arterio-venous shunt (in this case in the leg), being re-connected after each session.

THE INVESTIGATION OF URINARY TRACT DISEASE

Thanks to modern laboratory and X-ray techniques, surgical conditions of the urinary tract can now be diagnosed with considerable precision. Like every other system in the body, the surgeon proceeds through three logical steps in making a diagnosis. First, a detailed history is taken, second a careful clinical examination is carried out and third, if the diagnosis is still in doubt or requires confirmation, special investigations are performed.

Three important points must be emphasized in diseases of the urinary system:
1. It is wise to think of the whole urinary tract as a unit rather than as a series of independent structures since disease of any one part

Fig. 15.6. The apparatus used in peritoneal dialysis. Repeated lavage is carried out and waste products passing from the blood stream across the peritoneum are removed in the effluent fluid.

may often have effects elsewhere. For example, a tumour of the bladder may present because it is producing haematuria (blood in the urine); however, it may grow over and obstruct the ureteric orifice, produce hydronephrosis of the occluded kidney and the patient presents to the doctor not with bladder symptoms but with pain in the loin from his obstructed kidney (Fig. 15.7). As another example, a patient with tuberculosis of the kidney may not have any symptoms referrable to the kidney itself, but may complain only of frequency of micturition and dysuria (pain on passing urine) from secondary tuberculous infection of the bladder.

2. As a corollary to this, many of the principal symptoms of urinary disease, for example blood or pus in the urine, pain or frequency of micturition or passage of stones in the urine, may come from any part of the urinary tract and it is wise to tick off the organs one by one from the kidney down to the urethra. As an example, haematuria

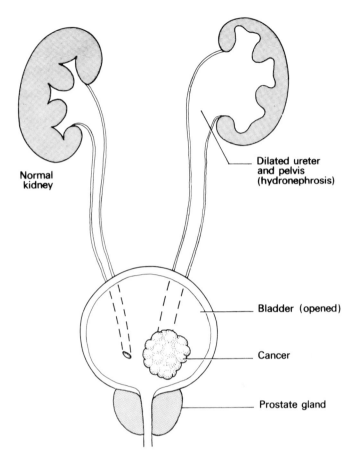

Normal
kidney

Dilated ureter
and pelvis
(hydronephrosis)

Bladder (opened)

Cancer

Prostate gland

Fig. 15.7. Carcinoma of the bladder producing a hydronephrosis as a result of ureteric obstruction.

may arise from the kidney (trauma, stone, tumour, tuberculosis), the ureter (stone or tumour), the bladder (trauma, cystitis, benign and malignant tumours), the prostate ('prostatic varices', which are distended veins over an enlarged prostate) or from the urethra (trauma). This is illustrated in diagram form in Fig. 15.8.

3. Patients can lead a normal life with only one kidney provided that this is reasonably healthy. However, many examples of urinary tract disease have bilateral renal involvement. Here the patient may present with not so much urinary symptoms as with the features of renal failure (*uraemia*)—lethargy, mental impairment, headache, vomiting and diarrhoea. It is obvious that unless disturbance of the urinary tract is thought of, the patient may well find himself in a clinic dealing with gastro-intestinal, neurological or even psychiatric illness!

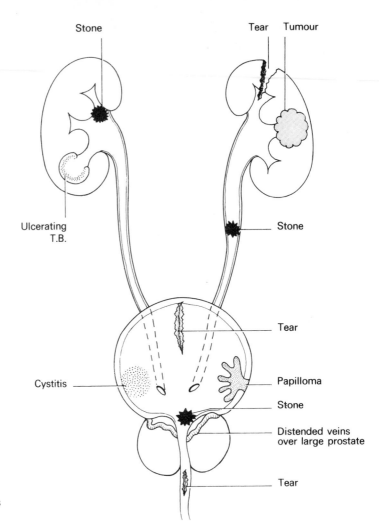

Fig. 15.8. Some important causes of bleeding in the urinary tract.

History

The majority of patients with surgical disease affecting the urinary tract present with one or more of the following symptoms:

1. Disturbance of micturition
2. Haematuria
3. Pain

Disturbance of micturition

Normal micturition (the act of urination) occurs three or four times during the day and depends to a large extent on the amount of fluid intake. It is rare for healthy people to have to pass urine at night (*nocturia*). Frequency, urgency to pass urine and *dysuria* (painful, difficult micturition) suggest urinary infection or prostatic obstruction, but note that patients with a perfectly healthy urinary tract but suffering from diabetes mellitus or diabetes insipidus may have very severe frequency.

Incontinence of urine may be due to damage to the bladder sphincter mechanism, enlargement of the prostate or 'overflow', when a chronically obstructed bladder trickles urine almost continuously. *Retention* of urine usually indicates obstruction of the bladder outlet. However, note that both urinary incontinence and retention may also be caused by diseases of the central nervous system, for example multiple sclerosis or spinal tumour, which interfere with the nervous pathways concerned with micturition.

Haematuria (blood in the urine)

Haematuria always calls for most careful investigation, and may be due to lesions anywhere along the urinary tract (see Fig. 15.8). Occasionally haematuria occurs in a patient with a perfectly normal urinary system but who has a bleeding tendency. The commonest cause of this is an overdose of one of the anticoagulants, for example heparin or dicoumarol.

Pain

A diseased kidney may give a dull aching pain in the loin which may cause the patient to complain of 'backache'. Obstruction of the pelvis of the kidney or of the ureter, especially by a calculus, results in typical ureteric colic, which is extremely severe, usually continuous, radiates along the course of the ureter into the scrotum or vulva and may make the victim roll about in agony. It is often accompanied by vomiting and sweating. Bladder pain is localised in the suprapubic region and is often accompanied by *dysuria* (pain on passing urine) or *strangury* (repeated painful attempts to micturate).

Examination

The general examination is important; renal failure may give rise to the typical uraemic picture of an anaemic, drowsy, dehydrated patient with a dry, brown tongue.

Local examination may reveal an enlarged kidney or renal tenderness, distension of the bladder or evidence of localised testicular disease. Rectal examination is extremely important because of the considerable information it gives about the status of the prostate gland.

Fig. 15.9. Tracing from a normal intravenous pyelogram.

Fig. 15.10. Cystoscopes. The uppermost photograph shows the telescope which slides along the shaft of the cystoscope. The middle instrument is the examining cystoscope, the lowermost the operating cystoscope, through which a ureteric catheter or diathermy probe can be introduced into the bladder.

Laboratory and X-ray examinations

Urine. It goes without saying that the first investigation of urinary tract disease is a full ward test of the urine, followed, if necessary, by chemical and bacteriological studies for protein, blood, white cells and organisms. For the latter, a midstream specimen of urine is required.

The blood urea is a useful test of renal function. The normal value is below 40 mg %; a value of 60 or 70 mg % indicates definite impairment of renal function. In severe uraemia the level may rise to 300 or 400 mg %.

The intravenous pyelogram (IVP) depends on the excretion of a radio-opaque dye by the kidneys after intravenous injection. The pelvis of the kidneys, the ureters and the bladder are outlined. A further X-ray of the bladder is taken immediately following micturition to give a measure of the amount of residual urine in the bladder (Fig. 15.9).

Patients with poor renal function (indicated by a raised blood urea) fail to excrete an adequate amount of the dye so that under these circumstances the procedure is useless. Some patients are sensitive to iodine and since the dye contains this material an IVP is contra-indicated.

Urethroscopy and cystoscopy. By means of these instruments the inside of the urethra and bladder can be directly inspected, together with the ureteric orifices (Fig. 15.10). Tumours and other lesions can be visualised and a biopsy taken for microscopic examination. If

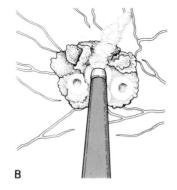

A   B

Fig. 15.11. Appearance of a bladder papilloma seen through a cystoscope (A). This can be treated by diathermy coagulation using a fine electrode threaded along the cystoscope (B).

necessary, diathermy coagulation can be performed. (Fig. 15.11). A fine ureteric catheter can be inserted into the ureter via an operating cystoscope so that a specimen of urine can be obtained from each kidney and by injecting radio-opaque dye through the catheter, the pelvis of the kidney can be outlined even if the organ is functioning so poorly that it cannot be demonstrated on an IVP (*retrograde pyelography*).

Micturating cystogram. The bladder can be outlined by injecting radio-opaque dye into its cavity via a fine catheter (cystography). X-rays taken during the act of micturition are useful in the demonstration of abnormal reflux of urine from the bladder into the ureters (vesico-ureteric reflux) which may be responsible for recurrent urinary tract infections. This technique can also be used to outline the outflow tract from the bladder.

Arteriography. In some cases an aortogram is necessary in the detailed investigation of a renal mass. It may be used, for example, to differentiate between a renal cyst and a carcinoma of the kidney (Fig. 15.12).

KIDNEY TRAUMA

The kidney may be injured by a direct blow in the loin (for example, a kick at football) or occasionally by a penetrating wound. The degree of damage varies from a slight bruise to complete rupture of the organ or avulsion of the kidney from its pedicle (see Fig. 15.8).

Clinical features

Following the accident, there is local pain and tenderness in the flank and a tender mass may develop in the loin. The clue to the

Fig. 15.12. An arteriogram in a case of renal carcinoma. Notice the extraordinarily rich blood supply of the tumour which occupies all but the uppermost part of the kidney. The catheter (which has been passed via the femoral artery, along the aorta and into the left renal artery) can be clearly seen.

renal damage is the presence of blood in the urine but it should be noted that occasionally the ureter is torn away from the kidney so that there may be severe internal bleeding without haematuria.

With modern high speed traffic accidents, it is not unusual for rupture of the kidney to be only a part of multiple injuries and it goes without saying that full examination must be carried out to determine whether there are accompanying fractures, chest injury, etc.

Treatment

Associated injuries will require appropriate treatment. Morphia is administered and shock treated if present by means of a blood transfusion. The patient is placed on a careful shock chart and each specimen of urine that is passed is saved so that it can be seen very readily whether the haematuria is increasing or getting less.

Fortunately, the great majority of renal injuries resolve with bed rest but nephrectomy, or partial nephrectomy, is required if signs of intra-abdominal bleeding continue. An emergency IVP is first taken to ensure that there is a functioning kidney on the other side!

HYDRONEPHROSIS

Hydronephrosis can be defined as an aseptic dilation of the renal pelvis and calyces. There may be an associated dilation of the ureter (hydro-ureter). One or both kidneys may be affected.

The causes of hydronephrosis fall into three large groups:

1. *Congenital.* This is found, as its name would imply, in children and young adults. Although no organic obstruction can be detected at the junction between the dilated pelvis of the kidney and the normal ureter, it is thought that some functional disturbances of peristalsis takes place across the smooth muscle fibres at this zone (Fig. 15.13).

2. *Obstructive.* Anything that produces a partial or intermittent obstruction of urinary outflow will produce hydronephrosis. This obstruction may be unilateral, (for example due to a stone in the ureter), or the block may involve the urethra, (for example a urethral stricture or prostatic hypertrophy) with resultant bilateral hydronephrosis.

3. *Associated with pregnancy.* Some degree of hydronephrosis occurs in pregnancy, the right kidney being rather more affected than the left. It is considered to be due in the main to relaxation of the ureteric muscle as a result of the high circulating level of progesterone. Pressure of the fetal head on the ureters may play some part by causing ureteric obstruction during the later part of the pregnancy.

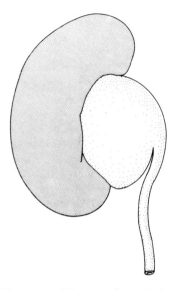

Fig. 15.13. Diagram of a typical hydronephrosis. Note the normal ureter and dilated pelvis.

Clinical features

Uncomplicated hydronephrosis may be symptomless, but more often the patient complains of a dull aching pain in the loin which is often mistaken for 'backache'. If both kidneys are severely affected, there may be the clinical picture of uraemia (see page 321). There may also be the symptoms produced by the underlying cause, for example the ureteric stone or the enlarged prostate.

The great dangers of hydronephrosis are its complications, which are as follows:

1. *Infection*—obviously the stagnant urine is very prone to infec-

tion and any carelessness in catheterizing such a patient may be disastrous. An infected hydronephrosis is termed a *pyonephrosis*.

2. *Stone formation*—phosphatic stones readily deposit in the infected stagnant urine of a pyonephrosis.

3. *Uraemia*—where there is extensive bilateral destruction of renal tissue. This destruction may be aggravated further by stone formation and infection.

4. *Hypertension*—secondary to renal ischaemia.

Special investigations

The urine is examined, but it should be noted that even if the hydronephrosis is infected, obstruction to the ureter may prevent pus from passing down into the bladder.

An intravenous pyelogram demonstrates the enlarged renal pelvis and the swollen, dilated, club-like calyces (Fig. 15.14). If renal func-

Fig. 15.14. Intravenous pyelogram of bilateral hydronephrosis due to prostatic obstruction. Note the very dilated calyces and ureters on each side.

tion is severely impaired, the kidney may not secrete dye and all that will be seen on X-ray is the outline of the distended kidney. In such a case a retrograde pyelogram may be required to show the exact anatomy of the hydronephrosis and to demonstrate any obstructive cause in the ureter. This is performed by passing a ureteric catheter up the ureter via an operating cystoscope.

Treatment

This is directed at removal of any underlying obstructive cause of the hydronephrosis. In the congenital group, a plastic operation at the pelvi-ureteric junction may save the kidney from progressive damage; the most popular operation is the Anderson-Hynes procedure (Fig. 15.15). A completely useless kidney, particularly if it is infected or almost replaced by a staghorn calculus, requires nephrectomy but obviously the surgeon must first satisfy himself that there is adequate function of the opposite kidney.

RENAL TUBERCULOSIS

With the general decline of tuberculosis in the Western world, involvement of the urogenital tract is also being seen with decreasing frequency.

Pathology (Fig. 15.16)

Tuberculosis of the urinary tract must obviously be secondary to a primary focus elsewhere, since the bacilli can only enter the body

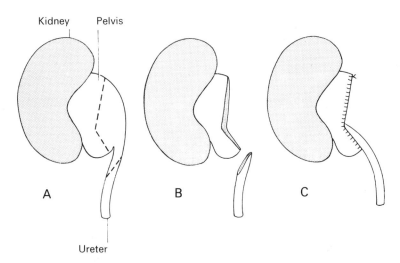

Kidney   Pelvis

A   B   C

Ureter

Fig. 15.15. The Anderson-Hynes pyeloplasty. A greater part of the dilated pelvis is excised together with the pelvi-ureteric obstruction. A plastic reconstruction of the pelvis is then performed.

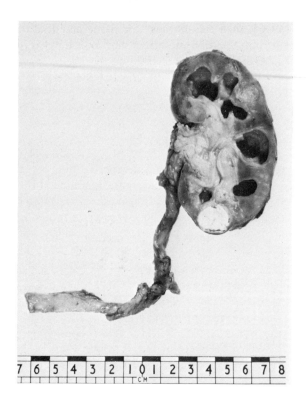

Fig. 15.16. Renal tuberculosis; an operative specimen. The pelvis is hydronephrotic and the renal substance is studded with tuberculous abscesses containing caseous material. This is especially well seen at the lower pole of the kidney.

either via the lungs or the gut. About one quarter of the cases have pulmonary tuberculosis but in many patients the original focus may be quiescent at the time of active renal disease.

Bacteria reach the kidneys via the blood stream and early lesions are found near the junction of the cortex and medulla of the kidney. These enlarge, coalesce and eventually produce extensive destruction of the renal substance. The tuberculous abscess, full of cheesy (caseous) pus, then ruptures into the pelvis of the kidney. The infection spreads by infiltrating the ureter and frequently involves the bladder in a tuberculous cystitis. In the male, the epididymis and seminal vesicles may become implicated. Thickening of the ureter may produce obstruction which can lead to tuberculous pyonephrosis and the useless bag of pus may eventually become calcified. Untreated, the opposite kidney often becomes involved, but this probably represents a separate blood stream spread.

The introduction of modern antituberculous drugs has modified the classical pathological picture of this disease. In most patients nowadays the disease process is arrested and healing takes place with the production of fibrous tissue. In early cases this merely produces a small scar in the kidney but if treatment is only commenced when the disease is advanced, then this fibrous scar tissue may lead to stricture formation within the pelvi-ureteric system and this results in secondary hydronephrosis. Fibrosis of the infected bladder may produce gross contraction on healing ('the golf ball bladder').

Clinical features

The patient is usually a young adult, often between the ages of 20 and 40. Frequently there is a history of present or previous tuberculosis elsewhere. In the early stages the symptoms are mild and may indeed be entirely absent. Usually the patient first complains of frequency of micturition which results from the tuberculous cystitis. There may also be pain on micturition, and the patient may notice either pus or blood in the urine. In more advanced cases, the pain and frequency of micturition becomes intense because of extensive involvement of the bladder and its diminished capacity from fibrosis. The constitutional symptoms of tuberculosis—fever, night sweats, loss of weight and anaemia—may then become manifest.

Examination is usually negative but the affected kidney may be tender and is sometimes palpable. The epididymis may become hard and thickened if diseased, and rectal examination may show thickening of the involved prostate and seminal vesicles.

Special investigations

Urine. The examination of the urine is all-important in making a diagnosis of tuberculosis of the kidney. Routine ward testing often reveals the presence of protein, pus and blood; the last two are easily confirmed by examining a drop of urine under the microscope. The reaction is usually acid. Ordinary techniques of culturing the urine for bacteria give no growth because the tubercle bacilli are delicate organisms which do not grow on ordinary agar plates; (for this reason one is always very suspicious of a urine which is acid in reaction, contains pus cells and yet is apparently sterile on routine laboratory examination—tuberculosis *must* be excluded). Early morning (and therefore concentrated) mid-stream specimens of urine are to be examined on at least three occasions; the bacteriologist spins down some of the urine and stains it with Ziehl-Nielsen's stain which involves washing the stained slide in acid. Most bacteria give up the stain under this treatment but the tuberculous bacilli are 'acid-fast' and, if present in sufficient numbers, can be seen under the microscope. The next step is to carry out a special culture of the urine on Lowenstein Jensen's medium, which is specially enriched and on which the delicate tubercle bacilli thrive. Whereas most organisms grow within 24 hours or so, these bacilli must be cultured for up to 6 weeks before they can be seen in colonies on this medium. Finally the urine is injected into a guinea-pig which is sacrificed after 6 weeks and, in most cases, will be found to have foci of tuberculosis within its body.

IVP. An excretory pyelogram will demonstrate the destruction of kidney tissue—there may be irregularity of the calyces or cavitation. Hydronephrosis may be evident and in late cases there may be no function of the destroyed kidney. Frequently calcification occurs in the tuberculous caseating pus and this shows up as patchy white spots on the X-ray.

Cystoscopy may reveal a decreased capacity of the bladder the wall of which may be inflamed and may show white tubercles. The ureteric orifices may be seen to be held rigidly open by fibrosis ('golf hole ureters').

Treatment

Specific chemotherapy must not be commenced until diagnosis has been confirmed by the bacteriologist, since, once undertaken, treatment must be continuous and prolonged. In the first instance streptomycin 1 gm, I.N.A.H. 400 mg and P.A.S. 15 gm are prescribed daily. Rifampicin is substituted if the organism is found to be streptomycin resistant. The urine is checked by culture each month and the treatment is continued until the urine has remained sterile for six months; this usually means about a year of intensive therapy. During this time sanatorium care is probably advisable so that the patient's general condition can be maintained and strict supervision of drug treatment carried out.

Surgery is only indicated in a minority of patients with advanced disease or where complications occur. A totally destroyed kidney, for example, may require nephrectomy. The damage produced by fibrosis may also indicate surgery. Thus late hydronephrosis with a totally destroyed kidney secondary to fibrosis of the ureter may require nephrectomy and a contracted bladder may require a plastic enlargement or transplantation of the ureters into an isolated segment of ileum draining as an ileostomy (see Fig. 15.25).

STONE IN THE URINARY TRACT

It is convenient to consider under one heading the topic of stone formation throughout the urinary system.

Predisposing factors can be grouped under three headings—inadequate drainage, excess of normal constituents in the urine, and the presence of abnormal constituents. It must be admitted, however, that many stones form without any apparent explanation so that obviously there are other factors of which, at present, we are quite ignorant.

1. *Inadequate drainage*

In any situation where urine stagnates, there calculi may deposit. This may be within a hydronephrosis, in a diverticulum of the bladder, or in the inadequately drained bladder which results from enlargement of the prostate or from a stricture of the urethra.

2. *Excess of normal constituents*

Kidney stones are especially likely to occur in tropical countries where dehydration results in an extremely concentrated urine. Patients with gout have an excess of uric acid in the serum which is excreted in the urine and which may be accompanied by uric acid stone formation. *Hyperparathyroidism* (see page 380) produces an increase in serum calcium and therefore urinary calcium; stone formation is the commonest manifestation of this condition.

3. *Presence of abnormal constituents*

Infection in the urine produces epithelial sloughs upon which stones may deposit, and this is particularly likely to occur in the presence of obstruction (e.g. pyonephrosis or chronic urinary retention). Any foreign body introduced into the urinary tract may form a nidus upon which calculi may form; thus stones may deposit on unabsorbable sutures inserted at operation or on a fragment of broken-off catheter tip. Patients have been known to introduce all sorts of strange objects into the bladder and most Hospital museums have stones with a centre made up of such things as hair pins. In the museum at Westminster Hospital we have a stone whose core is the rubber from a windscreen wiper. Another example of an abnormal constituent is *cystinuria*; in this condition the patient has an inborn defect in which the kidney tubules are unable to reabsorb the amino-acid cystine, which may then be deposited as cystine stones.

Patients who are immobilised on their backs for many months at a time, for example, long-stay orthopaedic cases or paraplegics, are particularly prone to develop calculi in the urinary tract. All three mechanisms that we have described may be at play; in the first place the urine stagnates in the kidney in the recumbent position and so we have the factor of inadequate drainage. Mobilisation of calcium takes place from the skeleton in these bed-bound patients and the excess is excreted in the kidneys. Finally, many of the paraplegics will have undergone repeated catheterisation, so that the third factor, purulent material in the urinary tract, may be present.

An important part of the nurse's duties in looking after paraplegic patients is prophylaxis against stone formation; this comprises regular moving of the patient, to promote urinary drainage, maintaining adequate fluid input, meticulous care of any catheter drainage system and regular testing of the urine for the presence of blood or pus.

Composition of urinary stones

The three common stones are phosphate, oxalate and urate (Fig. 15.17).

Phosphatic calculi are composed of a mixture of calcium, ammonium and magnesium phosphate ('triple phosphate stone'). These are hard, white, crumbly and rather like chalk. They are nearly always found in infected urine and produce a large 'staghorn' calculus which is found within a pyonephrosis.

Calcium oxalate calculi are hard with sharp spikes. These damage the urinary epithelium and the resultant bleeding usually colours the stone dark brown or black.

Uric acid and urate calculi are hard, brown and smooth. Pure uric acid stones are radio-translucent but, fortunately for diagnosis, most contain enough calcium to make them visible on X-rays.

Fig. 15.17. The three common varieties of urinary stone: left, a 'staghorn' phosphatic stone, middle, a smooth urate stone, right, a spiky oxalate stone.

Clinical features (Fig. 15.18).

Kidney. If the stone is embedded within the substance of the kidney, it may be symptom-free. If it is situated in the renal pelvis, the stone produces a dull loin pain. Impaction of the stone at the pelvi-ureteric junction, or its migration down the ureter, produces the dreadful agony of ureteric colic. The pain now radiates from the loin to the groin, is of great severity and is accompanied by restlessness, so that the patient is quite unable to lie still. There is often accompanying nausea, vomiting and sweating. Haematuria is frequently present and may be either obvious to the naked eye or may be detected under the microscope only; its presence is an extremely helpful means of clinching the clinical diagnosis.

Bladder. The typical triad of symptoms of bladder stone comprises *frequency* of micturition, severe *pain* (which is felt above the pubis,

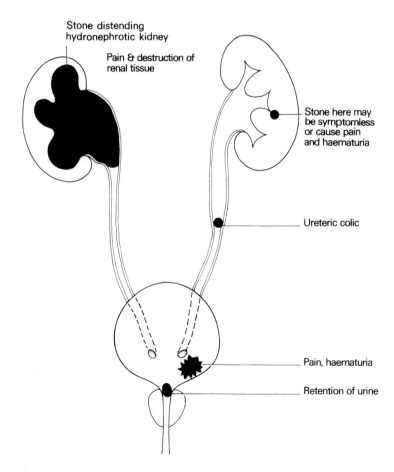

Stone distending
hydronephrotic kidney

Pain & destruction of
renal tissue

Stone here may
be symptomless
or cause pain
and haematuria

Ureteric colic

Pain, haematuria

Retention of urine

Fig. 15.18. Diagram of the effects of urinary calculi.

in the perineum or in the tip of the penis), and *haematuria*. Symptoms are particularly marked when the patient is in the upright position so that the stone lies over the bladder neck.

Urethra. The passage of a stone along the urethra may be accompanied by pain or may be hardly noticed. A large stone may impact and produce retention of urine, although this is surprisingly unusual.

Special investigations

The following laboratory and X-ray investigations are carried out in patients with suspected stone:
1. *The urine* is tested for the presence of blood.
2. *A plain abdominal X-ray* will show the presence of a stone in 90% of cases (Fig. 15.19).
3. *An intravenous pyelogram* will demonstrate the exact anatomy of the urinary system, e.g. the presence of associated hydronephrosis, although a completely obstructed kidney may show no function whatsoever (see Fig. 15.19).
4. *Cystoscopy* is used to visualise bladder stones.

When a stone is present, it is important to try to determine its aetiology; the urine is therefore cultured for bacteria and examined microscopically and chemically for the presence of cystine crystals. A serum calcium estimation is carried out and a value above 11 mg % (2.7 mmol/litre) is very suspicious of the presence of a parathyroid tumour. A high serum uric acid may be found with urate stones.

Complications of urinary stone

1. *Hydronephrosis*—this results from an intermittent or incomplete obstruction of the ureter by a stone.
2. *Infection*—(pyelonephritis, pyonephrosis).

Fig. 15.19. A plain X-ray of the abdomen reveals a large calculus in the right kidney (A). An intravenous pyelogram demonstrates the dilated pelvis of the right kidney and normal function on the left side (B).

A   B

Fig. 15.23. A pathological fracture through a secondary deposit in the femoral neck (arrowed). Notice a further deposit in the shaft of the femur. The patient had a renal carcinoma.

(Fig. 15.24). *Aortography* may be useful in doubtful cases. It demonstrates a typical tumour circulation and differentiates the avascular filling defect of a renal cyst (see Fig. 15.12).

A chest X-ray should always be performed for possible lung secondary deposits, which, if present, have a typical cannon-ball appearance.

Treatment

Nephrectomy is carried out provided there is no evidence of distant spread of the tumour.

TUMOURS OF THE RENAL PELVIS

Tumours arising from the transitional cell epithelium of the renal pelvis and ureter vary in malignancy from benign papillomas to invasive carcinomas.

Fig. 15.24. An intravenous pyelogram showing a left-sided renal carcinoma. The kidney is enlarged and there is gross distortion of the calyces.

Patients present either with haematuria or with hydronephrosis due to ureteric obstruction.

Treatment comprises nephrectomy combined with excision of the ureter, if this is involved.

The bladder

Anatomy

The urinary bladder of a normal subject is uncomfortably distended by half a pint (250 ml) of fluid. When fully distended, the adult bladder projects from the pelvic cavity into the abdomen, stripping the peritoneum upwards from the anterior abdominal wall. The surgeon utilises this fact in carrying out an extra-peritoneal incision into the bladder. The bladder lining is made up of transitional epithelium which, unlike any other epithelium, is completely resistant to continuous soaking with urine. The muscle coat is formed by a crisscross arrangement of involuntary muscle fibres which condense around the orifice of the bladder to form the *internal urethral sphincter.* The ureters enter the bladder posteriorly and the triangular area bounded by the ureteric orifices and the junction with the urethra is termed the *trigone*. In this area the mucosa is adherent to the underlying muscle, whereas elsewhere it is only loosely attached and is thrown into folds when the bladder is empty.

CONGENITAL ABNORMALITIES

Fortunately these are uncommon. The bladder may fail to develop normally so that the ureters and the trigone open directly on to the anterior abdominal wall, a condition termed *ectopia vesicae*. There is frequently an associated maldevelopment of the pubic bones, with failure of the pubes to meet at the symphysis. The child is, of course, completely incontinent of urine and may eventually die of ascending urinary infection. Malignant change may take place in the exposed bladder mucosa.

Treatment

The most satisfactory procedure is to implant the ureters, either into the colon or into an ileal loop with an ileostomy (uretero-ileostomy), combined with excision of the bladder mucosa (Fig. 15.25). Other surgeons attempt to reconstruct the bladder but in many cases this proves unsuccessful.

RUPTURE OF THE BLADDER

The bladder may be ruptured either into the peritoneal cavity or into the extra-peritoneal tissues. *Rupture into the peritoneum* may follow a penetrating wound (for example a bullet) or a crush injury to the pelvis when the bladder is distended. Occasionally the bladder may be perforated by a cystoscope or by a rigid catheter and rarely the over-distended bladder in acute retention may rupture spontaneously. *Extra-peritoneal rupture* is more common; the bladder may be penetrated by a fragment of bone in fracture of the pelvis, or is sometimes wounded during a hernia operation or in a vaginal repair of a cystocele.

Clinical features

If the bladder ruptures into the peritoneal cavity there results the typical picture of a peritonitis, with severe generalised pain and rigidity of the abdominal wall. Extra-peritoneal rupture is associated

A

Blood vessels

Small intestine

Stitches

Mesentery

Continuity restored

Stitches

Ureters implanted

Anterior abdominal wall

B

Fig. 15.25. Ureteric transplantation into an ileal loop.

with extravasation of a mixture of blood and urine into the pelvic tissues which produces a painful swelling rising out of the pelvis.

Treatment

An intra-peritoneal rupture is sutured and the bladder drained by means of a catheter. An extra-peritoneal rupture may be sutured, but if it is inaccessible at the base of the bladder then a suprapubic catheter is inserted to keep the bladder empty and to allow healing to take place.

CYSTITIS

Cystitis is a term applied to inflammation of the bladder. This may be either acute and chronic, affects any age, and may occur in both sexes, but it is extremely common in young women.

Aetiology

There must always be a cause for cystitis, but it must be confessed at once that in many patients, especially women, this cannot be found! Possible sources are:

1. The bladder itself—the presence of a stone, foreign body or ulcerating tumour.

2. Ascending from the urethra—this is by far the commonest cause in women. The short urethra may be traumatised during intercourse ('honeymoon cystitis') and may admit organisms from adjacent vaginal infection. The passage of a catheter without full aseptic precautions may infect the bladder and this is particularly dangerous if there is any obstruction to bladder drainage as the result of prostatic obstruction, urethral stricture, etc.

3. Descending infection—may occur from the kidney and this is particularly so in tuberculous cystitis secondary to renal tuberculosis. (Note also that the opposite may occur, that is to say, that pyelitis may result from an ascending infection of the kidney from the infected bladder.)

Clinical features

Acute cystitis is accompanied by frequency and pain on micturition. There may be haematuria and there may be obvious pus in the urine. The patient is often febrile and the bladder may be tender on suprapubic pressure.

Special investigations

It is essential that a mid-stream specimen of urine be sent to the laboratory at once for bacteriological examination. It is extremely bad practice to start any treatment until this simple step has been taken since if antibiotics are commenced it may then be quite impossible to determine the precise bacteriological diagnosis.

Treatment

This comprises specific antibiotic therapy determined by the bacteriological reports. Always keep tuberculosis in mind and in any suspicious case, specific tests for this are carried out (see page 331).

Once the acute infection is under control it is then necessary to try to determine whether there is an underlying cause—this will include carrying out an intravenous pyelogram and a cystoscopic examination of the bladder.

Bladder tumours may be benign or malignant. The former are papillomas, the latter, carcinomas.

Secondary invasion may sometimes take place from adjacent cancers of the rectum, ovary, uterus or prostate.

The benign papilloma forms a pedunculated growth which resembles sea-weed floating in the urine. A carcinoma, in contrast, is flat, solid, infiltrates the bladder wall and then ulcerates (Fig. 15.26). The malignant tumour may obstruct one or both ureters, producing hydronephrosis (see Fig. 15.7) or may obstruct the urethra with retention of urine.

Clinical features

Bladder tumours nearly always present with painless haematuria, although a malignant tumour which ulcerates and invades may also produce frequency, urgency and pain on micturition. Occasionally the patient may present with hydronephrosis due to ureteric obstruction, or with retention of urine due to the growth having involved the urethra.

Special investigations

Urine examination usually reveals blood, either to the naked eye or under the microscope. The skilled pathologist may be able to detect malignant cells in the urinary deposit.

Fig. 15.26. A benign bladder papilloma (A) contrasted with a carcinoma (B).

Ulcerated and sessile carcinoma   B   A   Branching papilloma

Ureteric orifice

An intravenous pyelogram may demonstrate a filling defect in the bladder and perhaps also ureteric obstruction or hydronephrosis.

Cystoscopy is the most valuable investigation since the tumour can be visualised and a biopsy obtained for microscopic examination.

Treatment

Most benign papillomas can be controlled by diathermy carried out through an operating cystoscope (Fig. 15.11). Since the lesion may recur, or others may appear the patient should be supervised by regular cystoscopic examinations.

The management of bladder carcinoma is difficult and the results are often poor. Occasionally a localised tumour can be excised by partial cystectomy. More extensive tumours are treated by high voltage X-ray therapy. If the growth does not respond, or if it recurs, then total cystectomy may be required with transplantation of the ureters, either into the colon or into an isolated loop of ileum, the urine then draining through an ileostomy stoma into a bag.

The male urethra

CONGENITAL ABNORMALITIES

The urethra may be mal-positioned during its development so that it may open anywhere along the lower aspect of the penis or, much more rarely, along its dorsal aspect. These abnormalities are termed *hypospadias* (Fig. 15.27) and *epispadias* respectively. The latter is usually associated with ectopia vesicae. These conditions require plastic surgical repair.

The other important congenital anomaly is the presence of urethral valves which can obstruct the flow of urine and result in chronic retention and uraemia in infants.

RUPTURE OF THE URETHRA

This most unpleasant injury can be classified into rupture of the bulb of the urethra, and rupture of the urethra within the pelvis in its membranous part (Fig. 15.28).

The bulbous urethra may be damaged by a direct blow, for example, falling off a tree astride a fence. It may also be torn by the surgeon during forcible dilatation or cystoscopy. There is severe pain in the perineum and bright red blood will be seen to drip from the external

Fig. 15.27. Hypospadias. The arrow points to the urethra, which opens along the inferior aspect of the shaft of the penis.

life—the condition of benign enlargement is therefore somewhat similar to the development of a nodular goitre or chronic mastitis.

As the prostate enlarges, the urethra may become obstructed. This obstruction may result in secondary hypertrophy of the muscle wall of the bladder. The obstructed bladder may become infected (especially after catheterisation) and bladder stones may form in the infected pool of stagnant urine. Back pressure on the ureters and kidneys may cause a progressive hydronephrosis and eventually renal failure (see Fig. 15.14).

Clinical features

The symptoms produced by an enlarged prostate may be divided into three broad groups:

1. *Disturbance of micturition*—the patient experiences increasing frequency and often has to get up from his bed several times at night to pass urine (nocturia). The stream becomes poor and hesitant and the whole act of passing urine may be converted into a long, slow, tedious dribble. Occasionally the congested veins over the enlarged prostate bleed, with resultant haematuria.

2. *Retention of urine*—this may be *acute* with sudden onset of severe pain, or *chronic*, in which the bladder gradually becomes distended and the patient develops dribbling overflow incontinence, with little or no pain. One Irish patient with this complaint told us that he was 'passing his urine wonderfully often'—a brilliant description of this situation.

3. *Uraemia*—progressive obstruction to the bladder outflow may result in renal failure so that the patient complains of headache, drowsiness, anorexia, nausea and mental deterioration.

Examination of the abdomen will reveal whether or not the bladder is distended. The prostate is assessed by rectal examination; the benignly enlarged gland can be felt as a rubbery swelling.

The patient is carefully examined for evidence of uraemia, characterised by a dried furred tongue, anaemia and mental confusion.

Special investigations

Patients with symptoms of prostatic enlargement should have the following studies performed:

The haemoglobin is estimated, since uraemia is often associated with anaemia.

The blood urea is measured—it should be under 40 mg% (7 mmol/litre) if renal function is normal.

The serum acid phosphatase is determined. This is useful in making a differential diagnosis from carcinoma of the prostate since in the latter situation it is raised above 3 units in 50% of cases.

A mid stream specimen of urine is sent to the laboratory for full examination and culture. Most patients with prostatic disease have a sterile urine unless infected by catheterisation.

An intravenous pyelogram gives useful evidence of kidney function, the amount of prostatic enlargement (which can be seen as a globular filling defect in the base of the bladder) and the amount of residual urine, which is studied by taking a further X-ray after micturition (Fig. 15.32).

Treatment

This depends on whether the patient is an elective case, due to troublesome prostatic symptoms, or whether he presents as an urgent problem of retention of urine. (This is dealt with on page 358.)

There are three routes of surgical approach to the prostate (Fig. 15.33).
These are:
1. Retro-pubic.
2. Transvesical.
3. Endoscopic (Transurethral).

Fig. 15.32. A very large prostate demonstrated on intravenous pyelography. The patient has just passed urine but there is still a considerable residuum in the bladder.

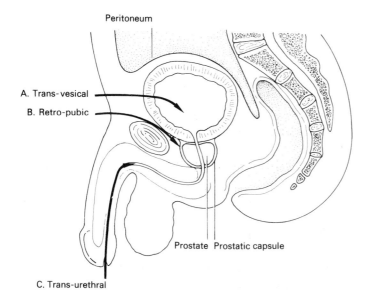

Peritoneum

A. Trans-vesical

B. Retro-pubic

Prostate Prostatic capsule

C. Trans-urethral

Fig. 15.33. The three approaches to the prostate.

1. The *retro-pubic prostatectomy* was devised by Terence Millin, after whom it is named. The capsule of the prostate is exposed by dissecting through the fatty tissue behind the pubis. The capsule is then incised, the enlarged prostate enucleated, a wedge removed from the posterior margin of the bladder neck to avoid stricture formation, and the prostatic capsule then sutured after the passage of a Foley self-retaining catheter. Since the inside of the bladder cannot be fully explored at this operation, the surgeon commences the procedure by carrying out a cystoscopy to make sure that he is not overlooking any calculi or a small tumour in the bladder, and to ensure that there is no stricture along the urethra.

2. The *transvesical operation* involves the enucleation of the prostate via an incision in the bladder. In the original operation no attempt at haemostasis was made, but a large tube was placed in the bladder to enable clots to escape freely. This operation had the advantage of speed and safety, but involved a long convalescence while the suprapubic fistula healed. Named after Sir Peter Freyer, it is now seldom performed. It was modified by Harris and by Wilson Hey, who introduced careful haemostasis followed by suture of the bladder, either with a urethral catheter alone, or with the addition of a small suprapubic catheter drainage.

3. *Endoscopic prostatectomy* is carried out with an operating cystoscope—either a diathermy loop (McCarthy) or else with a cutting punch (Thompson). The surgeon pares away slices of the prostate surrounding the urethra; this is particularly suitable for small fibrous prostates and for carcinoma of the prostate (see below). Following operation, a Foley catheter is left in place until bleeding ceases.

Post-operative care and complications

Prostatectomy is a common operation and a particularly challenging one to the nursing staff of a surgical ward. The patients are often elderly, frequently with pre-existing pulmonary or cardiac disease, who are then submitted to a major, unpleasant and uncomfortable procedure. As well as being on the alert for all .the usual post-operative complications there are a number of specific problems:

Fluid balance. A careful fluid chart is vital and is complicated by the fact that we must take into consideration the fluid that is being used in the bladder irrigation; this must, of course, be deducted from the amount in the urine drainage bottle to give the actual urinary output. The patient needs a high fluid intake to ensure diuresis and lavage to the bladder—yet he may be loath to drink. He may be tempted by being given his favourite drink and tea is usually welcomed by the average elderly Englishman. Intravenous supplement is required in most patients for the first day or two.

Prevention of infection. The raw prostatic bed plus the presence of an indwelling catheter makes infection a particular risk. Most surgeons cover the operation with a broad spectrum antibiotic, for example ampicillin or one of the sulphonamides, of which, sulphamethizole (Urolucosil) 0.5 gm 6 hourly or sulphatriad 1 gm 3 times daily are especially useful. The drug may need changing according to the sensitivity of any organisms grown in the urine. Particularly important is that a 'closed' system of bladder drainage is employed, the catheter emptying either into a sterile bottle below the level of an antiseptic solution or into a disposable bag (Fig. 15.34). If the system is disconnected for a bladder wash-out or any other purpose, this must be done under the strictest aseptic precautions.

Clot retention. It is everybody's duty to ensure that a continuous drip of urine takes place from the catheter post-operatively. If this stops it is due to one of the two causes. Either the catheter has been dragged down by the weight of the tubing into the urethra, or its lumen has been blocked by blood clot. The first is easily remedied by cleansing the catheter and replacing it in its proper position— but it should never be allowed to occur by ensuring that the catheter is soundly fastened by adhesive strapping to the thigh so that it lies

Fig. 15.34. Closed catheter drainage of the bladder. The Foley balloon catheter is strapped to the patient's thigh to prevent the weight of the tubing dragging on the bladder base.

at the correct level within the bladder. Clot retention is a much more serious state of affairs. Left untreated, the bladder rapidly fills with clot and the patient not only becomes severely distressed and in pain but also may become shocked from loss of blood. If diagnosed at once the situation can be remedied by washing out the catheter under full aseptic precautions. If this is unsuccessful, the patient must be taken back to the operating theatre and an attempt made to evacuate the clot using a wide bore metal catheter and a Bigelow evacuator (Fig. 15.35). If this fails the wound must be re-opened, the clot is cleared and a suprapubic tube inserted. Blood loss is replaced by transfusion.

CARCINOMA OF THE PROSTATE

Pathology

Cancer of the prostate is the fourth commonest cause of death from malignant disease in males in this country. It is rare below the age of 50 but becomes particularly common in the elderly.

The tumour is an adenocarcinoma, which arises from the glandular tissue of the prostate. Having spread through the prostate itself the tumour then invades adjacent organs—the bladder, urethra and, rarely, the rectum. It spreads into the lymph nodes along the iliac vessels and also by the blood stream, with a particular tendency to metastasize to the bones of the pelvis, spine, and skull. Deposits may also be found in the liver and lung.

Fig. 15.35. Bigelow's evacuator with metal catheters.

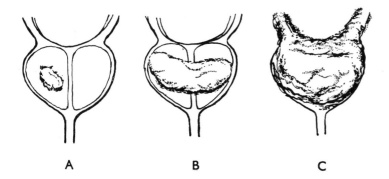

Fig. 15.36. The clinical stages of prostatic carcinoma, A, a hard nodule in the prostate; B, a mass obliterating the median sulcus; C, infiltration outside the prostatic capsule.

Clinical features

The symptoms of carcinoma of the prostate are usually identical to those of benign enlargement, but, in addition, the patient may present with symptoms due to secondary deposits, particularly pain in the back due to vertebral or pelvic involvement.

The diagnosis can usually be at least suspected by the surgeon when he examines the prostate per rectum. Instead of feeling the usual elastic gland, he notes that the malignant prostate is hard, irregular, and may infiltrate adjacent tissues. (Fig. 15.36).

Special investigations

The same investigations are performed as described under benign enlargement. The particularly useful finding in differentiating the malignant gland is the high serum acid phosphatase (above 3 units) which is present in about 50% of cancer cases. Some 25% have X-ray evidence of bony secondary deposits which, unlike most other secondaries, are usually osteosclerotic, that is to say, that they are more dense than normal bone (Fig. 15.37).

Treatment

Occasionally an apparently benign prostate is removed and found to contain a small focus of carcinoma. Under such circumstances, no further treatment is usually required. More often, carcinoma of the prostate is only discovered at a stage when it has already spread beyond its capsule and may well have involved other organs, particularly the pelvic cellular tissues, the base of the bladder, and perhaps also spread to the bones. Many of these patients respond to treatment with stilboestrol or to bilateral orchidectomy. The former treatment is usually preferred but orchidectomy is advised if the patient is unable to tolerate the stilboestrol or other oestrogens.

Fig. 15.37. A sclerotic deposit from a carcinoma of the prostate in the fourth lumbar vertebra.

The side-effects of these hormones include fluid retention, nausea and vomiting, gynaecomastia (enlargement of the breasts) and testicular atrophy.

Carcinoma of the prostate may produce urinary obstruction and this may be relieved by stilboestrol. If not, an endoscopic prostatectomy is indicated. (See page 356.)

URINARY RETENTION

A common surgical emergency is retention of urine. This may be *acute*, which is a painful condition (except when due to diseases of the central nervous system) or *chronic*, when the patient develops progressive obstruction which leads to dribbling overflow incontinence and which is painless.

It is first necessary to determine the cause of the retention and this may be either due to some *general* cause (with no organic obstruction to urinary flow), or to a *local* cause.

The commonest general cause is undoubtedly post-operative retention of urine. Indeed, this is the commonest of all causes of retention. It is well known to any experienced nurse how frequent it is for a patient following any surgical procedure (but especially an abdominal, pelvic or perineal operation) to be unable to pass urine in the post-operative period. This is due to a combination of the pain produced by straining, the difficulty in passing urine in the lying position, and perhaps also, in elderly patients, to some degree of prostatic obstruction aggravated by this situation.

Any disease or injury of the spinal cord may interrupt the reflex pathway of micturition, so retention of urine is commonly seen in patients with disseminated sclerosis, transverse myelitis or a spinal tumour, and is invariable in patients with paraplegia due to fracture of the spine.

Local causes are due to some obstruction of the urethra. Obstruction of any tube in the body must be classified into causes in the lumen of the tube, causes in its wall and causes pressing on the wall from outside. The urethra is no exception and so we have:

1. *Causes in the lumen*—calculus or blood clot (clot retention).
2. *In the wall*—urethral stricture.
3. *Outside the wall*—prostatic enlargement (benign or malignant), faecal impaction, pelvic tumour or pregnant uterus.

The diagnosis of the cause of retention is made on the history, examination and special investigations.

The history may reveal the typical progressive symptoms of prostatism, a story of urethral infection suggesting stricture, or associated leg weakness and numbness, indicating some neurological lesion.

Examination includes a rectal examination to determine the size and nature of the prostate, palpation of the urethra for stone or stricture, inspection of the urethral orifice to detect meatal stenosis or phimosis, and careful examination of the central nervous system.

Special investigations include estimation of the serum acid phosphatase which, if raised above 3 units, suggests carcinoma of the prostate, and X-ray of the pelvis, which may reveal a calculus at the bladder base or bony secondaries from metastatic carcinoma of the prostate.

In addition to establishing the diagnosis, the surgeon needs to know two other things about a patient with urinary retention before deciding on definitive treatment. These are:

1. *The general condition of the patient*—the average patient with retention of urine admitted to hospital is an elderly gentleman. Before proceeding to major surgery, his general condition must obviously be carefully investigated.

2. *The renal function*—the patient with retention of urine may potentially have damaged his kidneys by back pressure. This is assessed by the general condition of the patient and by estimation of the blood urea. Elevation above 40 mg% (7 mmol/litre) suggests renal impairment.

Management of urinary retention

Treatment naturally depends on the cause of the retention.

Post-operative retention

This can usually be overcome by giving the patient an injection of morphia and sitting him with his legs over the side of the bed. If this does not succeed, catheterisation may be required. The catheter can either be removed as soon as the bladder has been emptied, or, if the patient is particularly ill, can be left in place until the following day. Carbachol should not be used; it causes intense pain and there is risk of rupture of the bladder if any obstruction is present. Sometimes in a patient with an enlarged prostate retention of urine is precipitated by some other surgical procedure and can only be relieved by eventually proceeding to prostatectomy.

Patients with diseases of the central nervous system complicated by retention of urine are managed by means of indwelling self-retaining catheter.

The three common causes for an emergency surgical admission of a man with acute urinary retention are urethral stricture, benign prostatic hypertrophy, and malignant disease of the prostate.

Urethral stricture

A catheter cannot be passed through the narrowed urethra, which must be gently dilated with bougies under local or general anaesthetic. Following this, it is then possible to catheterise the patient and relieve the retention. Subsequently the patient must continue with regular urethral dilatations. Rarely the stricture is impassable and the patient then requires a temporary subrapubic cystotomy with insertion of a self-retaining catheter in the bladder. Once the oedema has been allowed to subside, it is then often possible to dilate the urethra after about a week to allow the suprapubic fistula to close.

Benign prostatic enlargement

The patient is catheterised under full aseptic precautions and prostatectomy can be carried out as soon as convenient if the renal function and general condition of the patient are satisfactory. If renal damage or the patient's poor general condition preclude operation, catheter drainage is continued until these can be improved. If the patient is in such poor health that operation will obviously never be possible, for example, a bedridden cardiac cripple, then he is best managed by a permanent urethral drainage, the catheter being changed weekly and urinary antiseptics being used should urinary infections occur. The modern plastic self-retaining catheter is far kinder to the patient than a leaking and odorous permanent suprapubic cystotomy tube.

Catheters and catheterisation

There are a large variety of urinary catheters, each subserving a useful function (Fig. 15.38).

Fig. 15.38. Urinary catheters. From above down: rubber, Foley balloon, Tiemann, coudé and bi-coudé gum elastic.

Jaques' plastic catheter is convenient for a single catheterisation, especially in the female, when it is not intended to leave a catheter in place. It can, if necessary, easily be sterilized by boiling, but it is usually available already sterilized and disposable.

Foley's balloon catheter is made of latex-rubber or polythene with a thin balloon which can be distended with sterile water injected through a side tube. A modification has a second side tube which can be used for bladder irrigation. This catheter is the most commonly used of the self-retaining catheters and, these days, is usually disposable and already sterilized by gamma irradiation.

Tiemann's catheter is made of hard rubber with a curved solid tip. This is used in male catheterisation when there is difficulty due to prostatic enlargement.

Gum-elastic catheters are semi-rigid catheters used in difficult cases of prostatic obstruction. They may have an olivary tip, a single bend (coudé) or a double bend of the tip (bi-coudé). The original gum-elastic material could not be boiled and had to be sterilised in formalin vapour. These catheters are now archaic and have been replaced by semi-rigid plastic material which can be boiled in the usual way.

Gibbon's catheter is a fine plastic catheter provided with plastic wings to attach the catheter to the penis. The long end of the catheter can be attached directly to a drainage bottle. This catheter is particularly useful in long-term catheterisation of paraplegic patients.

Whatever the catheter used, the strictest aseptic precautions must be employed. The operator wears a mask and sterile gloves. The urethral meatus is thoroughly cleansed with an antiseptic such as Hibitane or Cetrimide, sterile towels are employed and the catheter passed, if possible, by a no-touch technique using a sterile pair of forceps. If drainage is to be continued the catheter is immediately connected to a sterile drainage system (see Fig. 15.34).

The testis

Anatomy

Each testis is contained by a white fibrous capsule, the *tunica albuginea*, and each is invaginated anteriorly into a double serous covering termed the *tunica vaginalis*, just as the intestine is invaginated anteriorly into the peritoneum. Along the posterior border of the testis lies the *epididymis*, which is divided into an expanded head, a body and a tail (Fig. 15.39A).

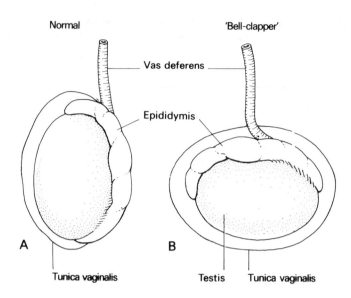

Normal   'Bell-clapper'

Vas deferens

Epididymis

A   B

Tunica vaginalis   Testis   Tunica vaginalis

Fig. 15.39. A, The anatomy of the normal testis; B, The 'bell-clapper' deformity in which the testis hangs within the tunica vaginalis. It is this variant that may undergo torsion.

The testis is supplied by the testicular artery, which arises from the aorta at the level of the renal vessels. Its venous drainage is via the *pampiniform plexus* which joins to form the testicular vein. On the right this drains into the inferior vena cava, on the left into the renal vein. The lymphatic drainage of the testis obeys the usual rule; it accompanies the venous drainage and thus passes to the para-aortic lymph nodes at the level of the renal vessels.

The testis is made up of coiled seminiferous tubules, each about two feet in length. These tubules drain posteriorly into about a dozen fine efferent ducts which pass into the head of the epididymis. The epididymis itself is made up of a considerably convoluted tube which drains into the vas deferens.

Development of the testis

This is important and the key to several features of clinical interest.

The testis arises from the posterior wall of the abdomen in the fetus and links up with a tube termed the *mesonephric duct* which is to form the epididymis and vas. From the third to ninth month of fetal life the testic migrates down the posterior wall of the abdomen and then along the inguinal canal until it reaches the scrotum, just before birth. A prolongation of peritoneum called the *processus vaginalis* projects into the fetal scrotum; the testis slides behind this and is thus covered on its front and sides by peritoneum. The processus becomes obliterated at about the time of birth, leaving the testis covered by the tunica vaginalis.

Three important abnormalities of the testis must be differentiated from each other:
1. Retractile testis.
2. Ectopic testis.
3. Maldescended testis.

The retractile testis is a normal organ which is drawn up into the groin by excess activity of the cremaster muscle which surrounds the spermatic cord.

An ectopic testis means one which is lying in an abnormal site (just as an ectopic pregnancy is one taking place in an abnormal site in the fallopian tube rather than in the uterus). A common anomaly is for the testis to emerge through the external ring and then, instead of descending into the scrotum, to come to lie in the superficial tissues of the groin. Other less common situations are in the perineum or at the root of the penis.

A maldescended testis lies in the normal course of descent anywhere from the abdominal cavity to the inguinal canal. The vast majority represent some local defect in development. Unilateral undescended testes are four times as common as bilateral.

Most, if not all, testes which *are* going to descend do so within the first few months of life.

Diagnosis

A retractile testis is a common condition and often the parents think that one or both testes have failed to descend. However, careful manipulation enables the infant's testis to be coaxed into the scrotum.

If the testis is easily palpable in the groin, then it is lying in an ectopic position and not in the inguinal canal where it is usually impalpable, or, at the most, in a thin boy, detected as a vague tender bulge.

Treatment

The child with retractile testes is perfectly normal, and all that is required is reassurance of the parents.

The ectopic or maldescended testis must be placed in the scrotum before the child reaches puberty if it is to function as a sperm-producing organ. The operation is therefore carried out when the child is about six or seven years of age and comprises mobilisation of the testis, removal of the coexisting inguinal hernia sac (the persistent processus vaginalis) and fixation of the testis within the scrotum without tension.

Left untreated the undescended testis will not produce sperm so that sterility will result in bilateral cases. In addition there is an increased risk of trauma, torsion and malignant disease in the maldescended testis.

TORSION OF THE TESTIS

Usually this is a torsion of the spermatic cord in a congenitally abnormal testis which is often hanging like a bell-clapper within a completely investing tunica vaginalis (Fig. 15.39B). It is probably impossible for a torsion to occur in a completely normal testis. Left untreated for more than a few hours, irreversible gangrenous change occurs in the organ.

Clinical features

Torsion usually occurs in children and adolescents. There is an acute onset of pain and the affected testis becomes swollen and extremely tender. The main difficulty is differential diagnosis from acute epididymitis. In the latter condition there is usually a pyrexia, a history of urinary tract infection, with pus cells and organisms in the urine, and the white cell count is raised. A useful factor in differential diagnosis is the age of the patient, since torsion of the testis is unusual after 20, whereas epididymitis is rare before that age.

Treatment

It may be possible in a very early case to untwist the torsion manually. If not, it is best to explore the testis if there is any doubt about the diagnosis, since every hour increases the likelihood of irreversible damage. If still viable, the testis is untwisted and sutured to the tunica vaginalis to prevent recurrence; if gangrenous, it is removed. In every case fixation of the other testis should be performed at the same time, since any congenital anomaly is likely to be bilateral and torsion of the opposite testis may therefore occur.

CYSTS WITHIN THE SCROTUM

There are two very common cysts associated with the testis. The first is a *hydrocele*, which is a collection of clear yellow fluid in the tunica vaginalis. This is usually without any obvious underlying cause, but it may be secondary to some inflammatory or malignant disease of the testis. The other condition is *cyst of the epididymis* which arises above and behind the testis and may contain either clear or milky fluid (Fig. 15.40).

Both types of cyst usually require surgical removal and it is important in hydrocele that the underlying testis should be carefully inspected to exclude any underlying testicular disease.

INFECTION OF THE TESTIS

Infection of the testis itself is unusual but may complicate mumps (*mumps orchitis*). A *gumma* of the testis due to late syphilis was once common, but is now extremely rare. Much more commonly the epididymis is affected as an ascending infection from the urinary tract, either due to gonorrhoea or to a coliform infection of the urine. Usually *acute epididymitis* resolves with antibiotic treatment. *Chronic epididymitis* may be due to tuberculosis, which is now becoming relatively uncommon, but is more likely to be due to a chronic phase of acute epididymitis which has not completely resolved following antibiotic treatment.

TUMOURS OF THE TESTIS

There are two main forms of malignant tumour of the testis—the seminoma and the teratoma.

The seminoma arises from the cells of the seminiferous tubules,

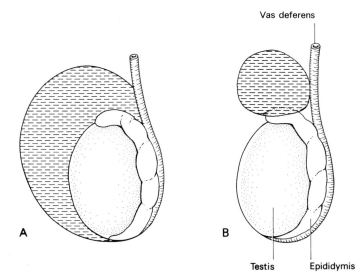

Fig. 15.40. A, Hydrocele. B, Cyst of epididymis.

usually in men between 20 and 40 years of age. The tumour is solid and white in appearance. About 10% arise in undescended testes.

The teratoma occurs in younger men, the peak incidence being 20 to 30 years. It is thought to arise from primitive germinal cells and has a markedly cystic appearance. Under the microscope the cells are very variable and the tumour may contain cartilage, bone, muscle, fat and other tissues.

Local spread of the tumour gradually destroys the testis. Lymphatic spread is to the para-aortic nodes on the posterior abdominal wall and in advanced cases there may be enlargement of the supraclavicular nodes on the left side of the neck due to thoracic duct invasion. Blood borne spread occurs to the lungs and liver.

The tumour usually presents as a lump in the testis which may rapidly enlarge in size and may be mistaken for an inflammatory condition. Some patients present with metastases—for example, a mass in the abdomen due to abdominal lymph nodes.

Treatment

This comprises orchidectomy, with radiotherapy to the paraaortic lymph nodes.

Penis

NON-RETRACTILE PREPUCE

It is extremely common for male infants in this country to be brought to the doctor or nurse because the parents notice that the prepuce cannot be retracted. In fact, the foreskin is non-retractile in 95% of infants at birth; 50% retract in the first year and the vast majority can be retracted by the third or fourth year as congenital adhesions between the glans and the prepuce break down (Fig. 15.41). Inability to retract the prepuce in the infant is no indication in itself for circumcision; indeed in the 'nappy' stage, the prepuce protects the delicate glans and the urethral orifice from the excoriation of ammoniacal dermatitis, which is liable to occur if the child's diapers are not frequently changed and are allowed to remain wet. Forcible attempts to retract the foreskin simply injure the tissues and the resultant scarring may lead to a true phimosis.

Circumcision is an operation which dates back some 15,000 years and which is steeped in religious, mystical, medical, social, hygienic

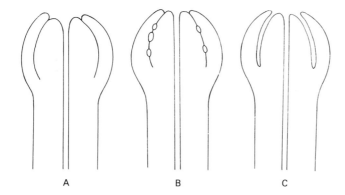

Fig. 15.41. The prepuce in the newborn baby is adherent to the glans penis (A). The adhesions gradually break down (B) until by the age of 3 or 4 the great majority of children have a prepuce which can be easily retracted (C).

and sexual traditions, misconceptions, myths and customs. Our practice is to carry out circumcision if requested by the parents on religious grounds, in the occasional case where the prepuce cannot be retracted in a child over the age of 4, or when an organic phimosis is present.

PHIMOSIS

This is a condition of gross narrowing of the orifice of the prepuce (Fig. 15.42). It occurs rarely as a congenital lesion but may follow the scarring produced by attempts at forcible retraction of the prepuce (see above), or may result from chronic inflammation of the prepuce (*balanitis*).

In extreme cases it may produce obstruction to the urinary stream. *Treatment* is by circumcision.

Fig. 15.42. Gross phimosis in a baby. This has resulted from attempted forcible stretching of the prepuce.

PARAPHIMOSIS

A condition in which the foreskin becomes retracted around the glans, interferes with venous return and results in swelling of the glans and extreme pain. There is an important practical nursing point here; always ensure that the patient's prepuce is pulled forward again after the insertion of an indwelling catheter—if not, a paraphimosis may well follow.

Treatment

Once the lesion has become established it is often too tender to manipulate without an anaesthetic. However, when this is administered the prepuce can usually be pulled forward into position; if not, a dorsal slit of the prepuce may be necessary.

CARCINOMA OF THE PENIS

This tumour usually affects elderly subjects (Fig. 15.43) and is practically never seen in circumcised men. Its most frequent site is in the groove between the glans and the prepuce. The tumour gradually erodes the penis and spreads to the lymph nodes in the groins. Indeed it is haemorrhage from fungation of these nodes that is likely to be the cause of death in cancer of the penis. Surprisingly enough the tumour never seems to occlude the urethra sufficiently to produce retention of urine.

Treatment

The diagnosis must always be confirmed by microscopic examination of a biopsy specimen.

Radiotherapy may be used in early cases but amputation must be carried out when the urethra is involved. If the groin lymph nodes are involved, block dissection is performed. Inoperably fixed nodes are treated by palliative irradiation.

Fig. 15.43. An extensive carcinoma of the penis.

Chapter 16.   The endocrine glands

The thyroid

Anatomy

The thyroid gland is made up of the isthmus, which overlies the second, third and fourth rings of the trachea, and the lateral lobes, each of which extends from the side of the thyroid cartilage down to the sixth tracheal ring (Fig. 16.1). On its deep aspect lie the larynx and the trachea, with the pharynx and oesophagus behind and the common carotid and internal jugular vein on either side. In the groove between the trachea and oesophagus lies the recurrent laryngeal nerve, which runs up into the larynx to supply its intrinsic muscles. The parathyroid glands are each about the size of a split pea and lie on, or are buried in, the posterior aspects of each lateral lobe. They are usually four in number, a superior and inferior on either side.

Development

The thyroid develops from a bud which pushes downwards from the floor of the tongue. This outgrowth then descends to its adult posi-

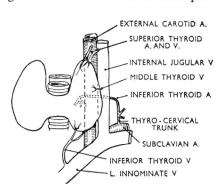

EXTERNAL CAROTID A.

SUPERIOR THYROID A. AND V.

INTERNAL JUGULAR V

MIDDLE THYROID V

INFERIOR THYROID A

THYRO - CERVICAL TRUNK

SUBCLAVIAN A.

INFERIOR THYROID V

L. INNOMINATE V

Fig. 16.1. The thyroid gland to show its immediate relationships and its blood vessels.

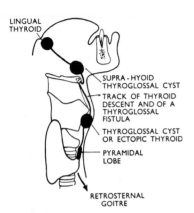

LINGUAL THYROID

SUPRA-HYOID THYROGLOSSAL CYST

TRACK OF THYROID DESCENT AND OF A THYROGLOSSAL FISTULA

THYROGLOSSAL CYST OR ECTOPIC THYROID

PYRAMIDAL LOBE

RETROSTERNAL GOITRE

Fig. 16.2. The descent of the thyroid, showing possible sites of ectopic thyroid tissue or thyroglossal fistula. The arrow shows the further descent of the thyroid which may take place into the retrosternal position.

tion in the neck. Normally it loses all connection with its origin which is commemorated, however, by the little pit termed the *foramen caecum*, which lies at the junction of the middle and posterior thirds of the tongue.

Congenital anomalies

The embryological line of descent of the thyroid from the base of the tongue to its normal position in the neck may be the site of fistula or cyst formation (Fig. 16.2). A *thyroglossal fistula* appears as an orifice in the midline of the neck which discharges watery fluid. A *thyroglossal cyst* forms a round cystic swelling in the midline of the neck which typically moves upwards when the patient protrudes the tongue, because of its attachment to the track of the thyroid descent.

Rarely the thyroid fails to descend properly into the neck and such a patient may present with a lump at the foramen caecum on the dorsum of the tongue, and which represents the whole of the thyroid tissue (*lingual thyroid*). On some occasions the thyroid descends beyond its normal station into the superior mediastinum so that the whole of the thyroid is situated within the chest (*retrosternal thyroid*).

THYROID PHYSIOLOGY

The function of the thyroid gland is to manufacture, store and secrete two iodine-containing hormones, *thyroxine*, amounting to about 80% of the hormone secretion, and *triiodothyronine*. These hormones are stored in the colloid contained within the follicles of the thyroid gland. The thyroid hormones are linked to protein in this colloid (*thyroglobulin*). The hormones are liberated into the bloodstream mostly bound to protein, although small amounts of both hormones are in their free active form. The rate of manufacture of the thyroid hormones and of their secretion into the blood is regulated by the thyroid stimulating hormone (TSH) secreted by the anterior lobe of the pituitary.

The thyroid hormones increase the metabolic activities of all the tissues of the body.

Hyper- and hypo-thyroidism

When the thyroid activity is normal the patient is said to be in a *euthyroid* state. If the thyroid is secreting an excess of thyroid hormones, the patient is said to be suffering from *hyperthyroidism* (or *thyrotoxicosis*), whereas if a subnormal secretion of thyroid hormone is taking place the condition is termed *hypothyroidism* or *myxoedema*.

Patients with hyperthyroidism show some or all of the following clinical features:

1. Central nervous system—the patient is irritable, nervous and demonstrates tremor of the outstretched fingers.
2. The skin—is moist and hot, the patient prefers winter to summer because she is so hot and sweaty in the warm weather.
3. The thyroid—this is usually enlarged but not invariably so. It may be highly vascular, which can be demonstrated by feeling the thrill of blood rushing through the thyroid when this is gently palpated.
4. The cardiovascular system—a rapid pulse is almost invariable and typically the sleeping pulse is also raised. There may be *auricular fibrillation* and, indeed, the patient may present with heart failure.
5. Alimentary system—the patient's appetite is increased and yet weight is lost. Diarrhoea is an occasional feature.

Many patients with thyrotoxicosis demonstrate *exophthalmos*. This is due to oedema and an actual increase in the mass of fat within the orbit and in the extrinsic muscles of the eye. Its cause remains unknown but the appearance is very typical (Fig. 16.3).

Hypothyroidism produces almost the complete opposite in the way of physical signs. Congenital hypothyroidism or *cretinism* is a condition in which the child is born with little or no functioning thyroid. He is stunted and mentally defective, with puffy lips, a large tongue and a swollen abdomen.

In the adult, hypothyroidism or myxoedema usually affects women and most often occurs in the middle aged or elderly. This patients have a slow deep voice, are overweight and apathetic with a dry coarse skin and thin hair (Fig. 16.4). They usually feel cold even in hot weather, have a slow pulse and are constipated.

Tests of thyroid function

The sleeping pulse rate. This is a simple and reliable test. A great difficulty in the clinical diagnosis of hyperthyroidism is its differentiation from an acute anxiety state. However, such patients when sleeping will have a normal pulse rate while patients with hyperthyroidism continue to have a rapid pulse even when asleep.

Laboratory tests of thyroid function fall into two main groups. The first measures the amount of iodine taken up by the thyroid gland, since this is usually increased in hyperthyroidism and depressed in myxoedema. A small dose of radioactive iodine is injected intravenously and its uptake into the thyroid measured by means of a Gamma ray detector; the count is proportional to the activity of the thyroid. The second group of tests measures the amount of thyroid

Fig. 16.3. Marked exophthalmos in a girl with severe thyrotoxicosis.

Fig. 16.4. Myxoedema. The patient is apathetic, the skin is thickened and coarse, and there has been loss of hair. This patient responded dramatically to treatment with thyroxine.

hormones circulating in the blood stream in the protein-bound form. This is normally raised in thyrotoxicosis and depressed in myxoedema, although false high values may be obtained in patients who have taken medicines such as cough mixture which contain iodine. A direct estimation can also be made of the serum level of thyroxine (the T4 level) and this is the most accurate of the laboratory tests in current use.

TYPES OF THYROID ENLARGEMENT

The clinical examination of a patient with enlargement of the thyroid gland falls into two phases. In the first place the physical characteristics of the gland must be determined to see whether it is smoothly enlarged, nodular, or infiltrating and invading adjacent tissues. Second, we must determine the endocrine state in order to see whether the patient is hyper-, hypo- or eu-thyroid.

A synthesis of these two phases gives a simple clinical classification of the vast majority of thyroid swellings.

(Note that *'goitre'* is an old world that simply means 'any sort of thyroid enlargement'.)

The common conditions are:

1. A smooth, non-toxic enlargement of the thyroid gland; this is the *'physiological'* goitre. It is particularly found in mountainous areas in which the water and diet are low in iodine; examples are in Switzerland, the Himalayas, Ethiopia and, in England, Derbyshire (hence the term 'Derbyshire neck'). Lack of iodine results in a raised secretion of the thyroid-stimulating hormone of the pituitary with consequent thyroid enlargement. A similar situation may occur when there is increased requirement of thyroid hormone, which accounts for the enlargement of the gland which may occur during puberty or pregnancy (Fig. 16.5).

2. A nodular, non-toxic gland; this is the commonest thyroid abnormality found in this country, there being either a solitary or multiple nodules present (Fig. 16.6).

3. A smooth, toxic goitre. This is termed *primary thyrotoxicosis* or Graves' disease.

4. A nodular enlargement of the thyroid in the presence of toxicity; this is termed *secondary thyrotoxicosis* and is due to a previous nodular non-toxic gland becoming toxic.

5. Smooth enlargement of the thyroid with myxoedema, usually in a middle-aged female, is the condition known as *Hashimoto's disease.*

6. An invasive enlargement of the thyroid is probably due to *malignant disease* (Fig. 16.7). Note that carcinoma of the thyroid is relatively unusual but must be suspected in any solitary nodule in the thyroid gland.

Fig. 16.5. 'Physiological goitre'. This young girl's thyroid became diffusely enlarged at puberty.

Fig. 16.6. A large nodular but non-toxic thyroid.

Fig. 16.7. An extensive carcinoma of the thyroid gland which is invading surrounding structures.

Outline of treatment of goitre

NON-TOXIC ENLARGEMENT

In endemic areas of goitre, the incidence of this condition has been greatly reduced by adding traces of potassium iodide to the table salt. In early stages of smooth enlargement, the condition may be reversible by administering thyroxine. However, if the physiological enlargement has failed to regress on this treatment and is producing symptoms of pressure on the trachea (Fig. 16.8) then partial thyroidectomy is necessary.

The single nodule in the thyroid or the non-toxic nodular enlargement will not improve on iodine or thyroxine treatment. In elderly patients with a long-standing goitre without symptoms it is probably best to leave well alone, but in nearly all other circumstances operative treatment is advisable for the following reasons:

1. Cosmetic appearance—often the patient is concerned about the appearance of her swollen neck.
2. There may be compression of the trachea and there is the risk of haemorrhage into a thyroid cyst which may produce acute airway compression.
3. Just as every solitary lump in a woman's breast is best removed, it is similarly wise to advise excision of any solitary thyroid nodule, since a small proportion of these prove to be carcinomatous.
4. There is a small risk that any nodular enlargement of the thyroid may undergo either malignant change or become toxic ('secondary thyrotoxicosis').

TOXIC GOITRE

The available methods of treatment in thyrotoxicosis are:
1. Medical treatment—antithyroid drugs.
2. Thyroidectomy after the patient has been rendered euthyroid by drug treatment.
3. Radioactive iodine.

Fig. 16.8. X-ray of the thoracic inlet. The air-filled shadow of the trachea is displaced well over to the left by a nodular goitre mainly involving the right lobe.

Medical treatment

This usually comprises carbimazole (proprietary name Neomercazole) which is given in a dosage of 10 mg three times daily, combined with sedation and bed rest in the acute phase of thyrotoxicosis. There is rapid regression of symptoms and the patient begins to feel better within about two weeks. Unfortunately, there is a high relapse rate after ending treatment, even if this is prolonged for two or more years. Medical treatment alone is usually confined to the management of primary thyrotoxicosis in children and adolescents.

Toxic effects include skin rash, fever and agranulocytosis in which the polymorph white cell count in the blood drops almost to zero. The first symptom of this is a sore throat in which the normal commensal bacteria in the mouth begin to invade the tonsil region. Patients on carbimazole must be warned to discontinue treatment immediately if this occurs and to report to hospital. Antibiotic therapy is commenced, fresh blood transfusions are given if necessary and the patient is barrier nursed until the bone marrow recovers.

Drugs and surgery combined

The majority of adult patients in this country are treated by preliminary carbimazole until euthyroid and then given iodine (potassium iodide 60 mg three times daily for about ten days) to reduce the vascularity of the gland, following which they are submitted to subtotal thyroidectomy; a small amount of thyroid tissue, about enough to fill a teaspoon, is left on either side.

Radioactive iodine

From the patient's point of view this treatment is miraculous! All she has to do is to swallow a glass of water containing the tasteless radio-iodine. There is no need to take tablets continuously, nor are there the risks of operation. It usually takes two or three months before the patient is rendered euthyroid and if seriously toxic it may be necessary to give carbimazole during this period.

There is a theoretical risk of carcinogenic change in the irradiated gland (although no case has yet been reported) and, because of this, it is current practice not to use radio-iodine in patients under the age of forty-five. It is not employed in young women who may become pregnant during treatment, since there is a danger of affecting the thyroid of the fetus.

The greatest disadvantage of this treatment is the production of hypothyroidism which increases in incidence with the passage of time and rises to nearly 13% after 10 years. When this occurs, thyroxine is used as replacement therapy.

Complications of thyroidectomy

Partial thyroidectomy is a common operation and the majority of cases make an uneventful recovery. However, there are a large number of possible post-operative complications which may occur, so that nurses on a surgical ward must always be on their toes when they are looking after thyroidectomy cases.

It is convenient to group these complications into three categories:
1. *The complications of any operation*
   Especially:
      Haemorrhage.

Wound infection.

Post-operative pulmonary collapse and chest infection.

2. *Hormonal disturbance*

(of the thyroid itself and the adjacent parathyroid glands).

Thyroid crisis.

Myxoedema (due to extensive removal of thyroid tissue). Late recurrence of toxicity (inadequate operation in the toxic gland).

Tetany (due to damage or bruising of the parathyroid glands).

3. *Damage to related anatomical structures*

Recurrent laryngeal nerve injury with vocal cord paralysis.

Injury to the trachea.

Pneumothorax due to injury of the dome of the pleura.

Some of these complications require further consideration here.

Haemorrhage

Haemorrhage immediately after thyroidectomy is a dangerous condition, since bleeding into the tissues of the neck may compress the trachea. The situation must be dealt with at once by removing the skin and subcutaneous sutures, in the ward if necessary, in order to decompress the neck. The patient can then be transferred to the theatre, any bleeding points secured and the wound re-sutured. Blood loss may require transfusion replacement.

Thyroid crisis

An acute exacerbation of thyrotoxicosis may occur immediately after operation but this complication is now extremely rare because of careful pre-operative preparation. It is thought to be due to massive release of thyroxine from the hyperactive gland during surgery.

Treatment comprises heavy sedation, intravenous iodine and cooling the patient by means of ice packs.

Hypoparathyroidism

Accidental removal of the parathyroids or their bruising during operation will be followed by the development of tetany a few days post-operatively, with typical tetanic spasms affecting hands and legs. This may be precipitated by inflating a blood pressure cuff around the arm (Trousseau's sign). The serum calcium falls from its normal 10 mg (2.5 mmol/litre) to below 6 mg% (1.5 mmol/litre).

In addition to frank tetany, (occurring in about 1% of cases), milder degrees of hypoparathyroidism may occur, and present months or even years later with mental depression, skin rashes or bilateral cataracts.

Treatment. Tetany is treated by giving 10 ml of 20% calcium gluconate intravenously. This is followed by calcium lactate 15 gm daily by mouth.

Recurrent laryngeal nerve injury

The recurrent laryngeal nerve lies in the groove between the oesophagus and the trachea, in close relationship to the inferior thyroid artery as this vessel passes forward into the posterior aspect of the thyroid gland (Fig. 16.9). Here the nerve is at risk of damage during thyroidectomy.

If only one nerve is damaged the patient develops slight hoarseness, which may gradually fade because the opposite vocal cord compensates by passing across the midline during speech. However, if both recurrent laryngeal nerves are injured, there is almost complete loss of voice and also serious narrowing of the airway, so that a permanent tracheostomy may be required. It is estimated that the nerve is injured in about 2% of thyroidectomies. Following operation, it should be routine practice to examine the vocal cords by means of a laryngoscope. Full movements of the cords during phonation means that the nerves are intact; damage to the nerve is shown by paralysis of the cord on the affected side.

CARCINOMA OF THE THYROID

Cancer of the thyroid is fortunately an unusual condition and accounts for about 400 deaths yearly in England and Wales. It is roughly three times more common in women than in men, may arise in a pre-existing goitre, and may follow irradiation of the neck in childhood.

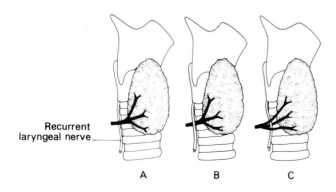

Recurrent laryngeal nerve

A   B   C

Fig. 16.9. The close relationship of the recurrent laryngeal nerve to the thyroid gland and the inferior artery. (A) The nerve is usually deep to the artery but (B) may be superficial to it or (C) passed through its branches.

Thyroid cancers fall into two main groups:

1. *Well-differentiated tumours* which, under the microscope, may have either a *papillary* or *follicular* appearance. The first is arranged in a frond-like pattern, the second resembles normal thyroid tissue. Quite often both types occur in the same tumour.

2. *Anaplastic carcinoma*, which is undifferentiated and is made up of masses of rapidly growing cancer cells.

Such important differences occur between these two groups that they might almost be considered as separate diseases.

The well-differentiated tumours occur in young adults, adolescents or even children. They are slow-growing, although they may spread to the regional lymph nodes and, as a late affair, by the blood stream to the bones, lungs etc. The anaplastic carcinomas, in contrast, occur in the elderly (see Fig. 16.7). Rapid local spread takes place, with compression and invasion of the trachea and involvement of the recurrent laryngeal nerve, resulting in hoarseness. There is an early lymphatic spread to the nodes in the neck and dissemination via the blood stream to the lungs, skeleton and the brain.

Treatment

The well-differentiated carcinoma presents as a localised mass in the thyroid and is treated by total removal of the affected lobe of the gland. If adjacent lymph nodes are involved these too are excised.

Many well-differentiated tumours take up radioactive iodine and it is possible to treat recurrences or metastases by this means.

The thyroid cells are under the control of the anterior pituitary and this applies also to the well-differentiated cells in thyroid cancer. It has been shown that giving thyroid will suppress the thyrotrophic hormone of the pituitary, and there have been remarkable examples of regression of thyroid cancer when large doses of thyroxine are given.

The anaplastic carcinomas may be treated by radical thyroidectomy but usually these patients present with an already inoperable mass in the neck. Palliative radiotherapy may give temporary relief and tracheostomy may be required for obstruction of the airway.

Prognosis

This is very different in the two groups of cases; the well-differentiated tumours may be associated with long survival, even in the presence of lymph node deposits, whereas patients with anaplastic tumours generally have a very poor outlook.

This is an uncommon disease which has, however, received considerable attention because it was demonstrated some years ago that in this condition the patient produces antibodies to her own thyroid tissue. This was the first of the group of conditions termed 'the autoimmune diseases'.

The patient is usually a middle aged female with an enlarged thyroid gland and evidence of hypothyroidism. Under the microscope the thyroid is diffusely infiltrated with lymphocytes and fibrous tissue. About 90% of these patients can be shown to have antibodies in their blood which react against thyroglobulin.

Biopsy may be necessary to confirm the diagnosis. The condition is treated by thyroxine, the maintenance dose of which varies between 0.1 and 0.3 mg daily.

The parathyroid glands

Anatomy

The parathyroid glands are four in number, each about the size of a split pea, which usually lie in two pairs behind the lateral lobes of the thyroid gland. The inferior parathyroids may lie occasionally almost anywhere in the neck or even descend into the superior mediastinum (Fig. 16.10).

Physiology

The function of the parathyroids is to secrete *parathormone*, which maintains the normal plasma calcium level. If the calcium in the

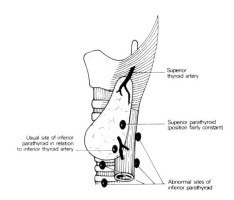

Fig. 16.10. The normal and abnormal sites of the parathyroid glands.

blood falls, the parathyroid glands are stimulated to secrete more hormone and vice versa. The exact mechanisms of the action of this hormone are not known. The most popular theory is that parathormone mobilises calcium from bones but it may also act by producing excessive excretion of phosphate from the kidney.

Tetany

Lack of parathormone produces a low serum calcium; this results in hyper-irritability of the skeletal muscles with spasms, the syndrome being termed *tetany*. This is liable to occur if the serum calcium falls below the normal level of 10 mg% (2.5 mmol/litre) to the region of 6 mg% (1.5 mmol/litre). The muscle spasms may affect any part of the body, but typically the hands and feet are involved. The wrist becomes flexed and the fingers are drawn together, rather fancifully like the hand of an obstetrician ('main d'accoucheur'). This spasm may be induced by inflating a blood pressure cuff around the arm (*Trousseau's sign*).

Parathyroid tumours

Parathyroid tumours are mostly benign adenomas; carcinoma may occur but it is fortunately rare. The importance of these tumours is that they produce an excessive secretion of parathormone. Occasionally this results from hyperplasia of the parathyroid glands.

The symptoms of excess parathormone secretion may fall under one or more of the following headings:

1. *Renal effects.* The commonest presentation of hyperparathyroidism is renal stone formation due to the excessive excretion of calcium in the urine.

2. *Bone changes.* There may be decalcification of bones with cyst formation and even spontaneous fractures. This condition is known as osteitis fibrosa cystica, which, as the name implies, means fibrosis and cyst formation in bone. It is also termed Von Recklinghausen's disease of bone.

3. *Features due to the high serum calcium.* These include lassitude, weakness, anorexia, loss of weight, and excessive thirst.

4. *Peptic ulceration.* Indigestion or duodenal ulceration is sometimes associated with a high serum calcium.

We can sum up the main effects as 'stones, bones, abdominal groans'.

The diagnosis is confirmed by estimation of the serum calcium, which is raised to 11 mg% (2.7 mmol/litre) or above. Other causes of a raised serum calcium include widespread malignant disease, sarcoid and excessive administration of Vitamin D. In these conditions the serum calcium falls to normal if a 10-day course of hydrocortisone is given (the cortisone suppression test).

Treatment. The parathyroid adenoma requires surgical removal. This can be rather difficult to find as the tumour may be small and may be lying in an ectopic position.

Hypoparathyroidism

This is usually secondary to surgery in the neck, especially thyroidectomy, and is considered on page 376.

The adrenal glands

Anatomy

The adrenal, or suprarenal, glands cap the upper poles of the kidneys and lie against the diaphragm. The left is related anteriorly to the stomach, whereas the right lies behind the right lobe of the liver and tucks itself on its inner side behind the inferior vena cava.

The adrenal gland is a good example of where two organs with entirely separate functions are fused into one anatomical structure. Other examples are the anterior and posterior lobes of the pituitary, and the insulin-secreting islet cells embedded in the enzyme-secreting glandular tissue of the pancreas. If the adrenal gland is cut across it will be seen to comprise a golden yellow *cortex* and a dark red central *medulla*. The latter is derived from the neural crest of the embryo, which also gives rise to the sympathetic ganglia. The cortex is derived from mesoderm. These two parts of the gland have entirely separate origins, functions and diseases and it is therefore also necessary to consider them quite separately.

THE ADRENAL MEDULLA

Physiology

The medulla of the adrenal gland is made up of large cells which stain yellow with chromic acid; for this reason they are termed *chromaffin cells*. Stimulation of the sympathetic nerves causes these cells to secrete adrenaline and noradrenaline into the blood stream. *Adrenaline* increases the heart rate and the cardiac output and, because of this, raises the blood pressure. Another effect is to mobilise sugar from the liver and thus to increase the blood glucose level.

Noradrenaline particularly acts by producing constriction of peripheral blood vessels.

Tumours of the adrenal medulla

From the surgical point of view the adrenal medulla is of importance because a number of rather unusual tumours may arise within it. These are:

1. Ganglioneuroma
2. Neuroblastoma
3. Phaeochromocytoma
4. Secondaries (a somewhat unusual site for deposits from carcinoma of the breast and bronchus).

Ganglioneuroma

A benign tumour which may arise from cells in the sympathetic ganglia or, in 15% of cases, in the cells of the adrenal medulla.

Neuroblastoma

A highly malignant tumour of sympathetic ganglion cells which occurs in young children. There is early dissemination to lymph nodes, the skeleton and the liver.

PHAEOCHROMOCYTOMA

Although this tumour is rather rare it is of considerable importance because it represents a cause of severe hypertension which can be cured surgically. It is a physiologically active tumour of chromaffin cells which secretes noradrenaline and adrenaline. Ninety per cent occur within the adrenal glands themselves but 10% arise elsewhere in the sympathetic chain and it is useful to note that 10% are malignant and 10% are multiple. For this reason it has been given the nickname of 'the ten per cent tumour'.

Any age may be affected, but the tumour is particularly found in young adults.

Clinical features

These are produced by the excess of circulating adrenaline and noradrenaline. The most important feature is the hypertension, which may be paroxysmal or sustained. This may be accompanied by palpitations, headache, blurred vision, fits and papilloedema. The intense constriction of peripheral blood vessels may produce episodes of pallor and there may be attacks of profuse sweating.

The excess secretion of adrenaline may produce hyperglycaemia with glycosuria; indeed about 10% of these patients have diabetes.

Special investigations

It is possible to measure the level of adrenaline or noradrenaline excreted in the urine. Most laboratories measure the major metabolite of these chemicals in the urine which is vanillyl mandelic acid (abbreviated to VMA).

The high blood pressure produced by phaeochromocytoma is brought down to normal by giving phentolamine, which is a noradrenaline antagonist.

If we are pretty certain that a tumour is present, attempts are then made to localise it to one or other adrenal, or to other parts of the sympathetic chain, by carrying out an aortogram or by outlining the retroperitoneal tissues for x-ray examination by insufflation with carbon dioxide.

Treatment

Having localised the tumour, surgical excision is carried out. This must be done with considerable care since manipulation of the tumour during the operation releases adrenaline and noradrenaline into the blood stream. The gross hypertension which may result is countered by intravenous phentolamine. Immediately after removal of the tumour the blood pressure may fall to very low levels and it may be necessary to counter this by blood transfusion and by a noradrenaline drip, which may have to be continued for a day or two after the operation (Fig. 16.11).

THE ADRENAL CORTEX

Physiology

The adrenal cortex is essential to life because of the important hormones which it secretes. Unless these are replaced, the adrenalectomised patient will certainly die. These hormones are varieties of chemicals called steroids and it is interesting that this chemical structure is also the basis of cholesterol, bile salts and the sex hormones.

The steroids secreted by the adrenal cortex overlap in their action, but they can be divided into three main groups:

1. *The glucocorticoids*—these regulate carbohydrate metabolism, protein breakdown and the mobilisation of fat from tissue stores. Most important of these are *cortisone* and *hydrocortisone*.

2. *Sex hormones*—of both the male (androgenic) and female (oestrogenic) varieties.

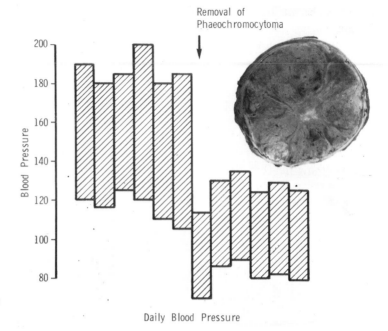

Removal of
Phaeochromocytoma

Fig. 16.11. Daily blood pressure
readings before and after excision
of a phaeochromocytoma. Note
the dramatic fall in pressure
after surgery. The inset shows the
cut surface of the tumour.

Daily Blood Pressure

3. *Mineral corticoids*—these regulate salt and water metabolism.
The most important of these is *aldosterone* which acts to retain
sodium and water and to regulate potassium excretion by the kidney.

It should be noted that representatives of these groups may overlap in their action. Thus although cortisone is an important member
of the glucocorticoid group, it also affects salt and water metabolism
and has androgenic effects (acne and excessive hair growth) if given
in large amounts.

The secretion of hormones by the adrenal cortex is under the
control of the anterior lobe of the pituitary, which produces adreno-
corticotropic hormone (ACTH), a specific stimulant to the adrenal
cortex. If excess cortisone is produced, there is what is termed a 'feed-
back' mechanism which inhibits the output of ACTH in an attempt
to reduce cortisone secretion.

Hyperadrenocorticism

Overaction of the adrenal cortex, with excessive secretion of its
hormones, may be due to a number of causes: hyperplasia of the
gland, a functioning tumour of the cortex (either a benign adenoma
or a malignant carcinoma) or occasionally the condition may be
secondary to a pituitary tumour producing an excess of ACTH.

The clinical pictures produced by hyperfunction of the adrenal cortex can be attributed to excess of each of its three groups of hormones:

1. Cushing's syndrome—glucocorticoid excess.
2. The adrenogenital syndrome, or virilism—due to excess androgen production.
3. Conn's syndrome or primary aldosteronism—oversecretion of aldosterone, the important mineral corticoid.

CUSHING'S SYNDROME

This syndrome was first described by Harvey Cushing of Boston, one of the pioneers of neurosurgery. It results from an oversecretion of adrenal corticosteroids and is also reproduced exactly by patients who are receiving large doses of cortisone (Fig. 16.12). The majority of cases are due to hyperplasia of the adrenal cortex, but some are due to benign or malignant tumours and rarely to a tumour of the anterior lobe of the pituitary.

Fig. 16.12. Cushing's syndrome. Note the 'Moon-face'.

Fig. 16.13. A large adenoma of the adrenal cortex.

Clinical features

The syndrome usually affects young adults, females much more often than males. The appearance is quite typical. The patient is obese, but the fat is distributed centrally, mostly over the trunk, face and neck, giving the typical 'moon face'; the arms and legs are, in contrast, relatively thin. The skin of the face is red, acne is common and there is often an increased growth of hair on the face so that the unfortunate woman may have to shave each day. Ugly red striae appear on the abdomen, exactly like the 'stretch marks' which follow pregnancy. The periods cease, the blood pressure is increased, the bones become thinned (osteoporosis) and diabetes is common.

Special investigations

The raised level of steroid production can be measured by estimating the excretion of ketosteroids in the urine. X-rays of the abdomen after injection of carbon dioxide into the retroperitoneal space may enable the radiologist to localise the adrenal tumour. The adrenals can also be outlined by aortography. An X-ray of the skull may sometimes reveal an enlarged pituitary fossa, which suggests the presence of a pituitary tumour.

Treatment

Bilateral adrenalectomy is performed for bilateral hyperplasia and the patient is then maintained on cortisone. In cases of adrenal tumour, the affected gland is removed (Fig. 16.13).

The rare examples which are due to pituitary tumour may respond to hypophysectomy.

THE ADRENOGENITAL SYNDROME

This syndrome results from an oversecretion of androgens by the adrenal cortex and can be divided into a congenital and an acquired type:

1. *The congenital form* appears to be due to a failure of the adrenal cortex to synthesise hydrocortisone. The pituitary therefore produces an excess of ACTH which results in hyperplasia of the adrenal cortex and hypersecretion of cortical androgens.

2. *The acquired variety* in children is always due to a tumour of the adrenal cortex, usually malignant. In young adults it may be due either to a tumour or to hyperplasia of the gland in examples of Cushing's syndrome where androgen production is excessive.

Clinical features

These fall conveniently into three groups, depending on the age of onset.

1. *Congenital.* In this variety, the newborn female has an enlarged clitoris and is often mistaken for a male (female pseudo-hermaphrodite). The child initially grows rapidly, but the epiphyses fuse early, so that eventually the youngster is stunted. There may be episodes of acute adrenal insufficiency especially precipitated by stress or infection.

2. *Childhood.* In the female there is virilisation and in the male child precocious sexual development (the 'infant Hercules'). The changes have been summed up as 'little girls become little boys and little boys become little men'.

3. *Adults.* In the male feminisation is seen, but this is extremely rare. The condition is commoner in females, who show the features of Cushing's syndrome together with amenorrhoea, excessive hair growth and atrophy of the breasts.

The diagnosis is confirmed in the laboratory by determining the excretion of 17-ketosteroid in the urine, which is greatly raised in this condition.

Treatment

In infancy treatment comprises the administration of cortisone. This suppresses the excess ACTH secretion which, in turn, cuts down the excessive excretion of androgens. In the acquired variety the adrenals are explored; if a tumour is present this is removed or if both glands show hyperplasia, bilateral adrenalectomy is performed with subsequent cortisone maintenance.

CONN'S SYNDROME

This is a rare disease produced by an aldosterone-secreting adenoma of the adrenal cortex. There is sodium retention and a fall in serum potassium, which results in muscular weakness. There is associated hypertension and it is the association of a raised blood pressure with a low potassium that gives rise to suspicion of this condition. The tumour is small, benign, and its removal cures the condition.

ADDISON'S DISEASE

This is a disease, first described by Thomas Addison of Guy's Hospital in 1849, of chronic insufficiency of the adrenal cortex. It may result from atrophy of the gland or its destruction by tuberculosis or malignant disease.

Clinical features

The sexes are equally affected. There is gross muscle weakness, low blood pressure and pigmentation of the skin from melanin deposition, which also occurs within the mouth.

Special investigations

Deficiency of the cortical hormones is reflected by a decreased sodium and chloride, together with potassium elevation in the plasma. The urinary excretion of steroids is also grossly diminished. Note that a similar picture (although without the pigmentation) is seen in patients following bilateral adrenalectomy who are not receiving sufficient steroid cover.

Treatment

This comprises the adequate replacement of cortisone.

Adrenalectomy for breast cancer

This is considered in Chapter 17.

The pituitary gland

See Chapter 10.

Treatment

Breast feeding is discontinued and the breast emptied of milk either by expression or by means of a breast pump. If seen within 24 hours of the onset of the symptoms, the infection is likely still to be in its spreading cellulitic phase and, at this stage, antibiotic treatment may abort the infection before abscess formation takes place. Since the majority of infections are acquired in hospital, the staphylococci are almost certain to be penicillin resistant and therefore it is necessary to use erythromycin or methicillin (celbenin). However, if infection is already established for several days, it can be assumed that tissue breakdown is already occurring with abscess formation. Antibiotic treatment at this stage will simply produce a chronic abscess walled off by dense fibrous tissue, a condition which has received the nicknames of 'antibioticoma' or 'penicillinoma'. In these circumstances it is surgical drainage that is necessary, not antibiotics. A small incision is made into the centre of the abscess, the finger used to break down any loculi and a soft drain inserted. The drain is subsequently shortened each day until the abscess cavity has healed from below upwards.

"CHRONIC MASTITIS"

This is the commonest by far of all conditions affecting the breast. In spite of its name, it is not an inflammatory condition at all. Many more scientific terms have been given to it, of which the best is *fibroadenosis*, but most people use the older and less accurate term.

Pathology

Any organ in the body which undergoes cyclical changes of proliferation and regression is prone to abnormalities of this process; these organs are the thyroid, prostate, ovary and breast. Since these cyclical changes only occur in the breast during the woman's menstrual life, the disturbances of chronic mastitis are seen between the age of about 30 and the menopause. The breast tissue is yellowy white, of rubbery, nodular consistency and may contain cysts. Under the microscope there is an increase of the connective tissue between the glandular elements, hyperplasia of the glandular tissue, formation of cysts, which vary from microscopic size to several inches in diameter, and infiltration by lymphocytes. It is, in fact, this infiltration of white cells which cause the early pathologists to label the condition 'chronic mastitis' in the mistaken belief that it was some sort of chronic inflammatory condition.

The patient usually complains of aching in one or both breasts, especially before the periods. A lump may be noticed in the breast or the patient may sometimes complain of discharge from the nipple, which may be blood stained, yellow or green. Examination may show a generalised lumpiness and granularity of both breasts or a mass confined to one sector of the breast which, for some unknown reason, is especially likely to be the upper, outer quadrant (Fig. 17.2). Less commonly there may be one or more cystic masses in the breast which may be of considerable size. Quite often the lymph nodes in the axillae are enlarged and rubbery.

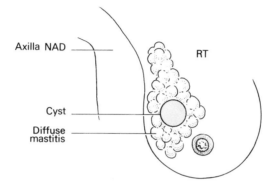

Fig. 17.2. Diagram of the typical findings in a patient with diffuse chronic mastitis and an associated cyst.

Management

Chronic mastitis is a harmless condition and there is no evidence that it predisposes to cancer of the breast. If the patient presents with diffuse granularity or nodularity in the breast and with no localised mass, nothing more is required than reassurance. However, if a discrete lump is discovered in the breast, then it is vitally important to make sure that this is not a cancer. The lump is removed and submitted to microscopic examination; if benign, no further treatment is needed, but if a tumour is found then appropriate surgery is carried out (see below).

If the surgeon thinks that the lump is a cyst, it is a common practice to perform aspiration under local anaesthesia (Fig. 17.3). If the fluid obtained is not blood stained (it is usually yellow, brown or green in colour) and if the lump disappears completely, we can be quite sure that the cyst is perfectly benign. If no fluid is obtained then, of course, excision of the lump must be carried out.

It is a wise saying that 'no lady should have a lump in the breast' and the diagnosis of any discrete lump in the breast must always be elucidated.

Fig. 17.3. Aspiration of a large cyst of the left breast. The mass disappeared completely and it did not recur.

BENIGN TUMOURS OF THE BREAST

There are two common benign breast tumours, the duct papilloma, and the fibroadenoma.

Duct papilloma

This arises from the epithelium lining one of the main breast ducts. The usual complaint is of bleeding from the nipple and the surgeon examining the patient may find a small lump adjacent to the nipple, pressure on which produces a bloody discharge. In other cases he may be unable to feel the lump but pressure on one spot causes a discharge of blood.

Treatment comprises excision of the lump or of the affected segment from which the blood can be expressed. Of course it is important to submit the tissue to microscopic examination because in some cases the same signs and symptoms can be produced by an intraduct carcinoma.

Fibroadenoma

This is a benign encapsulated tumour made up of fibrous tissue which surrounds proliferating epithelial ducts (Fig. 17.4). It commonly occurs in young women, often in their teens, and presents as a highly mobile firm lump in the breast, so mobile, in fact, that it receives the nickname of a 'breast mouse'. Sometimes in middle aged or elderly women a very large lobular fibroadenoma occurs which may even ulcerate through the overlying skin by pressure necrosis and mimic an advanced malignant tumour (Brodie's disease of the breast). Occasionally, sarcomatous change may occur.

Fig. 17.4. Fibroadenoma of the breast. This is easily enucleated from the adjacent breast tissue.

Treatment. Remembering our aphorism that 'no lady has a lump in the breast', all fibroadenomas should be removed and submitted to examination under the microscope to confirm the diagnosis and to ensure that a small carcinoma has not been misdiagnosed as a benign lesion.

CARCINOMA OF THE BREAST

Cancer of the breast is an immensely important subject. It is the commonest cause of death from malignant disease in women in the United Kingdom and accounts for approximately 10,000 deaths per year in England and Wales (Fig. 17.5). In the population as a whole, it is only exceeded in frequency by carcinoma of the lung, the large intestine and the stomach. About 1% of cases occur in males. Any age may be affected but the condition is rare below 30, and the

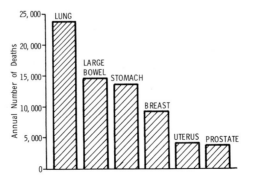

Fig. 17.5. Histogram of the common causes of death from cancer in England and Wales. Note that cancer of the breast is the fourth commonest for the sexes combined and the commonest cause of cancer deaths in women.

majority of patients present between the ages of 40 and 70. There is no definite evidence of any predisposing factors, although there is a familial tendency, it is less common in orientals and less likely to affect women who have had pregnancies in their teens. There is no association with the contraceptive pill. Any part of the breast may be involved, although the tumour is particularly likely to be found in the upper outer quadrant.

Pathology and spread

Carcinoma of the breast usually arises from the glandular epithelium, although occasionally it arises in one of the milk ducts to form an intra-duct carcinoma. An unusual variety is termed *Paget's disease of the nipple* which is believed to be an intra-duct carcinoma of the breast which invades and ulcerates the nipple by extending along the main ducts from the primary tumour to become implanted in the epidermis (Fig. 17.6).

Tumour spread may occur as follows:

1. *By direct extension* first expanding through the breast substance, then involving the overlying skin, which is first dimpled over it, and may then become ulcerated (Fig. 17.7). The fibrous reaction around the tumour may produce retraction and elevation of the nipple (Fig. 17.8). Eventually, deep extension involves pectoralis major and even the chest wall itself.

2. *Lymphatic spread.* The main lymph channels pass directly to the axillary and internal mammary lymph nodes. The former may be palpated in the armpit but the latter cannot be detected clinically. Later spread occurs to the lymph nodes above the clavicle, to the groin and to the opposite axillary nodes. Obstruction of the dermal lymphatics of the skin of the breast leads to cutaneous oedema which is pitted by the orifices of the sweat ducts. This gives the appearance of orange peel ('peau d'orange') (Fig. 17.9). This lymphatic invasion

Fig. 17.6. Paget's disease of the nipple. The nipple is reddened and ulcerated.

Fig. 17.7. Carcinoma of the breast which has involved and ulcerated the overlying skin. The tumour is also invading the underlying pectoralis major muscle.

Fig. 17.8. Carcinoma of the right breast. Note the elevation and retraction of the nipple. The skin is tethered to the underlying tumour mass.

produces daughter skin nodules and eventually the whole chest wall may become a firm mass of tumour tissue rather like a suit of armour ('cancer en cuirasse') (Fig. 17.10).

3. *Blood spread.* The tumour may invade the small blood vessels of the breast, allowing tumour cells to disseminate widely by the blood stream. These deposits are especially prone to grow in the lungs, liver (see Fig. 5.5) and bones. The skull, vertebral column, pelvis, ribs, upper end of the femur and upper end of the humerus are especially likely to be involved. There is no mystery about this; these bones are the sites where red bone marrow persists in the adult, so that they have a particularly good blood supply and thus favour tumour growth. The brain, the ovaries and the adrenal glands are also frequent sites of tumour deposits.

4. *Trans-coelomic.* In advanced disease, tumour seeding may occur over the pleural and peritoneal surfaces, accompanied by the development of a pleural effusion (see Fig. 5.6) and ascites respectively.

Fig. 17.9. 'Peau d'orange' due to lymphatic obstruction in an extensive carcinoma of the breast.

Fig. 17.10. 'Cancer en cuirasse'. This patient has already had a mastectomy for a carcinoma of the left breast. She now has an extensive tumour of the right breast involving the skin of the chest wall.

Clinical features

The commonest mode of presentation is for the patient to notice a painless lump in her breast or to have this detected during the course of a routine medical examination. Occasionally a pricking discomfort is noticed in the lump or the patient discovers recent indrawing of the nipple or a blood-stained discharge therefrom. A small proportion of patients present with symptoms produced by secondary deposits. A woman may discover a clump of enlarged nodes in the axilla, for example, or may complain of back-ache from spinal deposits, a pathological fracture, or breathlessness from involvement of the lung and pleura.

On examination, the surgeon may detect nothing more than a localised small lump in the breast and, without removal for microcopic examination, he may be unable to determine whether the lump is benign (a cyst, area of chronic mastitis or a fibroadenoma) or malignant. Signs which suggest malignant disease are retraction of the nipple, fixation of the skin to the underlying tumour, enlarged nodes in the axilla, or evidence of deposits elsewhere, for example enlargement of the liver, pleural effusion or ascites.

Note that only recent nipple retraction is significant, because the nipple may have been indrawn since birth or following a previous breast infection. If the retraction is recent it is significant; if of long standing, it can be discounted.

Special investigations

The chest is X-rayed and a radiographic skeletal survey is taken of the bones likely to be the sites of secondary deposits—skull, spine, pelvis, upper end of the femur and upper end of the humerus (the ribs, of course, will be visualised on the chest X-ray). Recently it has been shown that scanning of the bones following the injection of radioactive fluorine is an even more accurate way of detecting bony deposits than conventional X-rays but this technique can only be carried out in a number of special centres.

Clinical staging

Having carefully examined the patient, the surgeon can then place the tumour into one of the following stages:

Stage   I—the lump is confined to the breast

Stage II—in addition the axillary lymph nodes are enlarged

Stage III—the tumour is invading the skin and/or the underlying muscles; the axillary nodes may also be fixed to surrounding tissues

Stage IV—distant metastases are present

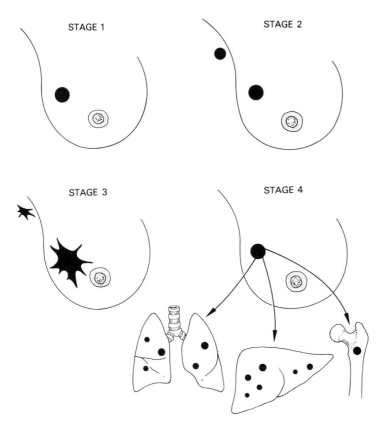

STAGE 1 STAGE 2

STAGE 3 STAGE 4

Fig. 17.11. The clinical staging of breast cancer.

This classification (Fig. 17.11), although useful, is fairly rough and ready. For example, although lymph nodes may not be palpable in the axilla, microscopic examination may subsequently reveal that they contain tumour deposits. Conversely, axillary nodes which are palpable may prove free from tumour. Although the tumour may appear clinically to be in Stage I, subsequent investigations by X-rays may reveal undetected bony deposits so that, in fact, we are dealing with a Stage IV case.

Treatment

This must be divided into 'curative' and 'palliative'.

When the disease is apparently confined to the breast tissue alone, or has only involved the axillary lymph nodes with no evidence of further spread, the surgeon hopes to be able to eradicate the disease and achieve a 'cure', (such patients fall into Stages I and II of the classification given above). Unfortunately, a proportion of these cases will already have microscopic metastases elsewhere in the body at the time that surgery is undertaken, and, inevitably, recurrence will eventually take place.

There is an enormous variation in the treatment of these early cases of breast cancer in different centres throughout the world. Some surgeons advise wide local removal of the tumour ('*lumpectomy*'). Others carry out a *simple mastectomy* in which the whole of the breast tissue is excised. In other centres, this procedure is combined with removal of the axillary lymph nodes, an operation which is termed '*extended simple mastectomy*'. In the long established operation of *radical mastectomy* the surgeon removes not only the breast and the axillary lymph nodes, together with wide sweep of overlying skin, but also the underlying muscles (the pectoralis major and pectoralis minor). In one or two hospitals the so called '*super-radical*' mastectomy is carried out, in which the internal mammary chain of lymph nodes is removed by resecting the anterior aspects of the ribs. Finally, some surgeons go so far as to advise, in addition, removal of the *opposite* breast at the time of the initial mastectomy. There is no uniformity of opinion as to which of these operations gives the best results, or indeed whether they should be combined with either pre- or post-operative radiotherapy. Fortunately, careful clinical trials comparing the various methods are now being carried out and within the next few years we should be able to state, quite clearly, which technique gives the most satisfactory results, both with regard to survival of the patient and, of great importance, the least disturbance of function. Obviously the more radical the treatment the more chance the patient may have of developing stiffness of the shoulder from scar formation and oedema of the arm from lymphatic interruption. Perhaps here we should state our own present practice, which is, in most instances, to carry out an extended simple mastectomy without post-operative radiotherapy.

Stage III cases

Once the tumour is invading surrounding structures, surgical clearance becomes impossible. Local radiotherapy often produces palliative regression although a 'toilet' operation may then be advisable to remove residual diseased tissue.

Stage IV, and recurrences after previous mastectomy

A solitary distant deposit, for example in one bone, or local recurrence in the scar following mastectomy can be controlled by radiotherapy treatment. Where dissemination is widespread, sex hormones or 'hormone surgery' are used. It is known that a proportion of breast tumours appear to be dependent for growth upon the hormone environment. Unfortunately it is at present impossible to determine whether a particular patient will or will not respond to therapy without trying it. Taking patients as a whole, it is found that about one third show objective response to such treatment (the tumour mass actually becoming smaller or disappearing), a third feel better or lose their pain, although we cannot measure shrinkage of the tumour (subjective response) and a third show absolutely no response at all to this therapy.

The possible methods of hormone treatment which are available include:

1. *Androgens*, which are usually employed in pre-menopausal patients (Durabolin 50 mg intramuscularly weekly).

2. *Stilboestrol* in post-menopausal patients (5 mg three times daily).

3. *Oophorectomy* (removal of the ovaries) particularly in pre-menopausal and early post-menopausal patients.

4. *Bilateral adrenalectomy* which is usually combined with bilateral oophorectomy, if this has not already been performed.

5. *Hypophysectomy* (removal of the pituitary gland) which may be performed either by a cranial operation, an approach through the nasal route, or by implanting radioactive material through a cannula under X-ray control.

In patients who fail to respond to hormone therapy, or who relapse after initial response, some temporary relief may be obtained by means of cytotoxic drugs (see Chapter 5).

THE CARE OF THE MASTECTOMY PATIENT

Women fear mastectomy probably more than any other commonly performed operation and it is the duty of the nursing as well as the medical staff to do as much as possible to allay the patient's anxiety and to make her stay in hospital as comfortable as possible. The words 'amputation of the breast' are cruel and should never be used. It should be explained to the patient that if the surgeon decides that the breast needs removal, this entails only removal of the breast substance and that the patient will wake up post-operatively with a linear scar across the chest wall. Some women are under the misconception that mastectomy must obviously leave a gaping hole where the breast has been removed and do not realize that they are to be left with quite a neat scar. It is worth pointing out to the patient that the mastectomy wound is easily disguised by the clothes and that the modern prosthesis worn within the brassiere enables the patient to wear evening dress, bathing costume etc. without anybody knowing that a mastectomy has been carried out.

At one time, the post-operative care of the mastectomy patient was bedevilled by the collection of blood or serum under the large skin flaps. Fortunately, this has now been overcome by the use of suction drainage by means of a low-pressure pump (Fig. 17.12). Suction should be continued until no further haemo-serous aspirate is obtained, usually about 3 days following operation. As a result of this, primary healing can be anticipated in the majority of cases. From time to time, (and this particularly applies to mastectomy for cancer in the male), the surgeon finds that there is inadequate skin for closure and in such cases a split skin graft from the thigh is required from the time of operation. The surgeon can usually anticipate this need, in which case the patient is warned before operation and the thigh prepared as a donor site by preliminary shaving and skin disinfection.

It was once the custom to torture the patient immediately postoperatively by insisting on violent exercise to the shoulder on the side of the mastectomy. This was due to the mistaken view that a few days of rest would result in stiffness of the shoulder. Of course, quite the reverse is true. It is a general principle throughout surgery that *damaged tissues should be placed at rest until healing has taken place*. Once this has been effected, then active movement will rapidly restore full function. Following mastectomy, the patient should be encouraged to use the elbow, wrist, and hand on the affected side but to keep the shoulder still, either by resting the arm on the pillow or (as in our practice) by supporting the arm in a

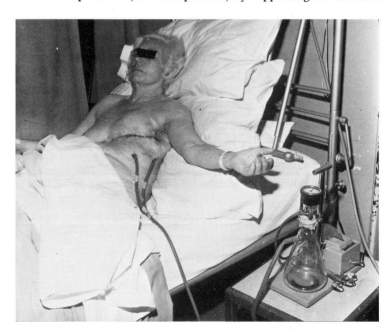

Fig. 17.12. Suction drainage following mastectomy; a Robert's pump is being used.

collar and cuff sling for a few days. Gentle movement is allowed after a week and, once the wound has healed, full movement of the shoulder is rapidly restored. With extended simple mastectomy, it is extremely rare for a patient to have any significant shoulder stiffness or oedema of the arm in the post-operative period. There is no hurry to remove the sutures. Following the mastectomy, the wound is sutured under a good deal of tension and early removal of the stitches may be followed by unpleasant gaping of the wound. It is our practice, therefore, to leave the sutures in place for 3 weeks.

SCREENING FOR BREAST CANCER

There are a number of ways of screening the adult female population in an attempt to diagnose breast cancer at an early stage. These include teaching women to examine themselves at regular intervals, regular medical examinations at 'Well Women Clinics' at the time of cervical smear examinations, thermography and mammography.

The majority of lumps are indeed diagnosed by the patients themselves, and self-examination once monthly is a reasonable suggestion to make to one's patients. Examination by a doctor will detect tumours at any early stage but is naturally time-consuming, expensive and would need to be repeated at least at yearly intervals. Many women, in addition, fail to attend such screening programmes. Thermography depends on the fact that breast cancer emits slightly more heat than normal breast tissue, and this can be picked up on a sensitive recording device. However, similar changes may be given by a variety of benign breast lesions, and in practice, this has proved of little value. Mammography produces a soft tissue X-ray of the breast and minute cancers of the breast can be detected as a small area of density which often shows specks of calcification. Once again, there are the disadvantages of time, expense, and failure of patients to attend for screening or who subsequently default from further appointments. At present an extensive trial in New York is taking place which should provide important data as to whether or not prognosis could be improved by such elaborate screening programmes. If it is shown to be so, then obviously further efforts must be made to introduce such screening programmes into this country regardless of their cost in time and money.

Chapter 18. The skin and its adnexae

Structure and function

Fig. 18.1. The structure of the skin. Note the clearly defined epidermis and the dermis and the adnexae to the skin—the hair follicle, sebaceous gland and sweat gland.

The skin is the largest organ of the body and extends over an area of about 1.5 sq. metres. It continues with the mucous membranes of the body's orifices (nose, mouth, anus, urethra and vagina) and is modified to form the conjunctiva and the ear drum. It is made up of two components, the epidermis and the dermis (Fig. 18.1).

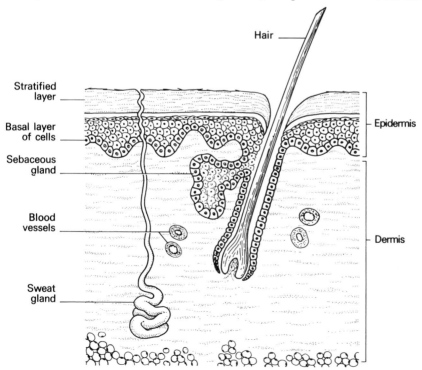

Hair

Stratified layer

Basal layer of cells

Epidermis

Sebaceous gland

Blood vessels

Dermis

Sweat gland

The epidermis is avascular and is formed by a stratified squamous epithelium. This is derived from a single layer of cells termed the basal layer or germinal layer. This continually proliferates cells which become flattened as they pass to the surface, and eventually die, so that the surface layer itself, the *stratum corneum* or horny layer, is made up of dry, flat, dead cells without obvious nuclei. These are continuously flaking away and are being replaced by further cells from below. The stratum corneum is especially thick over the palms of the hands and the soles of the feet, but becomes thickened at any place where the skin is subjected to prolonged and heavy friction.

The dermis is made up of fibro-fatty tissue containing the *sweat glands*, formed by coiled tubes which pass by thin ducts through the dermis to open onto the surface of the epidermis, the *hair roots or follicles*, which are, in fact, downward prolongations of the epidermis, and the *sebaceous glands* which discharge their fatty secretion, sebum, into the hair follicles from which they develop as outgrowths.

Sweat glands are universally distributed over the body, especially over the hands, feet and face. Hair follicles (and therefore their accompanying sebaceous glands) are absent over the palm of the hand and sole of the foot.

The skin has truly remarkable properties and functions, and is far more than being merely the outer wrapping of the body. It is extremely tough and waterproof and, as we have already noted, is able to thicken in areas exposed to excessive stress. By variations in blood flow through the skin and the amount of sweat production, the skin acts as an organ of body temperature regulation. Because of the rich supply of nerve endings in the dermis, it functions as an extensive sensory organ for perception of heat, cold, touch, and pain. Vitamin D is synthesized in the skin by the action of the ultraviolet rays of the sun. Finally, by producing melanin pigment as required, the skin can protect itself from excessive exposure to the sun by becoming pigmented—surely it is one of the most versatile of all the organs of the body!

Skin bacteriology

The skin is constantly being contaminated with bacteria and this is especially so among doctors and nurses in hospital where contact with infected wounds, ulcers and other septic foci is almost inevitable. However, the skin has quite remarkable powers of disinfecting itself, so that within an hour of soiling the healthy skin has got rid of the contaminants and is left with only two types of resident bacteria, the *Saphylococcus albus* and *diphtheroids*, both of which are rarely pathogenic and may actually themselves produce antibiotics which destroy invading organisms. The other mechanisms of skin auto-disinfection are desiccation (most bacteria require a moist environment in order to grow) and also the antibacterial effect of fatty acids derived from skin lipids.

Cleansing of the surgeon's and nurse's hands and of the patient's skin in the area of the operation is designed not to remove the harmless skin commensals but to clear away possible contaminants. This can be carried out effectively either by a vigorous scrub with soap and water or by the application of 0.5% chlorhexidine or iodine in 70% alcohol solution.

Skin infections—boils, carbuncles, cellulitis—see Chapter I.

SEBACEOUS CYST

A sebaceous cyst is a retention cyst produced by obstruction of an orifice of a sebaceous gland. The cyst can occur, therefore, on any part of the skin except those areas devoid of sebaceous glands—the palms of the hands and the soles of the feet. They are particularly common on the scalp (which was the site of the most famous sebaceous cyst of all, that of King George IV, removed by Sir Astley Cooper of Guy's Hospital in 1821), the face, the lobule of the ear and the scrotum. It is an easy diagnosis to make (Fig. 18.2); a

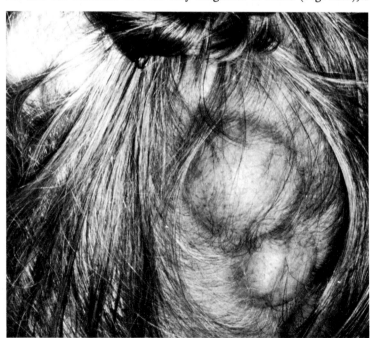

Fig. 18.2. Sebaceous cysts of the scalp.

soft elastic swelling, which is adherent to the skin and which may
show the typical punctum of the obstructed duct at the apex of
the cyst. Sometimes sebaceous material can be seen oozing from it.
The lump may be quite tiny but occasionally reaches 5 cm or more in
diameter before the patient seeks medical advice. The cyst contains
cheesy, whitish-yellow material with an unpleasant smell and this is
the inspissated secretion of the sebaceous gland.

Complications

Left untreated, the cyst is very likely to become infected and may
ulcerate. The ulcerated surface may even resemble a fungating
carcinoma and yet is, of course, still perfectly benign. For this reason
it receives the name 'Cock's peculiar tumour', named after Edward
Cock, a surgeon at Guy's Hospital in the 19th Century. It should be
noted that malignant change does very rarely occur in a sebaceous
cyst to form a sebaceous carcinoma.

Treatment

Sebaceous cysts should always be removed in order to prevent complications. When small, this can be done easily under a local
anaesthetic. If infection has taken place, incision and drainage is
required, followed subsequently by excision of the capsule wall.

    A number of other common cysts occur in the skin and subcutan-
eous tissues. These include:

Fig. 18.3. An implantation
dermoid of the index finger
which followed a puncture injury.

IMPLANTATION DERMOID (Fig. 18.3)

Occasionally a puncture injury may implant a fragment of epithelium into the subcutaneous tissues; growth and degeneration
of these cells results in a cystic swelling. Because of its origin, the
typical implantation dermoid is found on the index finger of a
needle-woman!

EXTERNAL ANGULAR DERMOID

Epithelial cells may become buried along the lines of fusion of the
skin in embryonic life. The commonest place for this to happen is at
the outer border of the eyebrow where the processes going to form
the forehead and the face fuse together. It is very easy to diagnose
this typical little cyst which begins to form in early childhood.

Ganglia are among the commonest of all superficial cysts. They arise from a joint capsule or a tendon sheath and occur especially around the wrist joint, the dorsum of the foot, the anterior aspect of the fingers or along the peroneal tendons on the lateral side of the ankle. The cyst is thin walled and contains a sticky mucoid colourless fluid which exactly resembles Wharton's jelly in the umbilical cord.

Treatment

If the cyst is troubling the patient it should be excised under a general anaesthetic, using a tourniquet to produce a bloodless field. In the old days treatment comprised rupturing the cyst with a blow from the family Bible, but unfortunately recurrence invariably followed this traumatic experience.

Fig. 18.4. A ganglion of the wrist.

PILONIDAL SINUS

The definition of a sinus is a blind track lined with granulation tissue which opens on to a surface; one of the best examples of this is a pilonidal sinus (Fig. 18.5).

The majority occur immediately above the anus in the cleft between the buttocks. The name is derived from the hair which is contained within the sinus, the word meaning 'nest of hair'. Pilonidal sinuses are also found in the clefts between the fingers in barbers (Fig 18.6) and, rarely, in the umbilicus, the perineum, between the toes and in the folds of skin on amputation stumps.

The origin of the pilonidal sinus has been the matter of some controversy but it is now agreed that the sinus forms from implantation of hair into the skin—this fits in with sinuses which develop on the hands of barbers and on the feet of men working in abattoirs,

Fig. 18.5. Multiple pilonidal sinuses. The three small needles have been placed in the orifices of the three hair-containing sinuses. From these, a long track extends headwards and opens as a discharging abscess, which is marked by the larger needle.

Fig. 18.6. A hair-containing pilonidal sinus between the fingers. The patient was a barber.

where the hair comes from the client and from the animals respectively. Once the hair has become implanted it sets up a foreign body reaction which produces a chronic infected sinus. The pilonidal sinus is symptomless until it becomes infected, following which recurrent abscesses occur; these either require drainage or discharge spontaneously.

Treatment

If there is an acute abscess present, this must be drained. In the quiescent phase the track is excised or laid open and allowed to heal by granulation. This may take a considerable time and it is the nurse's duty to ensure that the wound heals soundly from its depth upwards to the surface. If the epithelium is allowed to bridge over the defect, a persistent cavity will form and healing will be delayed. Further recurrence is prevented by keeping the surrounding skin free from hair by frequent cleaning and by rubbing with fine sand paper.

THE NAILS

The nails are the site of a number of common surgical conditions.

PARONYCHIA

A paronychia is an infection of the nail fold, usually of the finger but also quite commonly of the great toe as a complication of ingrowing toe-nail (see below). It is the commonest infection of the hand and makes up about one third of all such infections. The infecting organism is nearly always the *Staphylococcus aureus*, which most commonly invades through a tear in the nail fold ('hang-nail'). The nail fold becomes red, swollen and tender and pus may become visible.

Treatment

If seen at an early stage before pus formation has occurred the infection may subside with antibiotic treatment combined with immobilisation of the finger in a splint and a sling to the arm. If pus is present, however, surgical drainage is required through a small incision which may need, in addition, removal of the base of the nail if the pus is tracking beneath it.

Chronic paronychia may be seen in women who have their hands constantly soaked in water but may also occur as the result of fungus infection of the nail and also in patients with poor peripheral circulation, for example, Raynaud's phenomenon. The affected finger must be kept dry. If fungal infection is present, this is treated with oral griseofulvin.

INGROWING TOE NAIL

This condition is nearly always confined to the great toe. It results from a combination of tight shoes and the habit of cutting the nail downwards into the nail fold so that the sharp cutting edge of the nail grows into the side of the nail-bed with resultant ulceration and infection.

Treatment

If seen before infection has occurred, the patient is advised to cut the nail transversely rather than downwards into the nail fold and a wisp of cotton wool is tucked daily into the side of the nail-bed. These simple steps, combined with the wearing of sensible, wide shoes, enable the nail to grow up out of the fold.

If acute paronychia is present, the nail will require avulsion in order to allow drainage of pus to take place. If the nail continues to give trouble, it should be obliterated by excision of the nail base (Zadek's operation) which prevents regrowth of the nail (Fig. 18.7).

ONYCHOGRYPHOSIS

Any of the toe nails may be affected by this 'ram's horn' deformity of the nail, but the hallux is the commonest site. It usually occurs in the elderly and may follow trauma to the nail-bed.

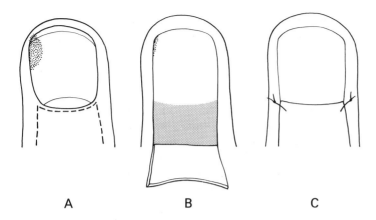

A   B   C

Fig. 18.7. Zadek's operation. A, the skin incisions to expose the nail base; B, the skin flap is reflected, the nail has been avulsed and the nail base (cross-hatched) from which the nail develops has been completely excised; C, the skin flap is now stitched back over the excised nail base.

Treatment

Mild examples can be kept under control by trimming the nail with bone cutting forceps. If the nail is simply avulsed recurrence invariably occurs and the only adequate surgical treatment is removal of the nail and excision of its base to prevent further growth (Zadek's operation).

LESIONS OF THE NAIL BED

There are a number of relatively common conditions which affect the nail-bed. These are:

Haematoma

A crush injury to the terminal phalanx may result in a tense painful haematoma under the nail. This may be accompanied by fracture of the underlying bone. The clot should be evacuated by drilling through the insensitive nail either with a dental drill or a red hot wire. Surprisingly enough a small haematoma may develop without the patient remembering any injury and this may closely mimic a subungual melanoma.

Subungual exostosis

This is a bony lump lying under the nail, usually of the great toe, especially in young adults. The exostosis may ulcerate through the overlying nail to produce an infected granulating mass. An X-ray reveals the exostosis and treatment comprises removal of the nail and the underlying bone nodule.

Melanoma

The nail-bed is a common site for malignant melanoma (see page 413).

Glomus tumour

The nail-bed of the fingers and toes are common sites of this extremely painful lesion, which is a benign tumour arising from a subcutaneous glomus body. These are tiny arteriovenous communications in the skin which are concerned with temperature regulation. The tumour comprises a plexus of blood vessels and nerves which, although tiny, is exquisitely painful on pressure. It is benign and the treatment is surgical excision.

TUMOURS OF THE SKIN AND SUBCUTANEOUS TISSUES

A wide variety of tumours are found in the skin and subcutaneous tissues. The explanation for this is the presence of numerous structures—not only the skin itself but also nerves, fat, blood vessels, sweat glands, etc. from any of which growths may arise.

BENIGN TUMOURS

Papilloma is a common benign tumour, situated on a stalk and often pigmented with melanin. Rarely it may undergo change into a squamous cell carcinoma (see below).

Senile Keratosis. This is a small, hard, scaly tumour which occurs particularly on the face and hands of the elderly; again, this may rarely undergo malignant change.

Seborrhoeic Keratosis is common in the elderly and occurs as a yellowish or brown raised lesion on the face, arms, or trunk. It is often multiple. Because of its pigmentation it is a differential diagnosis from a melanoma.

Verruca Vulgaris. This is the common wart and results from a virus infection of the skin. It is found on the fingers, hands and especially on the sole of the foot (plantar warts). Often it disappears spontaneously but if troublesome a wart may be removed by repeated applications of silver nitrate or may be curetted away under local or general anaesthetic.

SQUAMOUS CELL CARCINOMA

This is a malignant tumour of the skin epithelium (epithelioma) and is particularly likely to appear in the elderly male, especially in skin areas exposed to the sunshine, for example the face and the

Fig. 18.8. An enormous squamous carcinoma of the temporal region. It has invaded the facial nerve and produced a facial paralysis.

backs of the hands (Fig. 18.8). It is common in white men who live in sunny, tropical areas. Not only sun, but anything that chronically irritates the skin may predispose to this malignant change so that squamous cell carcinoma may arise in a chronic varicose ulcer, an unhealed burn or the sinus discharging over an area of chronic osteomyelitis. Such malignant change in a chronic ulcer is termed a *Marjolin's ulcer*. Exposure to irradiation or to pitch, tar or soot also predispose skin to malignant change.

The tumour presents as a typical malignant ulcer with raised everted edges and a central scab. Spread occurs by local infiltration and then by lymphatic drainage to the regional lymph nodes, but blood spread is seen only in very late cases.

Treatment

This comprises either wide excision or radiotherapy and depends rather on the site of the lesion. Involvement of the regional lymph nodes is an indication for their surgical excision.

BASAL CELL CARCINOMA (Rodent ulcer)

This is an extremely common tumour which occurs particularly in elderly males. The vast majority occur on the face above a line which joins the angle of the mouth to the external auditory meatus. Occasionally multiple tumours may be found. Predisposing factors are exposure to sunlight or irradiation and, just like the squamous cell carcinoma, the tumour is particularly common in white-skinned subjects in sunny tropical regions.

The tumour has a typical appearance of pearly nodules over which fine blood vessels are seen (Fig. 18.9). Its edges are raised and rolled. As the nodule enlarges slowly its centre ulcerates and becomes

Examination

The *general examination* of the eye demands little beyond a good light, aided by a magnifying lens, to inspect the front of the eye, and an ophthalmoscope, for looking through the pupil and examining the posterior structures (the 'fundus' of the eye). The light should be directed from the side to avoid dazzling the patient; and, if he is still reluctant to open his eyes adequately, the lids can be withdrawn gently by a finger (one lid at a time).

The *visual acuity* (Fig. 19.4) is then tested for each eye, first without glasses, and then with any distance-glasses he may possess. This is normally done by using letters of standard shape and size called Snellen's types, at a distance of six metres (to exclude all but a negligible amount of focusing). Vision is expressed as a fraction of the normal, the smallest letter usually visible without effort is thus '6/6'; if the patient can only see the letter twice its size, his visual acuity is '6/12'; while the largest letter usually displayed (ten times its size, and which thus should be comfortably visible to the normal-sighted at sixty metres distance), designates a visual acuity of '6/60'. Still poorer vision is indicated by his capacity to count fingers ('C.F.'), see hand movements ('H.M.') and finally just to perceive light ('P.L.'). Near vision is similarly tested by a card being graded sizes of print.

The under surface of the upper lid can easily be inspected by *everting the lid* over a finger or glass rod (Fig. 19.5); this is most easily done by standing behind the patient, who is told to look at the floor, and then pulling the upper lashes forwards and upwards,

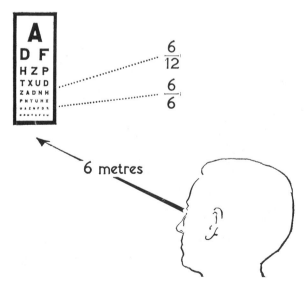

Fig. 19.4. Testing visual acuity.

Nearly all conjunctivites clear away within a week or so (like sore-throats), and treatment is barely necessary; but a broad spectrum antibiotic (such as chloramphenicol or neomycin) is justified if a frank infection is present. It should be remembered that by far the best and safest eye-lotion is a normal flow of tears (which contain their own antiseptic), and that most of the medicaments inserted into the eye do more harm than good. If the conjunctivitis persists, this may be due to the continued presence of an allergic irritant (such as pollens or cosmetics), or constant re-infection from a neigh-bouring inflammation, as in the lash roots (a *blepharitis*) or tear-sac (a *dacryocystitis*), or from a distortion of the lid margins (an *entropion* or *ectropion*).

Blepharitis

This is a very common eye-nuisance (Fig. 19.8), and generally is a sequel to a dry seborrhoeic skin (the Meibomian glands being simply enlarged sebaceous glands). Such patients tend to have reddish lid margins which become redder (and variably irritable) in smoky atmospheres, and when physical reserves are depleted (as after 'flu or a 'night-out'). The most effective treatment of this (as of simple allergic conjunctivitis) is the use of steroid drops, which will normally suppress the inflammation and therewith the symptoms, inserting these as often as necessary; they can be effectively combined with an antibiotic (e.g. prednisolone with neomycin drops) against any secondary bacterial infection. However, they must be used with caution, since they may promote the damaging corneal ulcers due to the herpes simplex virus, and they may also aggravate a simple glaucoma (although this is rare before middle age, by which time the

Fig. 19.8. Ulcerative blepharitis.

Fig. 19.9. External stye.

blepharitis is usually less troublesome). Such a blepharitis may lead to an accumulation of pus within an isolated eyelash follicle, an *external stye* (Fig. 19.9), or down a Meibomian gland, as an *internal stye*. Whereas the former (like any furuncle elsewhere) clears in a few days, irrespective of treatment, the Meibomian infection may leave a distended Meibomian cyst, (Fig. 19.10) which requires surgical evacuation (Fig. 19.11).

Fig. 19.10. Meibomian cyst.

Fig. 19.11. Evacuation of meibomian cyst.

Dacryocystitis

This is also fairly common, especially in middle-aged women, infection having passed up the nasolacrimal duct from a nasopharyngitis. Very occasionally the inflammation is acute, causing a tender swelling medial to the inner angle of the eye. Far more commonly it simply produces a gradual obstruction to the drainage of tears, which increasingly dribble onto the cheek, particularly in cold winds.

The treatment of such a watering eye first entails syringing of saline through the lower canaliculus (Fig. 19.12). This shows whether there is a nasolacrimal duct obstruction, and in the early stages may in fact clear the blocked passage; astringent drops or lotions (such as zinc sulphate $\frac{1}{2}$ per cent) may then help to reduce the watering. If the epiphora is sufficiently troublesome and has not yielded to several syringings, an operation may be justified; ideally this should be a dacryocystorhinostomy (Fig. 19.13), fashioning a new opening between the sac and the middle nasal meatus, but in the old and feeble, especially where regurgitation of pus is the main trouble, a dacryocystectomy may suffice to ease the symptoms by simply removing the source of conjunctival re-infection. Probing the naso-lacrimal duct is of value only in the absence of established infection—as in infants when the duct has failed to open-up after birth.

Fig. 19.12. Syringing the lacrimal sac.

Fig. 19.13. Dacryocysto-rhinostomy.

Entropion

A rolling inwards of the lid margin can cause a conjunctivitis, since the in-turned lashes will then abrade the underlying conjunctiva and cornea. In tropical countries it is usually caused by scarring of the under-surface of the upper lid, as the sequel to a common and damaging infection called trachoma; but in temperate countries it is usually a spastic entropion of the lower lid, in people who are consistently screwing-up their eyes (Fig. 19.14). Both types require an operation; in the cicatricial entropion in order to straighten the buckled tarsal plate (an epilation of the ingrowing lashes will bring temporary relief), and in the spastic entropion to re-orientate the spastic fibres of the orbicularis muscle.

Fig. 19.14. Spastic entropion.

Ectropion

An outward rolling of the lower lid margin (Fig. 19.15), is conversely the sequel to a weakened orbicularis muscle, as after a facial palsy,

Fig. 19.15. Atonic ectropion.

Fig. 19.16. Corneal ulcer. (This ulcer, in the upper cornea, is so severe that pus has collected in the lower part of the anterior chamber.)

allowing a stagnant lake of tears to collect behind the lid. These soon become infected, causing a chronic conjunctivitis (which itself aggravates the ectropion). Surgical re-ajdustment is again indicated.

A severe conjunctival infection may spread to involve the cornea, or the cornea may be directly abraded (as by an in-turned eyelash, a twig, or a foreign-body), provoking a *corneal ulcer* (Fig. 19.16). The pain is then more severe, the sight may be blurred, and the ulcer can sometimes be seen as a faint opalescence on the corneal surface; otherwise its presence can be made evident by inserting a drop of fluorescein, which turns the abraded or ulcerated area bright green. A little antibiotic ointment, followed by a firm pad to keep the upper lid splinted over the damaged cornea, will allow most simple abrasions to heal within a day or two. But some ulcers may be very slow in healing (especially the dendritic ulcer, caused by the herpes simplex virus); and if antibiotic or antiviral drops, atropine and a pad prove insufficient, cautery with carbolic acid may be needed, or even suturing together of the eylids or a corneal graft. When the ulcer has healed, a corneal scar remains, which if extensive, may impair the sight. Most corneal scars clear to a limited extent in time. But dense scars may persist and so reduce the vision that a corneal graft is justified—replacing a disc of the scarred cornea with a similar disc of cornea from a bequeathed eye (Fig. 19.17). Although technically exacting, this operation has become a straight-forward procedure in experienced hands, and a dramatic improvement in vision may be gained.

Inflammation of the inner eye

This usually involves the whole uveal tract; and therefore is labelled a *uveitis*, or simply an *iritis*, when only its anterior segment is apparently affected. In an "acute iritis" the eye is again red and pain-

Fig. 19.17. Corneal graft (A). The disc of scarred cornea excised and replaced with a clear disc (B), which is sutured in place (C).

ful, but the pain is a constant ache (not just the grittiness of a conjunctivitis) and the congestion is largely restricted to the blood-vessels around the cornea (nearest to the iris-root). The iris itself may be visibly affected, with festooning of the pupil (Fig. 19.18) where adhesions have tethered the pupil margin to the underlying lens. An iritis is serious, since an inflammatory exudate is retained within the eye, so impairing the vision; and this damage to sight may be permanent, if the inflammation is not checked—mainly by treatment with steroids such as prednisolone, (as drops, ointment or tablets) supplemented by atropine, to keep the pupil dilated.

When the brunt of the inflammation falls on the posterior segment of the uveal tract, the choroid, there is no pain or congestion, but only a variable blurring of sight. Such a *choroiditis* is often unrecognised until, years later, the classical scars are noticed through the ophthalmoscope.

Uveitis may stem from many causes. It often is associated with rheumatism elsewhere in the body or generalised infections (as

Fig. 19.18. Acute iritis.

syphilis or tuberculosis); but in the majority of cases no underlying cause can be found.

One other affection of the interior of the eyeball may cause a painful, red eye—the strangulated eyeball of an *acute glaucoma* (Fig. 19.19). Acute glaucoma is the sequel to a blockage to the exit passages of aqueous humour, so that this cannot escape from the eyeball into the veins outside, and the pressure within the eye then rises till the eye becomes very hard. The vessels around the iris-root again becomes congested, but appearing dusky in colour (unlike the brick-red circumcorneal congestion in an acute iritis), and through the waterlogged cornea the interior of the eye appears greenish (hence the word 'glaucoma'); and the sight is progressively blurred. Immediate treatment is necessary to relieve the pressure, by constricting the pupil with eserine or pilocarpine drops, by reducing the secretion of aqueous with Diamox tablets, and by sucking water out

Fig. 19.19. Acute glaucoma.

of the eye through reducing the osmotic pressure of the blood with a draught of glycerol or intravenous mannitol. Very occasionally the pressure remains high and a decompressing operation is needed.

FAILING SIGHT

Blindness in England is caused, in the main, by three diseases: cataract (23%), simple glaucoma and senile degenerations of the retina. These are all diseases of the elderly which gradually erode the sight, but whereas cataracts can be remedied, glaucoma can only be arrested, and retinal degenerations ruthlessly progress. Sometimes the loss of sight is more rapid, as after a detachment of the retina or damage to the optic nerves (an 'optic neuritis' is usually the first evidence of disseminated sclerosis, or the nerves may be compressed by a brain tumour). Occasionally it happens suddenly, as the sequel to a thrombosis of the retinal vessels or a haemorrhage within the eye.

Cataract

The lens of the eye is transparent, but in old age it tends to become white (in the same way that the hair tends to become white), and some degree of lens opacity or 'cataract' is found in most people of over sixty, although in the vast majority of these it never progresses to the point where it materially interferes with sight. Very occasionally cataracts may form in younger age-groups, usually as the sequel to inflammation, injury (by concussion, penetrating wounds, noxious drugs or radiation) or sometimes as a congenital blemish.

Cataracts are the commonest cause of failing sight in old age. When advanced, they are easily observed as a grey opacity within the pupil (Fig. 19.20); but in the earlier stages can readily be seen as an irregular silhouette with the ophthalmoscope (Fig. 19.21), or in the beam of the corneal microscope (the 'slit-lamp'). The only effective

Fig. 19.20. Mature cataract.

Fig. 19.21. The wedge-shaped opacities of a peripheral cataract standing-out as a silhouette when viewed through an ophthalmoscope.

treatment for a cataract is to extract it by operation (Figs 19.22, 19.23), and this is justified if the sight has become so impaired that reading and close work are rendered difficult. After removal of a cataractous lens, the retinal image is necessarily out of focus unless a similar lens, in the form of spectacles or a contact-lens (or, in exceptional cases, an intraocular lenticulus), is used as a replacement, and since these artificial lenses all introduce problems of their own (judgement of depth may become difficult and the two eyes may not readily work in unison, the spectacle lenses are large and heavy and the contact-lenses difficult to manage, and intraocular lenses are frequently damaging to the eye), an operation is rarely justified when only one eye is cataractous.

Fig. 19.22. Cataract extraction— the sutures are placed on the corneo-scleral incision, ready for closure, and the cataract lifted out by holding its capsule with forceps.

This operation, although the commonest in ophthalmology, and possibly the oldest in medical history, demands considerable experience because of the diversity of operative and post-operative complications, but overall about nine patients in ten recover normal reading vision.

Simple glaucoma

After middle-age a silting-up of the spaces through which the aqueous percolates out of the eye may lead to a very gradual increase in the intra-ocular pressure, as opposed to the rapid increase in pressure of an 'acute glaucoma' which follows sudden obstruction of the exit passages; and in time the more vulnerable cells in the retina (those towards the retinal periphery) become destroyed, so that the sight is gradually whittled away. As this erosion of vision is mainly off-centre, the central vision remains unaffected until most of the 'visual field' has been irreparably lost, and the patient who can still read the smaller letters, may yet be unaware that his peripheral sight has gone (Fig. 19.24).

Simple glaucoma is usually diagnosed by the excavated appearance of the optic disc (the front-end of the optic nerve, where it lies exposed near the centre of the retina Fig. 19.25). This is often discovered on a routine check with an ophthalmoscope, and then confirmed by finding that the pressure is raised (through a pressure-gauge placed against the cornea) and by plotting the field of vision with a perimeter (Fig. 19.6).

Fig. 19.23. Cataract extraction—the cataract can also be extracted by freezing it to the end of a probe.

Fig. 19.24. Field loss in simple glaucoma, as charted on a perimeter (Fig. 19.6). The black area represents the extent of vision lost in the right eye.

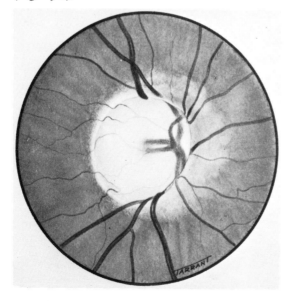

Fig. 19.25. Cupping of the optic disc from simple glaucoma.

The pressure can normally be kept below normal (which should prevent further erosion of the visual field) by measures similar to those used in acute glaucoma—Pilocarpine drops (usually 2%, t.d.s.), and Diamox tablets. Should these still fail to arrest the field-loss, the pressure may be reduced more radically by an operation which fashions a channel (a "sclerectomy") in the sclera at the corneal margin, through which the aqueous can drain away more freely into the lymphatics beneath the conjunctiva (Fig. 19.26).

Retinal degenerations

The large majority are simply dystrophies, and the result of ageing in a very specialised tissue, where dying cells cannot be replaced; there is no effective treatment, but since most dystrophies only affect the central area (the macula), these old people can still get about quite well, although reading may be rendered impossible. Other degenerative changes are the sequel to advanced diabetes or hypertension, and a host of other disturbances to the retina and choroid are equally revealed through the ophthalmoscope (Fig. 19.27).

Retinal detachment

This is relatively common, and causes a dramatic loss of sight. It is the sequel to a tear in the retina, either following injury to the eye, or from certain degenerative changes, such as occur in high myopia (short-sightedness) (Fig. 19.28). The retina peels off the wall of the eyeball like torn wall-paper in a room, and the retinal cells will soon die as they become separated from their nutrient blood in the choroid, unless the retina is replaced by operation. This usually involves indenting the overlying sclera, (usually by a tight encircling band of silicone) so that a fold of this is pushed forwards to meet the

Fig. 19.26. Sclerectomy—a segment of iris root is excised, and then a small piece of sclera is excised at the corneal margin, to allow the aqueous to escape beneath the conjuctiva.

Fig. 19.27. The fundus in senile macular dystrophy.

Fig. 19.28. Retinal detachment—the upper half of the retina has fallen forwards, following the development of the large U-shaped tear.

detached retina, and then glueing these together by applications of a freezing-probe (Fig. 19.29). If treated early enough the majority of retinas can be replaced, although some loss of sight will be permanent.

Thrombosis of the central retinal artery or vein

These are both fairly common causes of sudden loss of sight, or of part of the sight if only one of the arterial or venous branches is

Fig. 19.29. Retinal detachment operation. A tight strap encircling the eyeball indents the sclera, and to this ridge the detached retina can be made to adhere.

involved, and they usually stem from cardiovascular degeneration in the elderly. Immediate treatment very occasionally clears an arterial occlusion (if from spasm or embolus), and a limited recovery is likely after a venous block.

Haemorrhages in the retina

These are common sequels to various blood disorders (hypertension, diabetes, anaemia, leukaemia, etc.) but the haemorrhages are usually small, and, unless involving the macular area, unnoticed by the patient. Any of these may erupt into the vitreous, leaving the eye almost completely blind, and clearance of such a haemorrhage may be slow and incomplete.

SQUINT

Our eyes are kept parallel by a complicated reflex, established during infancy, in the interests of single vision; but when they fall out of alignment they are said to 'squint'. Usually they deviate along a horizontal axis (so that the eyes converge or diverge) but occasionally there is a vertical squint, with one eye looking above its fellow.

The simplest form of squint is that due to injury to any of the twelve muscles that govern the eye-movements, or of the nerves that motivate them. The affected eye cannot then rotate into the direction of this paralysed muscle, and the squint is increasingly obvious on attempting to look in this direction. Such *paralytic squints* are thus commonly the sequel to head injuries (especially with facial fractures), or tumours and haemorrhages within the brain, and they normally recover if the underlying damage is cleared. Thus all that is necessary in treatment is to cover the affected eye (usually by sticky paper over the appropriate spectacle lens) so as to prevent the double-vision that is inevitably provoked.

Much more frequently the squint starts in the first few years of life, when the child can no longer sustain the subconscious effort of holding the eyes straight under the stress of an illness (like measles), or of adaptation to an emotional situation (like the arrival of a younger baby). These are labelled *concomitant squints*, since the angle of deviation does not vary when the child looks in different directions. Once established, such squints tend to persist, since the vision of the squinting eye usually becomes suppressed (so as to avoid a tiresome double-vision), and the eye is then said to have become 'lazy'. Such childhood squints are usually convergent (Fig. 19.30), although divergent squints are not rare (generally arising in slightly older children).

Although in most children with 'cross-eyes', the convergence tends to become less marked in later childhood, such a natural cure is nearly always at the expense of spending the rest of their life with a lazy eye, in which full vision could have been restored (normally by sticking a patch over the spectacle lens of the master-eye and forcing the child to use the lazy eye (Fig. 19.31), if only this had been done in time—before the age of seven; for by the age of about ten, no further recovery of vision in the lazy eye can be anticipated.

Fig. 19.30. Convergent squint.

The treatment of the childhood concomitant squint entails the use of spectacles if the child is sufficiently long-sighted, since correction of this long-sightedness often reduces the degree of convergence), then patching the master-eye, if its fellow is becoming lazy. Orthoptic exercises will thereafter help to build-up the child's capacity for using the eyes in unison (as an incentive for the eyes to stay straight). If the squint is still marked, an operation is needed to align the eyes, usually by recessing the medial rectus muscle (dividing the insertion, and sewing it to the sclera about 5 mm

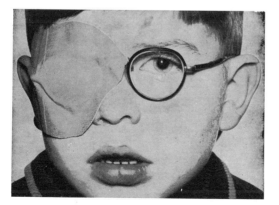

Fig. 19.31. Convergent squint—occlusion of the master-eye by elastoplast on the spectacles.

Fig. 19.32. Convergent squint operation—recession of lateral rectus. The muscle is cut free from its insertion (A), and sutured to the sclera 5 mm behind this (B).

further back) and resecting the lateral rectus (excising about 5 mm of its length) (Figs. 19.32, 19.33). Such a straightening operation may be needed when only a few months old, if the squint is sufficiently gross and constant that the eyes cannot hope to be used in unison otherwise; and it can equally be done at any time of life purely for cosmetic reasons. But, because it is only during the first few years of life that a lazy eye can only be taught to see again and the eyes to work in unison, and because a sudden squint may be the first evidence of other disorders' all squinting children should be seen be an eye-doctor as soon as the squint is noticed.

SPECTACLES

Failing sight need not be a sequel to organic changes in the eyeball, but may just be due to one of the four so-called Refractive Errors which result in an out-of-focus image on the retina, and which can be requited by spectacles.

Presbyopia is simply the result of the natural weakening of our focusing power (from the ciliary muscle) as we grow older, so that,

Fig. 19.33. Convergent squint operation—resection of medial rectus (the muscle is cut free from its insertion, and a segment of it, held in the clamp, is excised, before re-suturing).

by the age of about forty-five, the book must be held farther away from the eye than the normal reading-range. This can be compensated by weak convex spectacles, which will need to be strengthened a little every few years.

Sometimes the eyeball is rather shorter or longer than the normal: the short eyeball renders the eye long-sighted or *hypermetropic*, since some of the focusing power must be used-up in bringing the focus of the image forwards to the (abnormally forward-placed) retina. This leaves less of a reserve of focusing-power for near vision. Such patients will need the help of reading glasses before the usual age of forty-five (in other words, they have a premature presbyopia), and the effort of reading without glasses may cause eye-fatigue.

When the eyeball is too long, the eye is short-sighted or *myopic*, since, although near objects can be seen clearly, distant objects can only be brought to a focus on the (abnormally backward-placed) retina by wearing a concave spectacle lens. Such myopes do not experience eye-fatigue, but simply have a blurred view of the distance unless they wear glasses. Myopia tends to run in families, and starts usually in later childhood, increasing in degree until growth stops. Its progress is determined by one's heredity, and this cannot be influenced by wearing glasses, exercises, drugs, diet or any other fanciful remedies or restrictions.

The eyeball is never a perfect sphere, and apart from being a little too long or short, a little flattening, labelled *astigmatism*, is almost universal. Only very occasionally is this enough to cause headaches or slightly blur the retinal image and so justify special correcting spectacles.

It must be emphasized that the vast majority of headaches bear no relationship to refractive errors, and also that the eyes themselves can never be damaged by uncorrected or wrongly-corrected refractive errors. Spectacle lenses can be darkened, like sun-glasses, and very occasionally a genuine photophobia justifies this, but the vast majority of dark glasses are sought in the hope of protecting a frail psyche or concealing a guiltful one from the harsh or revealing light of day.

PRACTICAL NOTES ON TREATMENT OF EXTERNAL DISEASES

1. Toilet to the eye

Use lint swabs, (folded, with the fluffy side inward) soaked in normal saline. The unaffected eye is cleansed first (there is often some 'sympathetic' discharge in the fellow eye, and this warns the patient what to expect when his tender eye is touched). The patient is told to close the eye gently ('as if in sleep') and the upper lids are wiped gently from the nasal corner outwards. The patient is told to open the eye, and the lower lid margins are wiped likewise; this is repeated until all discharge is removed. The swab must not touch the eye itself.

2. Instillation of drops and ointment

Careful check of label (this is often helped by coloured labels: Red = pupil-dilators, Blue = pupil-constrictors, Orange = antiseptics). Warn the patient that the drop or ointment is coming, and ask him to look upwards. Pull the lower lid gently down and insert into the 'gutter' behind it (but not onto the cornea) one or two of the drops (Fig. 19.34) or squeeze in a small strip of the ointment. Ointment has the advantage of lingering rather longer before the tears wash it all away, and so exerting its effect longer, and also of being mildly lubricating to a roughened conjunctival surface; but the ointment itself is sometimes irritating, and it makes the sight blurry for a few minutes. When treating themselves, some patients find ointment the easier to insert.

Fig. 19.34. Insertion of eye-drops.

3. Eye irrigation

This is rarely necessary, unless there is a frank discharge that needs clearance, as routine bathing of the eye does not benefit the eye, and should normally be discouraged. When noxious chemicals have entered the eye, the head should be promptly submerged in a basin or pail of water, and the lids forcibly opened.

4. Removal of a foreign body

The patient should be recumbent or semi-recumbent, with good illumination. Examine, with a magnifying spectacle, to see if the foreign body is impacted on the cornea. If none is present, evert the upper lid, lest it is retained there (and whence it can readily be whisked away).

If there is an impacted corneal foreign body, insert a drop of local anaesthetic (e.g. amethocaine 1%). Attempt to dislodge it with twisted wisp of cotton wool. If (as is usual) this fails, excavate it with a fine, flattened needle. Insert antibiotic ointment and pad the eye. Refer the patient to an eye-surgeon if the eye is not white and comfortable the following day.

5. Syringing of tear-ducts

Insert a drop of local anaesthetic (amethocaine 1%). The patient should be recumbent or semi-recumbent, and good illumination is needed. Expose the lacrimal punctum by everting the medial end of the lower lid with the left forefinger. Insert Nettleship's dilator gently, passing it vertically downwards for about 2 mm then directing it medially and twisting it slightly for a further few millimetres. Then withdraw it. Insert a cannula, fitted onto a 2 ml syringe, filled with saline. Inject the saline. If the duct is patent, the fluid will enter freely, and its passage into the nose is usually confirmed by a gulp from the patient. Otherwise, it may flow back along the lower lacrimal canaliculus or squirt out of the upper one.

NOTES ON MANAGEMENT OF MAJOR SURGICAL CASES

Pre-operative

The patient is admitted the day before the operation to allow adjustment to hospital routine, general medical check (especially blood-pressure, urine, cough, etc.), and preparation of the eye. Some surgeons prefer the lashes to be cut (with fine scissors, smeared with

Vaseline to catch the severed lashes), and pre-operative cultures to be prepared (via a sterilised platinum loop which gently scrapes the lower trough (fornix) of conjunctiva, behind the everted lower lid, and transfers the scraping to a blood-agar plate). Prophylactic drops are then inserted, usually chloramphenicol 0.5% t.d.s. to both eyes. the scraping to a blood-agar plate). Prophylactic drops are then inserted, usually chloramphenicol 0.5% t.d.s. to both eyes.

A mild aperient may be given on the day before operation, and a sedative on the previous night. On the morning before operation the patient has a bath, long hair is combed and plaited, and male patients are encouraged to shave.

Premedication for cataract surgery usually starts about an hour before the operation. If he is having a local anaesthetic, guttae cocaine 4%, adrenaline 0.1%, homatropine 1% and chloramphenicol 0.5% are usually instilled every few minutes for twenty minutes, and then at ten-minute intervals until the operation. The eye is meanwhile covered with a pad. If a general anaesthetic is used, the cocaine is omitted. Similar drops are normally used before operations for retinal detachments. For glaucoma surgery, the homatropine and adrenaline are normally omitted, and pilocarpine included. But there are many variations practised.

The eye requiring operation is usually marked with a cross on the forehead; and this is also indicated on a label (along with the patient's name and age) fixed to his wrist.

Post-operative care

The patient will normally be returned to the ward, having the eye covered by a pad, a stiff cartella shield, and a bandage; after a local anaesthetic, two or more pillows are normally permitted. The locker should be placed on the side of his uncovered eye and the nurse should also approach his bed from this side. Care is needed that the patient does not knock his bandaged eye, move around unduly, cough or vomit.

The first dressing is normally done on the following morning; drops of antibiotic solution (and, after cataracts, atropine) are instilled. Thereafter the patient may wash his own face and feed himself (under supervision). Smoking should be curtailed (there is an added fire-risk from smoking in bed, with one eye bandaged). Patients are usually allowed to sit out of bed during bed-making directly after the first dressing, although carefully avoiding stooping or sudden movements, and to use the toilet on the third day; and all being well he may leave hospital a day or two later. Dark glasses are usually ordered after the eye-pad is discarded, since such eyes are light-sensitive, but these glasses can be discarded as soon as the patient is comfortable without them.

After glaucoma operations the regime is similar but less exacting. After corneal grafts and detachment operations the stay may be more prolonged, and strict rest in bed (even in a specific position) may be required, especially in detachment cases, according to the site and extent of the detachment. After squint operations, since the eyeball has not been opened, only a few days hospital stay is needed, simply for toilet to the eye and antiseptic applications.

Chapter 20. Diseases of the ear, nose and throat

THE EAR

Anatomy and physiology

The auricle or pinna is composed of cartilage, the closely adherent perichondrium, and skin. It is developed from six tubercles, and fistulae or other congenital abnormalities may occur if these tubercles fail to fuse.

The external auditory meatus, about one inch in length, is lined with skin which is supported by cartilage in its outer third and bone in its inner two-thirds.

The tympanic membrane or drum-head, commonly known as the 'ear-drum' (Fig. 20.1.) is composed of three layers—skin, fibrous tissue and mucous membrane—and is stretched across the medial end of the external auditory meatus.

The tympanic cavity, which contains the three ossicles—malleus, incus and stapes—communicates anteriorly with the nasopharynx via the *Eustachian tube* and posteriorly with the *mastoid antrum* and *air-cells* (Fig. 20.2). It is in close proximity to numerous anatomical structures including the facial nerve, internal carotid artery, sigmoid sinus and dura mater of the middle and posterior cranial fossae. Its detailed anatomy may be referred to in the standard anatomical text-books and, briefly, the function of its contents is to transmit vibrations of sound (which have been collected by the auricle and external meatus) from the tympanic membrane to the inner-ear or organ of Corti. This complex and incredibly difficult mechanical task is achieved with superb precision by the lever mechanism of the ossicles, the *malleus* moving with the tympanic membrane and in turn actuating the *incus,* whereby movement is imparted to the

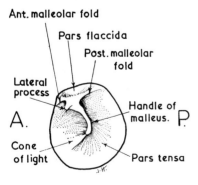

Fig. 20.1. The normal tympanic membrane (left).

Ant. malleolar fold

Pars flaccida

Post. malleolar fold

Lateral process

Handle of malleus.

A.

P.

Cone of light

Pars tensa

stapes, and thus eventually the fluids of the internal ear are set in motion, as the stapedial footplate is loosely sealed into the oval window.

CLINICAL EXAMINATION OF THE EAR

The ear is often examined in hospital clinics with the aid of the surgeon's head-mirror and small metal aural speculae into which may be fitted a pneumatic or Siegle's speculum—the latter enabling the examiner to vary the external air pressure on the tympanic membrane or drumhead and thus reveal small perforations. On the other hand the surgeon may choose to use an electric otoscope (auriscope) and certainly the latter is most convenient at the bedside.

Electric otoscopes require care and attention, and every effort must be made to ensure that the battery is well up to standard, the bulb is functioning and the speculum fits. Even then a poor view of the meatus and tympanic membrane may result, and in such cases the bulb holder may have become bent.

Assuming that a good instrument and a little tuition are available, a reasonably good view of the drum-head with its pearly lustre (Fig. 20.1) should be obtained without undue difficulty by the novice, though it is true that some external auditory canals are both narrow and tortuous and present problems to the most experienced observers.

Testing the hearing

Hearing tests range from the most simple to the most sophisticated, and in the first place many examiners make an approximate assessment of hearing acuity by asking the patient to repeat words which have been whispered or spoken at conversational level. Even in such a simple test as this precautions are necessary to avoid serious errors. The possibility of lip-reading must be excluded, and in the case of a patient with good hearing in one ear and moderate or severe deafness in the other, great care is necessary to exclude the better hearing ear from the test, not as one might suppose by blocking its canal, but by applying a continuous noise to it—in the clinic—by means of the Bárány noise apparatus (Fig. 20.3).

This important manoeuvre is known as masking and is used in different forms in many audiological tests.

Tuning fork tests are employed to detect not the degree but the type of hearing loss—Conductive or Sensorineural. *Conductive deafness* being present when some disorder prevents sound waves reaching

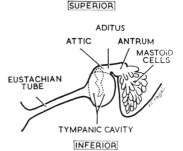

Fig. 20.2. The tympanic cavity showing its relationship to Eustachian tube and mastoid cells. The tympanic membrane and malleus are indicated by broken lines.

Fig. 20.3. Bárány noise apparatus.

Fig. 20.4. Conductive deafness is caused by an abnormality of the external or middle ear (shaded).

Fig. 20.5. Sensorineural deafness is caused by an abnormality of the inner ear or auditory nerve (shaded).

the inner ear (Fig. 20.4), and *sensorineural deafness* signifying a disorder of the inner ear or auditory nerve (Fig. 20.5).

Examples of some of the causes of conductive deafness are wax, middle ear disease and otosclerosis and of sensorineural deafness are Menière's disease, senile deafness and VIIIth nerve tumour.

In Rinne's test the tuning fork is normally heard better when it is held near the ear than when its base is applied to the mastoid process, though in conductive deafness the findings are reversed owing to the presence of some impediment to the normal magnification provided by the middle ear mechanism. In Weber's test the base of a tuning fork is held on the vertex and sound is heard in the more deaf ear in conductive deafness or the less deaf ear in sensorineural deafness.

In pure-tone audiometry a series of tones ranging from 125 c.p.s (cycles per second) to 12,000 c.p.s. are fed into the patient's ear by means of a headphone (Fig. 20.6). The volume of these tones can be varied by the operator whose object is to discover the threshold at which the patient can only just hear any particular tone. By this

Fig. 20.6. Audiometry. The patient is signalling that he can hear a test tone.

Fig. 20.7. Audiogram showing good hearing.

means a graph may be produced showing hearing loss by both air and bone conduction for a number of different frequencies (Figs. 20.7, 8 and 9). Such a graph is of great help in diagnosis and in estimating the degree of hearing-loss. Pure tone audiometry is practised widely, but in certain centres more sophisticated audiological methods such as speech, Békésy, impedance and evoked response audiometry are available.

Conditions of the auricle (pinna)

Congenital deformity may occur in the form of 'bat ears' in which the outstanding auricles are very unsightly and cause their owner to be the butt of much ragging in childhood. They are corrected surgically between the ages of four and six years. Other congenital anomalies are seen in the form of accessory auricle, fistulae around the ear or variations in the size of the auricle.

Fig. 20.8. Audiogram showing conductive deafness. Horizontal scale shows the frequency in cycles per second. Air conduction ×, bone conduction].

Fig. 20.12. Direct stream of solution along the roof of the external auditory meatus.

Fig. 20.13. Jobson Horne wool carrier. An invaluable instrument.

the usual method of removing wax, is an operation which almost any doctor or nurse is expected to carry out with skill, and attention must be paid to the following points:

1. *History.* Has the patient had a discharging ear? If any possibility of a dry perforation, do not syringe.

2. *Inspection.* If wax seems very hard always soften over a period of one week by using warm olive oil drops nightly.

3. *Towels.* Protect patient well with towels and mackintoshes. He will not be amused by having his shirt soaked.

4. *Lighting.* Use a head-mirror or lamp.

5. *Solution.* Sodium bicarbonate, 4–5 grammes to the pint, or normal saline, are ideal. Tap-water is satisfactory.

6. *Temperature.* This is vital. It should be 38°C (100°F). Any departure of more than a few degrees may precipitate the patient on floor with vertigo.

7. *Syringe.* A metal syringe is considered by some to be the most easily controlled, but others prefer rubber syringes of the Bacon type. In any case make sure that the nozzle is firmly attached to the syringe and is prevented from entering too far into the external meatus. Tympanic membranes have been ruptured by a deeply penetrating nozzle.

8. *Direction.* Direct stream of solution along roof of auditory canal (Fig. 20.12).

9. *Inspection.* After removal of wax, inspect thoroughly to make sure none remains. This advice might seem superfluous, but is frequently ignored.

10. *Drying.* Mop any excess solution from meatal canal. Stagnation predisposes to otitis externa.

Otitis externa is a diffuse inflammation of the skin lining the external auditory meatus and is characterised by irritation, scanty discharge and tendency to relapse. It has a predilection for certain persons, particularly those with a tendency to eczema and is not infrequently seen in Europeans visiting the tropics. There is usually a mixed infection with several types of microorganism, bacteria and fungi, and the bacteriology is investigated by submitting an aural swab for culture.

Aural toilet is carried out meticulously with the aid of the Jobson Horne wool carrier (Fig. 20.13) dressed with fluffed-out cotton wool, and following cleansing a dressing soaked in a solution such as 1.5 per cent hydrocortisone with neomycin is inserted with aural dressing forceps (Fig. 20.14) and left for 24 hours.

Following this initial treatment various medicaments in the form of ear drops may be advised and the patient is instructed to avoid scratching the ears and to prevent water from entering them. Repeated attention may be required.

Fig. 20.14. Keen's aural dressing forceps.

Malignant disease of the external auditory meatus may be first manifested by a bloodstained discharge from the ear. Intractable pain may be a feature of this relentless affliction and treatment is by radiotherapy or radical surgery in which an attempt may be made to remove the entire ear and temporal bone.

Conditions of the middle ear

Acute otitis media is a common condition in childhood and is most frequently associated with acute tonsillitis, common cold, influenza, measles (and other infectious diseases of childhood), sinusitis and enlarged and infected adenoids. The infecting organisms are usually streptococci, pneumococci or staphylococci which arrive in the middle ear via the Eustachian tube.

The symptoms are earache and deafness and the temperature may be high. Examination reveals a red or bulging tympanic membrane and if treatment is delayed the membrane may burst with the release of pus (sometimes blood-stained). The ear-discharge (*otorrhoea*) may in fact be so profuse as to drip out of the ear.

Treatment varies according to the severity of the infection. In the mildest cases analgesics such as aspirin may suffice but in most cases antibiotics, such as penicillin, are necessary and occasionally—in the case of a persistently bulging tympanic membrane—myringotomy is required (Figs. 20.15 and 16). In this operation, which is

LAT. SEM. CANAL

FACIAL N.

OVAL WINDOW

PROMONTORY

Fig. 20.15. Myringotomy. Coronal section of left ear.

Fig. 20.16. Myringotomy. The extent of the incision.

Fig. 20.17. A large central perforation as seen in the mucosal type of C.S.O.M.

carried out under general anaesthesia, an incision is made in the tympanic membrane with a sharp and delicate knife known as a myringotome.

Chronic otitis media may ensue in some cases of acute otitis media which do not undergo complete resolution. This is particularly liable to occur if nasal or pharyngeal sepsis persists, or if lowered resistance, owing perhaps to malnutrition or anaemia, is present. In the so called *mucosal* type of infection there is mucoid discharge from a central perforation of the tympanic membrane (Fig. 20.17) and in the *bony* type of disease there may be purulent evil-smelling discharge from a marginal perforation (Fig. 20.18). The latter form of *chronic suppurative otitis media* (C.S.O.M.) is sometimes associated with the formation of cholesteatoma—an accumulation of epithelial debris—or with aural granulations. Serious complications of middle-ear infection are more liable to occur in the course of this type of infection than in the mucosal form.

Treatment consists in the first place of local toilet, the eradication of sepsis from the upper respiratory tract and attention to the general state of health. Aural toilet is carried out two or three times daily, ideally by skilled personnel using a Jobson Horne wool carrier. Obviously such attention can only be obtained in clinics but the intelligent patient can often be taught to mop the ear with orange sticks dressed with fluffed-out cotton wool. After the ear has been thoroughly cleaned, various preparations in the form of ear-drops may be instilled.

Operative treatment is indicated when the disease progresses in spite of conservative treatment or when the infection is likely to be associated with dangerous complications.

The most simple form of treatment is known as suction clearance which is carried out under a general anaesthetic and with the aid of the operating-microscope. In other cases various forms of mastoidectomy are employed. In the first place there is the *cortical* operation in which a post-auricular incision is made and the mastoid air-cells opened and drained. The tympanic membrane and ossicles however are left without interference and after

Fig. 20.18. A perforation in Schrapnell's membrane in the 'attic' type of C.S.O.M.

recovery there may be little impairment of hearing. In *radical mastoidectomy*, which is employed in cases of more advanced disease, the incision may be post-auricular or endaural and the surgeon exenterates the mastoid cells and clears all diseased tissue from the antrum, aditus, attic and tympanic cavity together with remains of the tympanic membrane and ossicles, with the excepton of the footplate of the stapes.

In some cases the techniques of tympanoplasty are used in attempts to reconstruct the sound conducting mechanisms of the middle-ear by replacing the tympanic membrane with temporal fascia and by utilizing undamaged ossicles.

Complications of middle-ear infection

These are fortunately much less common than before the era of antibiotics but still occur from time to time and comprise the following (Fig. 20.19):

> Acute mastoiditis
> Meningitis
> Extradural abscess
> Petrositis
> Labyrinthitis
> Facial paralysis
> Lateral sinus thrombosis
> Brain abscess
> Subdural abscess

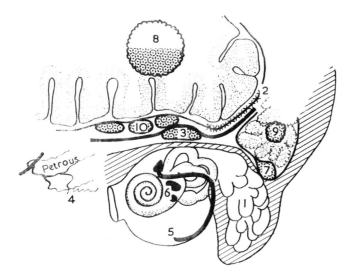

Fig. 20.19. The complications of middle ear infection. (1) Mastoiditis (2) Meningitis (3) Extradural abscess (4) Petrositis (5) Facial nerve paralysis (6) Labyrinthitis (7) Lateral sinus thrombosis (8) Temporal lobe abscess (9) Cerebellar abscess (10) Subdural abscess.

Acute mastoiditis is the result of extension of infection into the mastoid cells associated with bone necrosis and faulty drainage. There is persistent pain, pyrexia and sometimes swelling over the mastoid process. X-rays show loss of cell outline.

Meningitis is manifested by pyrexia, headache and neck rigidity. The C.S.F. shows characteristic changes and unless antibiotic treatment is given early and in adequate dosage other intracranial complications may ensue.

Extradural abscess or pus formation inside the skull but outside the dura mater sometimes occurs by direct extension from the mastoid cells and is characterised by severe pain.

Petrositis and Labyrinthitis are unusual, and as their names imply denote extension of infection from the mastoid to the petrous apex of the temporal bone and the labyrinth respectively. In the latter case there is, as one might expect, violent giddiness.

Facial paralysis may occur at any stage of middle ear or mastoid infection, acute or chronic, and when one considers the lengthy course of the facial nerve in the temporal bone and its close proximity to the middle ear and mastoid cells it is surprising that facial nerve paresis is not more common.

Lateral sinus thrombosis or thrombosis of the huge venous sinus which lies adjacent to the mastoid cells is of interest in that tremendous swings of temperature—often with rigors—are likely to occur.

Brain abscess and multiple subdural abscesses are the most sinister of all intracranial complications of middle ear disease. Nursing and medical personnel must be ever-watchful for such untoward symptoms as headache, apathy, drowsiness, malaise or nausea in patients suffering from any form of otitis media, for such patients may be quietly forming a brain abscess which will perhaps prove fatal unless recognised early.

The treatment of the various intracranial complications consists basically of antibiotics with, in some cases, mastoid surgery. Brain abscess, of course, calls for very special investigation including air-encephalography, angiography, electro-encephalography and radio-isotope studies and often neuro-surgical techniques, e.g. tapping through burr holes, are employed. (See page 137.)

Secretory otitis (glue ear) is frequently seen in young children and is undoubtedly due basically to inadequate Eustachian tube function. The Eustachian tube normally fulfils a most important role in that it enables the air-pressure within the middle-ear to adjust itself on swallowing to the external atmospheric pressure. If this function is interfered with—by, for example, enlarged adenoids, a partial vacuum forms in the middle-ear resulting in an effusion of fluid and resultant deafness.

Treatment is carried out under general anaesthesia. With the aid of the operating microscope a myringotomy is performed and the fluid which may be thin or viscous (glue) is sucked out. A grommet or Teflon tube (Fig. 20.20) is then inserted and the hearing usually returns to normal. The grommet functions as a 'stand-in' for the Eustachian tube by allowing equalization of air pressures on both sides of the tympanic membrane. Grommets often remain in place for several months and whilst in position it is customary for the medical adviser to render himself exceedingly unpopular by advising the grommets' young host not to enter the swimming pool.

Otosclerosis

This is a form of deafness which most commonly affects young females and is caused by fixation of the stapes in the oval window. There is a tendency for the deafness to occur in families and sometimes hearing loss is first noticed during pregnancy. Other symptoms are tinnitus (ringing in the ears), and paracusis or the ability to

Fig. 20.20. Tubes inserted through the tympanic membrane for the purpose of ventilating the middle ear. A Teflon tube and a grommet with wire attached.

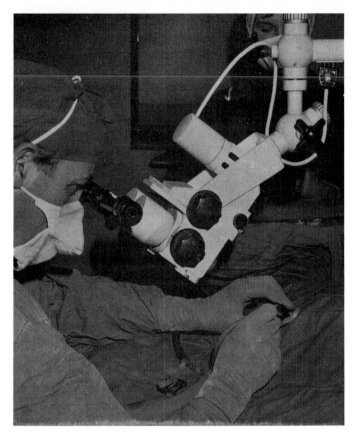

Fig. 20.21. A binocular operating microscope (in this case one of the Zeiss Otoscopes), is now being used for stapedectomy and for many other aural operations.

hear the spoken word more clearly in the presence of background noise. The diagnosis is confirmed by tuning-fork tests and audiometry, which show conductive deafness.

Treatment is by the operation of stapedectomy which is carried out with the aid of the operating microscope (20.21). Having reflected the tympanic membrane and opened the middle ear, the surgeon removes all or part of the fixed stapes replacing it with one of the forms of prosthesis shown in Fig. 20.22. One end of the prosthesis is fixed to the incus and the other end is able to move with some degree of freedom in the oval window thus forming the penultimate link in the vibrating chain—tympanic membrane—malleus—incus—prosthesis—organ of hearing (cochlea).

Earache (Otalgia)

Earache is associated with every inflammatory, and many other, conditions of the external ear and middle ear cleft, the most common *aural* causes of severe earache being furunculosis, acute otitis media and mastoiditis. Malignant disease of the external and middle ear may cause intractable pain and the victims of this appalling condition have sometimes been advised to undergo leucotomy in an attempt to control their suffering.

It is often forgotten that there are many causes of *referred otalgia*, i.e. the pain is felt as earache but the cause lies in some structure distant from the ear. These causes are obviously of great importance in diagnosis and are shown pictorially in Fig. 20.23. The conditions which most frequently give rise to referred otalgia are, impacted

Fig. 20.22. Three forms of stapes prosthesis used in stapedectomy. From above down, Teflon piston, steel piston, fat and wire.

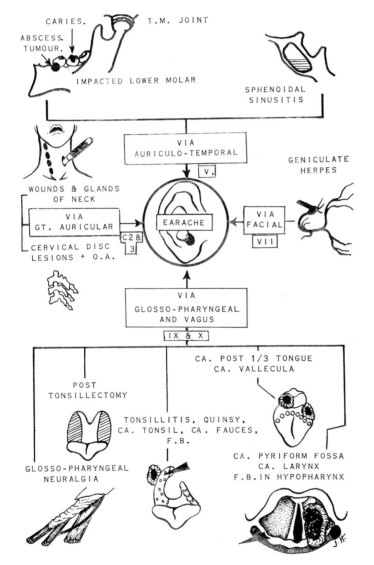

Fig. 20.23. Referred earache.

lower wisdom teeth, tonsillectomy (3rd–4th day post-operatively), temporo-mandibular joint disorders and malignant disease of the posterior third of tongue, vallecula, fauces, tonsil, lateral pharyngeal wall, larynx and hypopharynx.

THE NOSE, PARANASAL SINUSES AND NASOPHARYNX

Foreign body in the nose

Children between the ages of 1–4 years sometimes insert foreign bodies into one or both nostrils and even an intelligent child is unlikely to indicate that a foreign body is present owing to the fear of rebuke.

The rapidity with which symptoms develop depends to some extent on the nature of the foreign body, for example a vegetable object such as a green pea will soon produce a unilateral evil-smelling nasal discharge with excoriation around the nostril. On the other hand a more inanimate object, such as a small stone or glass bead, may remain in residence for weeks without upsetting its little host; eventually, however, a nasal discharge is likely to make its appearance.

Probably the chief danger lies in the attempts made by an unskilled person (e.g. grandma with a knitting-needle) to remove the foreign body, and such attempts, whilst very likely to push the latter yet deeper into the nasal passage, may even be the cause of a serious complication such as meningitis.

Always bear in mind the fact that a young child with a unilateral malodorous nasal discharge is very likely to be harbouring a foreign body, and expert attention is called for. In the case of a co-operative child the medical attendant may be able to extract the foreign body with ease but should the child be in any way refractory full general anaesthesia with an endotracheal tube is likely to be required.

Injuries of the nose

The nose is commonly injured in sport, traffic accidents and personal assault, and such injuries may result in lacerations of the skin, fractures of the nasal bones, deviation of the nasal septum or septal haematoma. *Epistaxis* (nose-bleeding), may occur as a result of even the most minor nasal injury.

The nasal bones may be splintered into many fragments but provided no undue deformity is present no active steps to reduce the fracture are required. On the other hand a very simple fracture may result in the nose pointing markedly in one direction or the other or being squashed against the face, and if such unsightly deformity occurs, reduction under general anaesthesia must be carried out when local oedema has subsided (3–5 days). The surgeon is likely to employ Walsham's forceps (Fig. 20-24) and provided the operation is not delayed for more than about 10 days no great difficulty in mobilising the fragments should be encountered.

If however the patient seeks attention weeks, months or years after the injury a major surgical procedure, involving re-fracturing of the nasal bones, will be required in an attempt to restore his or her former beauty.

Epistaxis (Nose-bleeding)

The causes of epistaxis are numerous and are usually classified as *local*—'spontaneous', trauma, post-operative etc., and *general*—hypertension, atherosclerosis, abnormal conditions of the blood (e.g. anaemia, leukaemia) etc.

Spontaneous epistaxis is most common in children, adolescents and young adults and usually arises from *Little's area* of the nasal septum (Fig. 20.25). Patients often seek relief on account of the recurrent nature of this disorder which is embarrassing in its tendency to occur at the most unexpected and inopportune moments (e.g. when just about to propose marriage).

The problem is met by cauterising Little's area with some caustic substance such as a bead of fused silver nitrate or with galvano-cautery after the mucous membrane has previously been treated with a topical analgesic solution.

Epistaxis associated with hypertension or atherosclerosis usually arises far back in the nose and may be serious.

The method of arrest of epistaxis depends to some extent on the cause but in the first place *pressure and posture* is usually tried. The patient, in a sitting position with the head flexed slightly forwards, presses with his finger against the bleeding side of the nose for 10 minutes. The mouth is kept open, swallowing is forbidden, and a

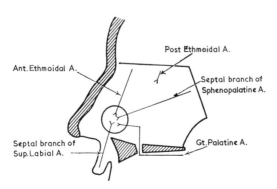

Fig. 20.24. Walsham's forceps.

Fig. 20.25. The blood supply of the nasal septum. Little's area is within the circle.

Post Ethmoidal A.

Ant. Ethmoidal A.

Septal branch of Sphenopalatine A.

Septal branch of Sup. Labial A.

Gt. Palatine A.

bowl—to receive dribble—is held under the chin. Epistaxis cannot always be treated with ease and security at home and elderly hypertensive patients should be regarded as candidates for hospital admission.

If pressure and posture fail to control the haemorrhage, resort has to be made to *anterior nasal packing*. The side which is bleeding is sprayed with a cocaine and adrenaline mixture (10 per cent cocaine, 1/1,000 adrenaline, equal parts) and the nose is packed with ½-inch ribbon-gauze which may be soaked in a solution according to the surgeon's directions e.g. bismuth, iodoform, paraffin paste.

With Tilley's forceps (Fig. 20.26) the ribbon is first passed along the floor of the nose to the back in a loop, and then built up in successive loops from the floor upwards (Fig. 20.27). The pack may be left for 24 hours, or longer if the patient is under hospital supervision and antibiotic cover. An inflatable bag is sometimes used in lieu of a gauze pack.

When nasal bleeding is arising from far back in the nasal cavities or from the nasopharynx, *post-nasal plugging* may be necessary. The plug consists of a tightly compressed ball of gauze about the size of a small walnut firmly secured by stitches to the centre of a piece of tape about 2 feet in length. It is inserted via the mouth with the aid of a soft rubber catheter which has been previously passed along the floor of the nose and afterwards secured to the 'leading' end of the tape (Fig. 20.28). Once the plug has been inserted the

Fig. 20.26. Tilley's nasal dressing forceps.

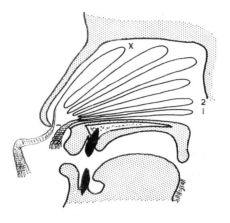

Fig. 20.27. Insertion of anterior nasal pack. 1 is the first loop, 2—the second, and X—the last.

leading end of tape is secured firmly to the side of the face with adhesive tape and the trailing tape emerging from the corner of the mouth is attached without tension.

Surgical methods e.g. ligation of the ethmoidal or maxillary arteries may have to be resorted to in an attempt to arrest epistaxis but such heroics are fortunately seldom necessary. At the same time epistaxis must always be treated with extreme respect as in some cases numerous blood transfusions are required and a fatal outcome has not always been avoided.

Disorders of the nasal septum

Deflected nasal septum, which is usually a result of trauma, is a common cause of nasal obstruction and in most cases may be corrected by surgery, with excellent results. In developmental cases a smooth S-shape deflection may be present but in the more common traumatic case there are sharp angular deviations or spurs.

The treatment is by the operation of *submucous resection* (S.M.R.) which is commonly carried out in adults but seldom in children,

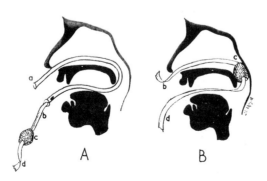

Fig. 20.28. Insertion of a postnasal plug (A) First stage (B) Second stage a. Catheter b. Leading tape c. Plug d. Trailing tape.

and the object of this delicate manoeuvre is to fillet out deflected cartilage and thin bone from between the two layers of muco-perichondrium (Fig. 20.29).

Surgeons vary considerably in regard to their preference of post-operative management and no single method of packing can be said to be 'right' or wrong'. One accepted method which has proved valuable over a number of years is to insert a glove-finger pack and a silastic splint in each nasal cavity at the conclusion of the operation. The packs are removed after 24 hours and the splints after 7 days.

Septal perforation is a troublesome complaint which may follow trauma, and very occasionally occurs post-operatively. It is associated with epistaxis and crusting in the nose and on rare occasions causes the patient to whistle softly with the nose on every breath.

Septal haematoma has already been mentioned as a possible result of trauma. Blood accumulates between the two layers of muco-perichondrium covering the septum and very severe nasal obstruction is caused. Surgical drainage may be necessary but in spite of every care a serious deformity of the nose may ensue.

Septal abscess forms, as might be expected, as a result of infection of a

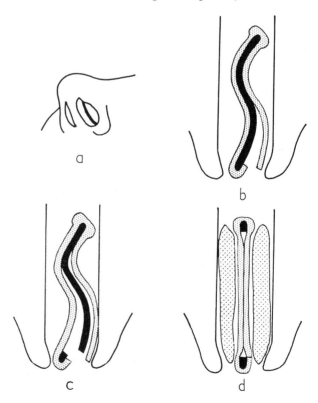

Fig. 20.29. Submucous resection of the septum. a. The incision. b,c,d. Diagrammatic transverse sections showing the separation of muco-perichondrium (stippled) from underlying cartilage and bone (black). In d, the packs (either side) have been inserted.

haematoma. It is likely to settle with adequate drainage and anti-biotic therapy but in the pre-antibiotic era it was a sinister condition which might herald fatal cavernous sinus thrombosis.

Infections of the nose and sinuses

The nasal cavities and sinus mucosa are of course infected (usually by a virus) whenever we have a common cold or one of the upper respiratory infections which occur in association with measles, German measles, etc. We do not, however, use the term 'sinusitis' unless there is in addition some form of obstruction to the sinus drainage, leading to specific symptoms. In the later stages of the common cold there is a secondary infection with bacteria causing a purulent nasal discharge for a varying number of days.

The correct treatment for the common cold is to keep warm, avoid contact with others, avoid antibiotics or local medicaments for the nose and throat, but take simple 'misery-relieving' preparations, such as soluble aspirin, in adequate quantity. Those unfortunate persons who are particularly liable to recurrent attacks of common-cold are often helped by a course of anticatarrhal vaccine administered at the end of the summer.

Acute maxillary sinusitis may arise during the course of a common cold or influenza, or it may occur as a result of diving or dental infection. The maxillary antrum becomes filled with pus, there is pain in the face and sometimes nasal discharge and obstruction. A tilted X-ray film may show a fluid level in the maxillary sinus (antrum) as shown in Fig. 20.30. Transillumination of the sinuses, in which the patient is seated in a blacked-out cubicle and has a bright light shone in the mouth, may demonstrate relative opacity of an infected antrum.

Treatment is by antibiotics such as penicillin, analgesics and the use of nasal decongestants such as 1–2 per cent ephedrine drops and in almost all cases the patient will, after a few days, have a very copious nasal discharge and lose his symptoms.

Chronic maxillary sinusitis used to be seen much more frequently in the pre-antibiotic era. The acute infection does not resolve and the patient continues to have a purulent nasal discharge associated with X-ray changes in the affected antrum. In such cases it is usual to carry out antrum puncture and lavage using a Lichtwitz trocar and cannula (Fig. 20.31). This minor procedure is usually carried out under local analgesia and once the surgeon has punctured the antrum via the inferior meatus of the nose, the sitting patient is instructed to lean forward over a bowl. Specimens for bacteriological investigation may then be aspirated and finally the antrum is

Fig. 20.30. X-ray of maxillary sinuses in tilted position. Note fluid level in left antrum.

irrigated with sterile normal saline by means of a Higginson's syringe.

Most surgeons prefer to carry out this manoeuvre under general anaesthesia if the patient is a child, and should this be necessary Walford's silver cannulae may be inserted and left in the sinuses for several days, during which time they may be irrigated frequently and painlessly (Fig. 20.32).

Sometimes the infection is particularly resistant and persists even after several 'wash-outs', in which case the next step in treating the adult patient may be the operation of *intranasal antrostomy*. In this operation an opening is made in the antro-nasal wall (under the inferior turbinate). In many cases the drainage opening will remain patent and enable the patient to wash out his own antrum with a curved (Rose's) cannula, after he leaves hospital.

There remain cases in which the membrane lining the antrum

Fig. 20.31. Lichtwitz trocar and cannula.

Fig. 20.32. Walford's silver cannulae have been inserted (under a short general anaesthetic) into the antra, which can now be irrigated painlessly several times daily.

is particularly unhealthy or for some reason it is necessary for the surgeon actually to look into the cavity—perhaps for the purpose of taking a biopsy. The operation of choice is the *Caldwell-Luc procedure*, sometimes known as radical antrostomy (Fig. 20.33) and in this case the maxillary sinus is approached via the buccal cavity.

Acute frontal sinusitis is fortunately much less common than maxillary sinusitis, though the predisposing causes (head-cold, influenza, diving, etc.) are similar. The pain is felt mainly over one eye and swelling over the affected area may occur. It is interesting to note that swelling of the face in maxillary sinusitis is hardly ever a feature, swellings of the face usually being of dental origin. X-rays are a valuable aid to diagnosis and resolution usually takes place with adequate antibiotic and decongestant treatment. It must be remembered however that, unlike maxillary sinusitis, frontal sinus infection is a potentially dangerous condition carrying the possibility of fatal complications (Fig. 20.34).

In some cases pain and swelling increase in severity when it may be necessary to drain the frontal sinus under general anaesthesia. An incision is made below the inner third of the eyebrow and the sinus opened with a hammer and gouge. Drainage tubes are inserted.

Recurrent and chronic infections of the frontal sinus may call for relatively minor procedures such as *submucous resection* of the nasal septum or *turbinectomy* in an attempt to improve drainage. On the

Fig. 20.33. Caldwell-Luc. A. An incision has been made in the mucoperiosteum of the right canine fossa B. A large window has been made in the anterior antral wall. An opening has also been made in the medial wall of the antrum providing free drainage into the nose.

Fig. 20.34. Complications of frontal sinusitis. 1. Osteomyelitis 2. Extradural abscess 3. Subdural abscess 4. Meningitis 5. Frontal lobe abscess. 6. Orbital cellulitis and abscess. 7. Cavernous sinus thrombosis.

other hand radical operations on the frontal sinus are very occasionally called for. These may be of the nature of *radical fronto-ethmoidectomy* in which a curved incision is made below the inner third of the eyebrow and carried down to a point medial to, and below, the inner canthus (Fig. 20.35). Diseased ethmoidal cells are cleared and a wide channel created to form a new fronto-nasal duct. An important practical point regarding the preparation for this operation is that the eyebrow should not be shaved, for if this is done the patient will present a lop-sided appearance for a very long time.

As an alternative to fronto-ethmoidectomy, *obliteration* of the sinus may be advocated. Techniques vary; some are directed to the removal of the anterior wall of the sinus, others to the raising of an osteo-plastic flap followed by the insertion of bone chips.

Tumours of the nose, sinuses and nasopharynx

Carcinoma of the maxillary antrum and ethmoids, which in its early stages gives rise merely to a persistent blood-stained nasal discharge and nasal obstruction, later will produce a grim clinical-picture, including swelling of the cheek, epiphora (overflow of tears), proptosis, double vision, erosion into the mouth and severe facial pain (Fig. 20.36).

X-rays and biopsy are needed to confirm the diagnosis and treatment is usually a combination of surgery and radiotherapy. The surgery may be simply a large fenestration of the hard palate after which the patient wears an obturator built on to this upper denture. This enables him to speak and eat normally and also allows the surgeon to inspect the operative cavity afterwards. In some cases more radical surgery, e.g. total maxillectomy, or even exenteration of the orbit, will be necessary.

Carcinoma of the nasopharynx, though rare in Europeans, is common in some parts of the world—notably South China. It is responsible for early enlargement of the cervical lymph nodes and by virtue of the proximity of the nasopharynx to the base of the skull there is an amazing tendency to involvement of cranial nerves—the second, third, fourth, fifth, sixth, ninth, tenth, eleventh and twelfth may be affected. Other symptoms include deafness as a result of involvement of the Eustachian tubes.

Treatment is by radiotherapy.

Nasal polypi

Nasal polypi are common and are usually associated with allergy. They arise as a rule from the ethmoid sinuses, but a single 'antrochoanal' polypus has its origin in the lining-membrane of the maxillary sinus and passes back into the narrow aperture between the nasal cavity and the nasopharynx—the choana (Fig. 20.37).

It is customary to remove polypi in the E.N.T. clinic or consulting room using topical analgesia and a nasal snare (Fig. 20.38). On the other hand, if the patient is of a nervous disposition or has other nasal problems which require attention e.g. deviated septum or turbinate hypertrophy, it is far better for him to be admitted, in

Fig. 20.35. Incision for radical fronto-ethmoidectomy.

Fig. 20.36. Carcinoma of the right maxillary antrum. The orbit has been invaded.

Fig. 20.39. Adenoidectomy. The curette is swept down the posterior wall of the nasopharynx.

THE TONSILS AND PHARYNX

Acute tonsillitis

Acute tonsillitis can occur at any age but is most common in children under 9. The symptoms consist of sore throat and dysphagia but very young children who do not know whereabouts the throat is to be found do not of course complain of sore throat. They just don't swallow anything. There may be earache, high temperature and a heavily furred tongue and often enormously enlarged and tender cervical lymph nodes. The tonsils are enlarged and may be covered with yellowish exudate, and sometimes present a speckled appearance, the so-called 'follicular tonsillitis'.

Swabs taken from the tonsils and cultured may disclose the presence of streptococci and treatment is with antibiotics, such as penicillin or ampicillin, rest, and aspirin mixtures. Disinfectant and antibiotic lozenges are of little value and may predispose to monilial infections.

The complications of tonsillitis include otitis media and quinsy. The former condition has been described.

Quinsy (Peritonsillar abscess) is a collection of pus arising outside the capsule of the tonsil and in close relationship to the soft palate. It is more common in adults than in children. The patient, already suffering from acute tonsillitis, becomes more ill and develops very severe pain and *trismus* (spasm of the muscles of mastication). He is thus unable to open his mouth or swallow and is consequently in a state of utmost misery. The quinsy may resolve with adequate antibiotic treatment or it may burst spontaneously into the mouth with immediate relief. On the other hand the medical attendant may decide to open it by making a small stab incision through the overlying palatal mucous membrane and inserting a pair of sinus forceps.

Pharyngeal ulceration

Ulceration and membrane formation may occur in the pharynx, buccal cavity or on the tonsils, and sometimes poses interesting and difficult problems for the diagnostician. The conditions responsible include such varied pathological processes as infectious mononucleosis (glandular fever), Vincent's angina, agranulocytosis, moniliasis (thrush), leukaemia, malignant disease and syphilis.

Tonsillectomy

Tonsillectomy is frequently indicated in cases of severe recurrent attacks of tonsillitis. One attack of quinsy is also a most important indication but other reasons for tonsillectomy such as focal sepsis are less certain. A commonly held fallacy is that large tonsils are of necessity unhealthy, but this is not so; the appearance of the tonsils is not regarded by specialists as being of particular significance when advising for or against tonsillectomy in any particular case but the frequency and severity of the attacks of acute tonsillitis undergone by the patient are all important in making a decision.

When the patient is admitted to hospital certain very important facts must be established. In the first place an attack of sore throat during the previous few weeks means that the operation may have to be postponed and secondly, if the question of abnormal bleeding or bruising tendency has not been already raised in out-patients, this matter must certainly be enquired about. If there is the slightest suspicion of such abnormality the patient must be fully investigated for haemorrhagic disorders. Simple tests for bleeding and clotting time are not sufficient.

The operation of tonsillectomy is almost always carried out under general anaesthesia. The 'guillotine' technique which calls for very great expertise and teamwork is employed in many centres with excellent results but it is probably true to say that the 'dissection' technique is more widely practiced.

The patient lies supine, the shoulders elevated on a small sandbag. A Boyle-Davis gag (Fig. 20.40) is inserted and the surgeon grasping the tonsil with special tonsil-holding forceps, then dissects it away from its bed using scissors or dissectors, and ulti-

Fig. 20.40. Boyle-Davis gag. (Used in tonsil dissection).

⅓ Sc

mately a tonsil snare (Fig. 20.41) to sever its last attachments. He then spends some time arresting haemorrhage using, for example, Wilson's forceps (Fig. 20.42) and Waugh's tenaculum forceps (Fig. 20.43).

Post-operative care calls for experience, knowledge and a good deal of common sense, and the responsibility for post-tonsillectomy cases must never be delegated to inexperienced nurses. As soon as surgery is completed the patient is turned over into a semi-prone position, often with a pillow crosswise under the abdomen and lower ribs. This posture is of great importance in preventing the inhalation of blood or secretions and must be maintained until the reflexes return and the patient starts objecting to, and finally spits out, his metal or rubber airway. He now passes into a phase of post-operative sleep and even during this stage should be kept lying on the side and not allowed to roll over on to his back. It is most important during this phase that the patient should be allowed to sleep peacefully and, in the author's experience of over 30 years, visiting in the immediate post-operative period is not only undesirable but hazardous. The safety of the patient must come before emotional considerations.

On waking, his pillows may be restored to him, and bland fluids such as orangeade administered. In adults pain may be severe and pethidine or morphine are justified but one golden rule applies in this connection. *Sedative drugs must not be given unless the patient has fully regained consciousness.*

During the post-operative period the patient is watched with the utmost care and any untoward event, e.g. haemorrhage from the nose or mouth, swallowing movements or rising pulse rate must be reported immediately, so that necessary action may be taken without delay. Needless to say any degree of respiratory obstruction will call for instant restoration of the air-way by the attendant.

Complications include haemorrhage, which may be reactionary or secondary. Reactionary haemorrhage occurs within a few hours of operation and it may be stated with confidence that during this period the patient's life is entirely within the hands of the nursing staff for if haemorrhage is recognised and treated promptly it should not be dangerous, but if there is any tardiness in its recognition, or procrastination and delay in its treatment, it may be fatal.

If, in fact, any of the signs of haemorrhage mentioned above—e.g. bleeding from the nose or mouth, swallowing movements, or rising pulse rate—are present, medical advice is obtained *immediately*, and the exact treatment will depend on the surgeon's assessment. It is likely to consist of the administration of a sedative such as papaveretum, and this may be combined with the removal of blood clot from

Fig. 20.41. (left) Eve's tonsil snare. (Used in tonsil dissection.)

Fig. 20.42. (right) Wilson's tonsil artery forceps (Used in tonsil dissection.)

the tonsillar fossa which is bleeding. Sometimes a swab soaked in 1/1,000 adrenaline solution is applied to the area for a short time, but if haemorrhage continues the patient will be returned to the operating theatre for ligation of the bleeding point.

Secondary haemorrhage is uncommon but may occur between the fifth and tenth post-operative days. Parents of post-tonsillectomy children should always be warned of the possibility, and are advised to notify the doctor or hospital without delay if there is any bleeding in the mouth or from the nose. As a rule all that is required is re-admission to hospital and careful observation and sedation for a few days.

Otitis media sometimes occurs as a complication of tonsillectomy. Referred pain in the ears is present at some stage after almost every tonsillectomy, a fact which is so well known that the unwary may fall into the trap of disregarding the complaint of 'earache' and omit to report it to the medical attendant. Thus otitis media may be missed.

THE LARYNX

The larynx may be regarded as the specially adapted upper extremity of the wind-pipe. Its functions are primarily to protect the lungs and secondarily to produce sound, and speech. It is essential for these requirements—valve and voice-box—that its structure should be rigidly supported and this is achieved by the strong thyroid and cricoid cartilages which surround its lumen and are seen shaded in Fig. 20.44B. The vocal cords, which are not really cords but folds, extend antero-posteriorly and are normally examined with a laryngeal mirror (Fig. 20.44A).

A proportion of patients cannot tolerate the mirror touching the soft palate and it may be necessary for the laryngologist to apply a topical anaesthetic to the patient's palatal and pharyngeal mucosa. In some instances it is necessary to carry out an even more direct examination, with perhaps biopsy, and for this purpose a general anaesthetic is administered and a laryngoscope passed—*direct laryngoscopy*. It is now a routine matter to employ in addition the operating microscope—*microlaryngoscopy*.

Fig. 20.43. Waugh's tenaculum forceps. (Used in tonsil dissection.)

Injuries of the larynx

The larynx may be injured by penetrating wounds, blows, hot or poisonous vapours, corrosive poisons or indwelling tubes (left for excessive periods).

Tracheostomy may be required as any injury of the larynx is likely to be accompanied by internal swelling—*glottic oedema*—and the

Fig. 20.44. (A) View obtained in mirror at indirect laryngoscopy A. Epiglottis B. Vocal cord C. Vestibular fold (false cord) D. Interarytenoid region E. corniculate cartilage F. Cuneiform cartilage G. Pyriform fossa H. Vallecula.
(B) Diagrammatic coronal section of the larynx showing the laryngeal sinuses between the vestibular folds above the vocal cords below.

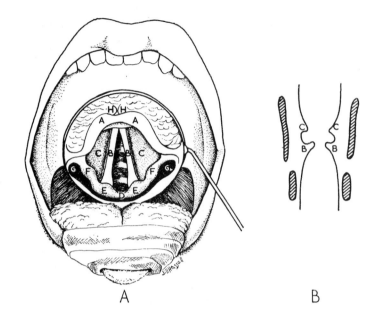

A   B

development of this sinister complication may result in asphyxial death unless prompt action is taken.

Infections of the larynx

Acute laryngitis is a not uncommon complication of upper respiratory infection and is predisposed to by shouting or excessive use of the voice, particularly if such an infection is present at the time. The voice becomes hoarse and may disappear completely and the most important part of the treatment is to ban the use of the voice by confining the patient to bed and prohibiting visiting. Bland inhalations of medicated steam such as Vap. Benz. or Pini are comforting, and reassure the patient that he has not been forgotten.

Acute epiglottitis is a localised infection, usually associated with *H. influenzae*, of the epiglottis, which becomes congested and oedematous. In the child the infection may kill within hours by respiratory obstruction and it is now thought that it may have been the cause of unexplained death in young children in the past.

A young child who develops stridor (noisy breathing) is in the shadow of death. Medical attention and hospital admission is required with urgency. Tracheostomy is likely to be necessary and ampicillin in heavy dosage often combined with steroids is employed in the treatment.

Laryngo-tracheo-bronchitis is also a serious condition of childhood and fraught with danger. Hospital admission with skilled nursing care, antibiotics, humidification oxygen therapy and occasionally tracheostomy will be required.

Laryngeal diphtheria is rarely seen in the British Isles thanks to immunization of the child population, but those of us who have seen it are not likely to forget its horror. The child is ill and presents the clinical picture of faucial diphtheria (membrane on fauces and tonsils). Stridor suggests the spread of membrane to the larynx and trachea and by the time this stage is reached even skilled treatment may not forestall death. Antitoxin and penicillin are administered in appropriate dosage and tracheostomy or intubation may be needed.

Chronic laryngitis is the term applied to those cases in which there is persistent hoarseness of voice perhaps as a result of habitual faulty voice production, over indulgence in alcohol or tobacco, or chronic upper respiratory infection.

Laryngologists never make a diagnosis of chronic laryngitis until all other causes of persistent hoarseness have been carefully excluded and in this connection it may be appropriate to mention that members of the medical and nursing professions should always be aware of the possible significance of hoarseness and advise an expert opinion when this symptom has been present for more than two or three weeks.

The reason for this golden rule is of course that carcinoma of the vocal cord (mentioned later) will perhaps cause no symptom other than hoarseness for many months and this type of malignant disease of the larynx is par excellence a form of cancer which, with early diagnosis and thorough treatment, can be completely cured in a high proportion of cases.

Tumours of the larynx

Benign tumours of the vocal cords occur rarely and cause hoarseness. They are removed at direct microlaryngoscopy and carefully scrutinised by the pathologist.

Carcinoma of the vocal cord, as already mentioned, causes hoarseness, and its presence is confirmed by laryngoscopy and biopsy. Early cases are given a full course of radiotherapy and carefully followed-up afterwards. Sometimes the disease fails to respond to radiotherapy, or, if diagnosis has been delayed, it may have spread within the larynx or trachea. In such cases *total laryngectomy* with or without removal of the cervical lymph nodes may be advised.

Removal of the larynx is a major procedure but owing to improved anaesthetic technique and modern antibiotics it is not associated with a high mortality as it was 30 years ago. Unhappily, like many other medical matters, it is bedevilled with popular fallacy, for example, that the patient will never speak again and become a permanent invalid unfit for any kind of work. In fact, the majority of patients, provided they possess 'guts', and are given good speech therapy and encouragement to use their new 'oesophageal voice' will be able to indulge in *any* occupation other than swimming; the latter being interdicted on account of the permanent tracheal stoma in the neck (Fig. 20.45).

Fig. 20.45. Some patients after laryngectomy need to wear a Colledge tube (left). The central figure is its introducer, and on the right is a Moure-Lombard tube, which is used during the post-operative period when dressings might obstruct the orifice.

Stridor

Stridor or noisy breathing has already been mentioned in connection with acute epiglottitis and laryngeal diphtheria. It may be associated with many conditions including the congenital cysts and webs of the larynx (which if present are apparent in neonatal life) multiple papillomatosis of the larynx of childhood, general weakness of the larynx, foreign body, tumours or vocal cord paralysis. The noise may be maximal on breathing in—*inspiratory stridor* (most common in laryngeal cases); or it may be more apparent when the patient breathes out—*expiratory stridor* (often heard in asthmatic attacks).

In any case stridor is a danger signal and must never be passed over lightly. Some of the conditions which cause it are rapidly fatal unless relieved by skilled and speedy intervention.

Vocal cord paresis

Paresis, (weakness) or paralysis (complete loss of function), of one or both vocal cords is caused by trauma or disease affecting the nerves which supply the vocal cord muscles, the recurrent laryngeal nerves.

The left recurrent laryngeal nerve is more commonly affected as it has a long course (into the thorax and back again to the larynx) and it may be involved in carcinoma of the bronchus or oesophagus, in enlargement of the mediastinal lymph nodes or following thoracic surgery.

In the neck either left or right recurrent nerve may be affected by surgery or carcinoma of the thyroid gland. If one vocal cord is paralysed the voice may be weak for a number of months though speech therapy can do much to improve matters. But if both cords are paralysed they move in to meet each other, as in phonation and the consequent reduction of the laryngeal airway is a matter of great danger. Tracheostomy may be necessary. The condition is often referred to as 'bilateral abductor paralysis' and some patients will continue to wear a tracheostomy permanently, speaking well with a K.C.H. speaking-valve in the tracheostomy tube. There have been devised several laryngeal operations (the most popular being Woodman's operation), for the purpose of drawing one of the vocal cords away from the mid-line and thus providing an airway and avoiding a permanent tracheostomy.

THE HYPOPHARYNX

The hypopharynx is that part of the pharynx which lies behind the larynx. It is in fact the upper part of the swallowing tube joining the back of the mouth or buccal cavity with the oesophagus, and because it is compressed between the cartilaginous box of the larynx (in front) and the cervical vertebrae (behind) it is slit-like in cross section. As there is more pressure on this flattened tube in its central part, most of our swallowed food and saliva goes down in the outer extremities sometimes known as the 'lateral food channels', but if we swallow a large hard object, for example a lump of undercooked potato, it has to occupy the central part of the food passage on its way down and pushing the larynx forwards causes considerable pain.

Foreign bodies

Fish, poultry and other bones (and sometimes unusual objects see Fig. 20.46) are often inadvertently swallowed, and in most cases scratch or tear the hypopharyngeal mucosa but pass down into the

Fig. 20.46. An object most commonly found on the chest wall, but in this unusual case firmly wedged in the cervical oesophagus. A *very* large oesophagoscope was required.

stomach and are eventually voided, occasionally causing consternation when reaching the anal canal. Sometimes, however, they become impacted in the hypopharynx or oesophagus, and unless removed may lead to perforation, parapharyngeal abscess or mediastinitis, and even fatal perforation of the aorta.

Patients who give a history of having swallowed a foreign body are x-rayed and even if no abnormality is disclosed, (many foreign bodies are radio-translucent), the patient is examined under general anaesthetic with an oesophagoscope.

Malignant disease

Malignant disease of the lateral food channel or its upper extremity —the pyriform fossa—occurs predominantly in men, and may reach an advanced stage over a number of months during which the symptoms and signs are seemingly relatively trivial e.g. slight discomfort in the throat and the appearance of a lump in the neck.

In women the disease is more commonly found in the lower and central part of the hypopharynx—the so-called post-cricoid region —and may be associated with a history of the Paterson-Brown Kelly syndrome extending over a period of several years. This syndrome, which was first described by Paterson and Brown Kelly in 1919 and again by Plummer and Vinson in America in 1940, is of interest and great importance as its early recognition and treatment may prevent the development of carcinoma at a later date.

The clinical picture is of dysphagia, soreness of the tongue, cracks at the corners of the lips, spoon-shaped finger nails and an iron-deficiency anaemia. Webs and strictures may occur in the mucous membrane of the post-cricoid region and precede carcinoma.

Treatment in the premalignant stage consists of vigorous anti-anaemia measures with iron preparations such as ferrous sulphate or gluconate regularly each day, often combined with ascorbic acid. The patient is kept under surveillance.

The treatment of malignant disease of the hypopharynx may involve very major procedures, combining removal of the larynx, hypopharynx, oesophagus and cervical lymph nodes. How is the patient then able to swallow? The stomach is freed and brought up through the thorax to be anastomosed with the back of the tongue and oropharynx. Needless to say there are some patients whose general condition will not support such radical measures and others in whom the disease is so advanced as to render its recurrence likely, even after heroic surgery.

Hypopharyngeal diverticulum (Pharyngeal pouch)

Hypopharyngeal diverticulum or pouch is an uncommon condition affecting those in middle and later life. The mucous membrane herniates through the muscular wall of the hypopharynx, and over a period of months and years forms a sac, at first behind and later at the side of the oesophagus pressing upon it and causing dysphagia. Other symptoms may occur in addition to difficulty in swallowing—regurgitation of undigested food long after it has been swallowed—and strange gurgling noises in the neck, in fact one patient's wife told the writer that often when her husband swallowed it sounded as though the chain had been pulled.

The condition is investigated by means of barium swallow X-rays (Fig. 20.47) and oesophagoscopy, and treatment consists of regular dilatation of the oesophagus in the case of a small pouch giving rise to minimal symptoms, or excision via the neck in more advanced cases. Sometimes Dohlman's method is employed in very frail subjects. It involves the removal by diathermy of the thin wall between oesophagus and pouch and is carried out endoscopically, thus avoiding an open operation.

A

B

Fig. 20.47. Barium swallow demonstrating a pharyngeal pouch. A antero-posterior, B lateral view.

TRACHEOSTOMY

Tracheostomy, or the making of an opening into the trachea is an operation which has many, and very varied, indications. These may be classified as follows: (1) conditions causing upper respiratory obstruction, (2) conditions necessitating protection of the lungs and (3) conditions causing respiratory insufficiency.

Upper respiratory obstruction includes such conditions as congenital stenosis, foreign body and trauma of the larynx, infections such as acute epiglottitis, laryngo-tracheo-bronchitis and diphtheria, malignant disease of the larynx and bilateral recurrent nerve paralysis. All these conditions are fairly obvious causes of severe respiratory obstruction and tracheostomy may be required with varying degree of urgency in an attempt to restore the airway and save life.

Protection of the tracheo-bronchial tree is perhaps a less obvious reason for tracheostomy but it is, in fact, often required in such conditions as coma due to barbiturate poisoning, head injuries, cerebral vascular catastrophes, neurological and traumatic conditions, and in other circumstances where inhalation of secretions may constitute a risk of drowning.

Respiratory insufficiency may occur in pulmonary disease, severe chest injury and of course in many of the conditions mentioned above such as coma, when tracheostomy is not only necessary to prevent inhalation of secretion but to provide a means of carrying out intermittent positive pressure respiration (I.P.P.R.) using a respirator.

Technique of tracheostomy

In past years tracheostomy was almost always performed under local analgesia but today it is more often carried out under a general anaesthetic after preliminary intubation.

The patient lies supine with the head hyperextended over a small sandbag placed under the neck. The surgeon may infiltrate the incisional area with 0.5 per cent Lignocaine and he may choose to make either a transverse collar, or a vertical incision over the trachea. He then dissects down between the small strap muscles and, clearing several layers of fascia, divides the isthmus of the thyroid gland and makes a window in the tracheal wall through which he inserts a tracheostomy tube (Fig. 20.48).

Tracheostomy tubes

The standard form of tracheostomy tube is of silver and there are several excellent patterns, e.g. the K.C.H. tube (Fig. 20.49) and the

Fig. 20.48. Tracheostomy. A. The incision is midway between the cricoid cartilage (c) and suprasternal notch (n) B. The investing layer of fascia covering the pretracheal muscles C. The thyroid isthmus D. The tracheal window.

Fig. 20.49. The K.C.H. or Negus tracheostomy tube. From left to right: introducer, outer tube, inner tube with 'speaking valve' and open inner tube.

Durham or lobster-tail tube (Fig. 20.50). When intermittent positive pressure respiration is necessary, or when the lungs are at risk from inhaled secretions some form of cuffed tube is essential (Fig. 20.51). In infants a most suitable tube is the 'Great Ormond Street' pattern (Fig. 20.52).

Fig. 20.50. The Durham tracheostomy tube (centre). Above is the 'lobster-tailed' inner tube and below—the introducer.

After-care in tracheostomy cases

Tracheostomy cases demand the most dedicated and skilled nursing care, and any lapse of attention or thoughtless action on the part of the attendant nurse may have a catastrophic result.

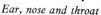

Fig. 20.51. A cuffed Portex tracheostomy tube.

Fixation of the tracheostomy tube is a matter of basic importance. The tapes securing the tube must not be too loose or too tight.

Aspiration must be performed regularly, using a sterile catheter attached to the sucker. Disposable gloves are employed and up to 1 ml of 5 per cent sodium bicarbonate solution may be run into the trachea if the secretions have become very tenacious.

Humidification of the inhaled air is essential for some days or even weeks after the establishment of a tracheostomy. The main function of the nose is to moisten and warm inhaled air and condition it so that it does not cause too traumatic an impact on the delicate mucosa of the pulmonary alveoli. The tracheostomised patient's nose has been by-passed, so humidification is necessary and constitutes a large subject in itself. There are several elaborate humidifiers available and these have largely replaced the steam-kettle of former days.

Tube-changing constitutes no problem when a silver tube with inner fitting is being employed. It may be necessary at first to remove the inner tube once or twice every hour for cleaning and sterilizing but at a later stage this manoeuvre may be carried out less frequently.

In the case of plastic tubes which have no separate inner lining, the whole tube may have to be removed if it becomes occluded with tenaceous secretions. This is a matter for experienced medical staff. In their absence complete blockage of the tube will require immediate action. Courage and resolution are necessary—the tube is removed and the track leading down to the opening in the trachea held open with a tracheal dilator until assistance arrives.

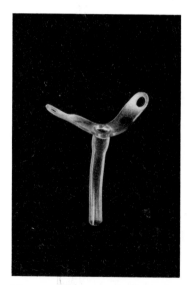

Fig. 20.52. Great Ormond Street pattern tracheostomy tube.

Chapter 21. Fractures

Trauma is the modern epidemic and a large percentage of the injuries seen in the Accident and Emergency departments of our hospitals are due to road accidents. Many details of the injured patient have been described in the previous chapters (skull fractures, Chapter 10; abdominal trauma, Chapter 14) and the systemic changes seen in the patients with multiple injuries and shock have been discussed in Chapter 3.

CARE OF THE INJURED PATIENT IN THE ACCIDENT DEPARTMENT

When a person injured in a road traffic accident is brought into the Accident Unit it is important to examine the patient's body as a whole. The Ambulance Staff always indicate the main injuries, but frequently fractures or soft tissue injuries are not immediately apparent. It is always useful to obtain information as to the cause of the accident to help both the nursing and the medical staff to assess the damage. Whilst the nurse on duty is summoning the Casualty medical staff to the injured person's assistance, she should make sure that (1) there is an adequate airway, (2) the position of the unconscious patient is correct. Ideally, he should be positioned on his side (Fig. 10.13), especially if he is vomiting, to prevent aspiration and further respiratory obstruction. (3) the shocked patient should be put into a head-down tilt position to maintain the blood pressure and stimulate blood circulation to the vital centres, and to assist venous return from the lower limbs. (4) excessive bleeding must be stopped by local pressure on the wound or by elevation of the limb. (5) the nurse should make her own assessment of the skeletal injuries

A   B

Fig. 21.1. Simple fractures of different types. A Undisplaced transverse and oblique fractures; B Comminuted displaced fracture with many fragments.

Fig. 21.2. A compound fracture. The overlying skin is broken.

in order to prevent further damage and to plan appropriate splints and plasters. When these essential procedures are completed the patient's fracture treatment may be planned.

FRACTURES

A *fracture* is a break in the continuity of a bone. There are many types of fracture (Fig. 21.1) but from the practical and treatment point of view they should divided into:

1. *Simple or closed fracture* where the bone is broken but the overlying skin remains intact.

2. *Compound fracture* where there is a wound in communication with the break contaminating the bone and producing the possibility of infection (Fig. 21.2).

Greenstick fracture (Fig. 21.3)

In the immature skeleton of a child the bone frequently bends, fracturing one cortex of the bone, but leaving the other intact. A green twig of a tree breaks in a similar fashion, hence its name.

Fig. 21.3. (left) A greenstick fracture of a child's radius.

Fig. 21.4. (right) A pathological fracture through a tumour deposit.

Pathological fracture (Fig. 21.4)

The skeleton may be infiltrated with secondary deposits from various carcinomas arising especially from the breast and lung. The bone is weakened at these sites and pathological fractures may result (see Fig. 15.23). Similar fractures may occur through benign tumours, the weak bone of osteoporosis and osteomalacia, and the bone disease of Paget.

Joint dislocation is the total separation of the two bones which articulate together (Fig. 21.5). The retaining ligaments are completely ruptured.

Joint subluxation is the partial and incomplete separation of these two bones with only partial rupture of the ligaments and the joint capsule (Fig. 21.6).

The dislocation or subluxation may become recurrent and a fracture may complicate this injury.

Fracture healing

Fracture healing depends upon a good blood supply and an adequate diet providing vitamins, protein and calcium salts. The process which heals bones is slow and the re-modelling which follows takes many months (Figs. 21.7, A & B). The blood present around the fracture site at the time of injury soon clots and then organises, with infiltration of granulation tissue. Calcium salts are laid down

Fig. 21.5. A The normal shoulder. B Anterior dislocation with the humeral head out of socket.

Humeral head Glenoid Coracoid Clavicle

Scapula

A

B

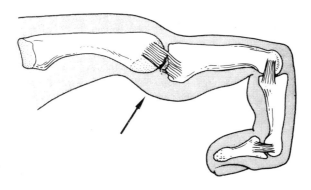

Fig. 21.6. Subluxation of a finger joint.

and at this stage a fluffy shadow around the fracture site will be seen on X-ray; this is called *callus*. Bone forming cells called osteoblasts then move in to the granulation and fibrous area and true bone is laid down between the bone ends and beneath the periosteum. Eventually subperiosteal new bone completely bridges the gap between the bone ends and re-modelling continues to strengthen the repair over the next few months.

Complications of fractures

These may be divided into early, intermediate and late.

Early

1. *Haemorrhage.* Excessive bleeding may shock the patient and in multiple fractures blood transfusion is essential to restore blood volume.

The blood loss in major fractures is greater than one would expect and average quantities are:

    a. Femoral shaft fracture, 1.0–1.5 litre (i.e. equivalent to 2 to 3 units of transfusion blood).

    b. Tibial shaft fracture, 0.5–1.0l.

    c. Major pelvic fractures 1.0–2.0l.

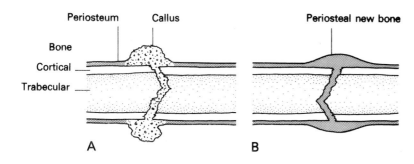

Fig. 21.7. Fracture healing and remodelling.

2. *Damage to large vessels.* In the supracondylar fracture of the child's humerus the sharp spike of bone may pierce the brachial artery (Fig. 21.8).

3. *Nerve damage.* The radial nerve winds around the back of the humeral shaft and may be damaged by fractures at this site. The result is a wrist drop with the extensor muscles of the forearm losing their innervation.

4. *Damage to viscera.* The lung may be penetrated by a rib fracture and the bladder and urethra pierced by fractures of the pelvis.

Intermediate

Fat embolism. In every fracture of a long bone the fat laden marrow cavity is disturbed and fat globules escape into the circulation. In a very small number of injured patients with multiple fractures the fat globules produce widespread areas of ischaemic damage. The brain is affected, with the patient becoming confused and later unconscious. The lung becomes consolidated and fine petechial haemorrhages are seen in the skin and the conjunctiva. The severe fat embolism syndrome is frequently fatal but vigorous treatment designed to avoid hypoxia and lung hypoventilation together with the addition of anticoagulants is frequently successful.

Pulmonary embolism. See Chapter 2.

Metabolic changes. In the injured patient salt and water is retained in the body for the first 48 hours. After this period excessive potassium

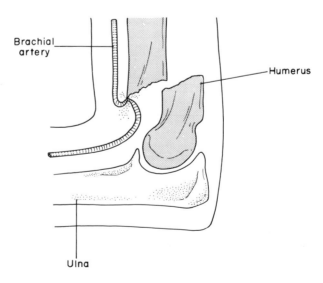

Fig. 21.8. Supracondylar fracture above the elbow with arterial damage.

excretion becomes a problem resulting in electrolyte and fluid imbalance. The management of fluid and electrolyte change is outlined in Chapter 2.

Late

Delayed union. In the lower limb 12 weeks is the average time required for the union of fractures strong enough to allow weight bearing. In the upper limb weight bearing is not a problem and the fractures are usually united satisfactorily to allow full function after 6 weeks. If union is seen to be progressing but is delayed beyond these times then it should be considered a 'delayed union'.

Non-union. The fracture remains unhealed and is painful and mobile. The limb functions poorly and eventually a false joint may develop at this non-union site.

Fracture healing may be disturbed by many processes. Essentially these fall into three groups:

1. Inadequacy of the blood supply. The lower shaft of the tibia is particularly vulnerable, and this is a site commonly affected by non-union.

2. Lack of immobilisation. The limb long bones unite faster if they are immobilised by either external plaster or internal fixation devices. Constant movement of the long bone results in a non-union state.

3. Interposition of soft tissues. In femoral shaft fractures muscle may be interposed between the bone ends and this usually results in non-union.

Mal-union. A very displaced fracture may well unite but it will produce deformity or angulation which if severe will interfere with function. Fractures cannot always be reduced anatomically but it is important to correct the alignment. The displaced but well aligned fracture will always remodel satisfactorily but the malaligned bone shown in Fig. 21.2 always produces deformity however well the remodelling process continues.

PRINCIPLES OF FRACTURE TREATMENT

1. Reduction

A fracture is frequently displaced and needs to be repositioned in good alignment with adequate bone contact. The bone ends may be manipulated to achieve this result, usually under a general anaesthetic. Traction on the peripheral part of the limb is necessary

Fig. 21.9. A tibial fracture is immobilised by a plaster cast from foot to mid thigh.

to disimpact the bone ends from one another before manipulation is successful. The reduction of most fractures is possible by closed methods of manipulation through the skin, but difficult fractures may require open operation to restore satisfactory position.

2. Fixation

The fracture is held in this reduced position by an external plaster of Paris cast or by internal metal fixation devices. Plaster casts must be carefully applied with soft padding protecting the skin. The plaster is manufactured in rolls which are soaked in tepid water and applied as bandages. The cast must be firm, but not tight, and should be moulded around the fracture site. If the cast immobilises the joint above and below the bone which is fractured then adequate control of the break is possible (Fig. 21.9.)

Dangers of plaster casts

If a tight plaster is applied to an injured limb, continued swelling of the tissues against the rigid cast may occlude the peripheral blood supply. The first signs of this compression are pain and swelling of the periphery with cold and pale skin. The fingers or toes then become numb and anaesthetic, and peripheral gangrene due to tissue death may occur. Any patient who has a plaster applied must be given instructions to ensure that he returns to the hospital or to his doctor if any of these worrying symptoms or signs develop. The orthopaedic surgeon ensures against this catastrophe by applying only a plaster backslab if considerable swelling is expected, or by splitting the plaster to allow expansion. A plaster must be padded adequately by application of thin rolls of cotton wool. This protection will usually prevent pressure sores where the plaster is liable to rub over bony prominences.

Sustained traction

Fractures of the shaft of the femur are surrounded by large muscle masses and it is initially difficult to reduce the fracture by simple manipulation. They are almost impossible to control by external plaster fixation. Strong traction, however, will align and reduce the fracture adequately and if the pull is maintained on the peripheral part of the leg the immobility will be adequate to allow the bones to unite. Skin traction (Fig. 21.10), will satisfactorily hold a limb in the correct position, but as 10 lbs. is the maximum which can be applied continuously, it is not enough to reduce the femoral

Spreader   Sticky plaster   Crepe bandage

6lbs.

Fig. 21.10. Skin traction.

fracture. Skeletal traction is necessary with a metal Steinmann's pin drilled through the bone of the upper tibia (Fig. 21.11). Twenty pounds can be comfortably applied to this pin and this weight is usually more than enough to maintain most fractures in good position.

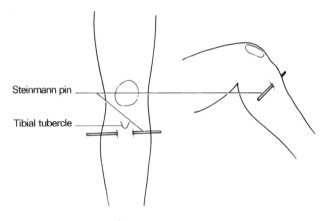

Steinmann pin

Tibial tubercle

Fig. 21.11. A Steinmann pin through the upper tibia enabling skeletal traction to be applied to a femoral fracture.

Internal fixation

The fracture may be stabilised with a plate and screws (Fig. 21.12) or a metal rod through the medullary canal (Fig. 21.41).

3. Rehabilitation

If a limb is put into a plaster of Paris cast the joints which are not immobilised must be exercised regularly and effectively. Sometimes the help of a physiotherapist is required, especially if the limb is swollen and painful.

It is important to remember that the shoulder frequently becomes stiff if an arm plaster is applied. Similarly, the knee may become a problem in a below-knee plaster applied to immobilise an ankle

Fig. 21.12. Internal fixation of a fracture by means of a plate and screws.

fracture. If the patient is in bed with skeletal traction to immobilise a femoral fracture then the nurse or physiotherapist must make sure that all joints are regularly mobilised, the chest is exercised and the patient is turned regularly to avoid the complications of a deep vein thrombosis and skin pressure problems.

PRINCIPLES OF TREATMENT OF A COMPOUND FRACTURE

The open or compound fracture is a potentially dangerous situation for infection may complicate the injury. If the bone becomes infected the resulting osteomyelitis may be resistant to treatment (page 526), and the bone union is severely delayed.

The patient with a compound fracture must be given tetanus prophylaxis and must be put on the appropriate antibiotic. Tetanus toxoid 0.5 ml is given routinely subcutaneously. Anti-tetanus serum is only rarely given (see page 12) in those wounds which are grossly contaminated. Penicillin 500 mg q.d.s. and ampicillin 250 mg q.d.s. is a satisfactory combination to use and should be continued for seven days. The wound is cleaned and dressed in a sterile fashion in the Accident and Emergency department and arrangements are made for exploration of the wound—usually under a general anaesthetic. At operation it is essential to remove dirt and debris from the wound and to excise the wound edges. All crushed and contaminated fat and muscle are removed and all crevices of the wound are explored and carefully debrided. After this careful wound excision and clearance the surgeon will suture the wound if he is certain of its cleanliness and if the wound edges will come together without tension. However, the grossly contaminated wound or one in which much skin and tissue is removed so as to make closure impossible will be left open and packed with a paraffin tulle-gras dressing.

The fracture is treated by reduction in the usual way and then stabilised by means of external plaster or by traction. It is important to avoid internal fixation initially for the metal may act as a nidus for infection. When the wound is well healed it may be possible to fix the fracture if necessary by some internal means as described above.

FRACTURES AND DISLOCATIONS IN THE UPPER LIMB

The clavicle

This bone is usually fractured by falls on to the outstretched hand. It is frequently severely displaced but it rapidly unites with conservative treatment.

Fig. 21.13. Figure-of-eight bandage to brace the shoulders in fracture of the clavicle.

Treatment

A figure of eight bandage applied as in Fig. 21.13 will brace back the shoulders, will tend to reduce the displacement and will hold the fracture comfortably. It is important not to apply the bandage too tightly, for pressure in the axilla will then become a painful problem. After a week or two in this bandage a simple sling will be required until the shoulder is comfortable enough to be mobilised.

Acromioclavicular separation (Fig. 21.14)

A direct blow to the shoulder whilst playing rugby is often responsible for this injury. There is tenderness and swelling at the

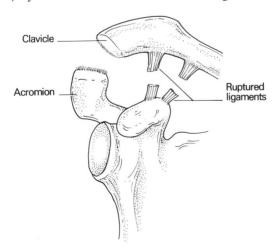

Fig. 21.14. Acromio-clavicular separation.

joint site and if there is wide separation of the two bones the lateral portion of the clavicle will be easily felt beneath the skin.

Treatment

Most separations are minor and will repair satisfactorily. A simple sling is applied until the shoulder is comfortable enough to be mobilised. If there is wide dislocation of the joint as shown in Fig. 21.14 internal fixation with a screw from the acromion to the clavicle will be necessary.

FRACTURES OF THE UPPER HUMERUS

The great tuberosity

Direct falls on to the shoulder may crack the great tuberosity (Fig. 21.15). Although this would appear a very minor injury the shoulder function may be interfered with for the tendon and ligaments constituting 'the rotator cuff' are damaged.

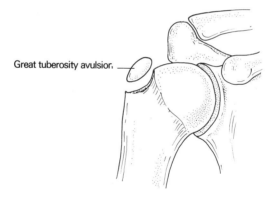

Great tuberosity avulsion.

Fig. 21.15. Avulsion fracture of great tuberosity of the humerus.

The surgical neck of the humerus (Fig. 21.16)

Again, falls on to the outstretched hand will fracture this site beneath the humeral head, especially in the elderly patient. Pain, bruising and extreme tenderness will be present around the shoulder, and joint function is grossly limited. Most fractures in this region are impacted with the shaft fragment tightly and stably thrust into the head of the humerus.

Treatment

The great tuberosity and the impacted humeral neck fractures should be rested in a simple arm sling until comfortable. The physiotherapist will then be asked to mobilise the shoulder at the

Fig. 21.16. Fracture of surgical neck of humerus.

earliest moment to prevent joint stiffness. The upper humeral fragments may be unstable and displaced, in which case open operation to reduce and internally fix the fractures with a nail may be required.

The shaft of the humerus

This fracture is frequently very displaced but rapidly comes into good alignment with a simple collar and cuff sling (Fig. 21.17). The radial nerve winds around the posterior aspect of the humerus

Fig. 21.17. Collar and cuff sling.

Fig. 21.18. Humeral shaft fracture.

in this mid-shaft region and may be damaged in fractures at this site (Fig. 21.18). A dropped wrist develops if the radial nerve is divided or more commonly pressurised by this injury. However, the paralysis is usually temporary.

Treatment

If the patient is sat up and allowed to stand erect with the arm in a collar and cuff sling, the pull of gravity will tend to reduce and align the fracture. A plaster 'U loop' may be added to give greater stability, but the point of the elbow must be left hanging free.

Shoulder dislocation

Rotational forces on the shoulder in falls and in sports injuries may dislocate this joint. Most of the dislocations are anterior but rarely the displacement of the humeral head is posterior or inferior. The shoulder joint may be considered a ball and socket joint, but as seen in Fig. 21.5 the glenoid socket of the scapula is very shallow and is deepened by a fibrous ring, called the labrum. In the anterior dislocation of the shoulder joint the labrum or capsule (or both) is torn severely anteriorly. If it repairs poorly then recurrent dislocation through this weakened area may occur.

Treatment

Traction is applied to the arm and with a sustained pull relocation is usually possible. The method described by Hippocrates—the Greek father of medicine—in the 4th Century B.C. is still considered the best. The surgeon's foot is placed in the axilla and this acts as a counter pull to the arm traction.

The supracondylar fracture

This particular injury proves to be the most troublesome fracture in the child because of the vascular complications which may ensue. The distal condylar fragment is displaced posteriorly and the sharp spike of the upper fragment irritates or in a few cases actually lacerates the brachial artery (Fig. 21.19). The pressure of haematoma and the vessel irritation may close the lumen of the brachial artery at this site and unless it is re-opened a pulseless and bloodless forearm and hand will result. The end result of this avascular periphery will be a Volkmann's contracture, in which the dead and fibrosed forearm muscles produce clawed and contracted fingers, and the death of the peripheral nerves will produce anaesthesia and trophic ulcers (Fig. 21.20).

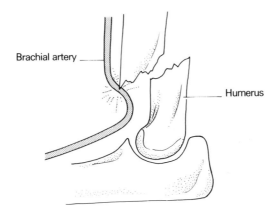

Fig. 21.19. A supracondylar fracture with vascular injury.

Fig. 21.20. Volkmann's contracture of the hand.

Treatment

When the child is first admitted to the Accident Unit the nurse should feel for the radial pulse. If it is absent, reduction of the fracture should be undertaken without delay. Under an anaesthetic the fracture is manipulated to a reduced position and a well padded backslab of plaster is applied with the elbow at a right angle. The reduction of the fracture usually restores the circulation but if it fails the brachial artery must be explored and decompressed. In a few cases arterial repair or grafting is necessary to restore the blood flow.

Dislocation of the elbow (Fig. 21.21)

Falls on to the hand are again usually responsible for this injury with the forearm dislocating posteriorly on the humerus.

Fig. 21.21. Posterior dislocation of elbow.

Treatment

Manipulation of the joint under an anaesthetic with traction on the forearm will easily reduce the dislocation. The elbow must be rested in a sling or a backslab, for an irritable elbow joint which is not rested following an injury reacts by producing joint stiffness. This is due to scarring or even calcification and ossification of the capsule (a condition called myositis ossificans).

The olecranon

The upper ulna is fractured by a direct blow or a fall on to the point of the elbow. The olecranon receives the insertion of the triceps muscle and this bone fragment pulls away from the ulna by the action of this muscle. Operative fixation is required for restoration of the normal anatomy and elbow function, and the screw fixation shown in Fig. 21.22 is effective.

The radial head

The radial head articulates with the humerus and the ulna at the elbow joint and fractures of this bone may interfere with rotation of the forearm.

Fig. 21.22. Fracture of the olecranon—internal fixation with screw.

Treatment

Minor displaced fractures are allowed to unite by resting the elbow in a sling for three weeks. If a substantial portion of the radial head is avulsed then it is best to remove the fragment and excise the damaged head remnant. If an irregular radial head fragment remains there is a risk of subsequent osteoarthritis in the elbow joint. The radial neck is still retained in an annular ligament and rotation persists.

Colles' fracture

This fracture is the commonest seen in the Accident and Emergency departments and is again sustained by a fall on to the outstretched hand, usually in elderly ladies. It is an impacted fracture of the lower radius within an inch of the joint line. The distal radial fragment is displaced and rotated posteriorly and the ulnar styloid is sometimes fractured and separated. The patient complains of pain and tenderness in the wrist, and there is frequently such displacement that a deformity, similar to a dinner fork, is noted (Fig. 21.23).

Fig. 21.23. Colles' fracture with displacement produces a 'dinner fork' deformity.

Treatment

The fracture must be reduced in all but the elderly or those in poor general health in whom operation is contra-indicated. A general anaesthetic is usually advisable but local regional anaesthesia may be undertaken.

Fig. 21.24. Reduction of a Colles' fracture by traction.

Fig. 21.25. Back-slab applied to the wrist following reduction of a Colles fracture.

Technique of Reduction The impacted fragment can be disimpacted by traction (Fig. 21.24). The radial fragment must then be manipulated so that the joint surface of the wrist joint comes into the correct alignment. A plaster backslab is then applied to maintain position (Fig. 21.25). A full plaster is not advisable at this stage for the wrist will continue to swell after reduction and pain and decreased circulation will result. Following the manipulation the fracture position is checked on X-ray and the patient should be seen again in 3 to 4 days to again check the position and to complete the plaster. Further check on X-ray is advisable at about the tenth day, for after this it will be very difficult to alter the fracture position if slipping should occur. The plaster is retained for approximately 6 weeks and the physiotherapist then mobilises the stiff wrist joint.

A *Smith's fracture* is a reverse Colles and its treatment is by manipulation in the reverse direction.

Scaphoid fracture (Fig. 21.26)

This small bone of the carpus is fractured in falls on to the wrist and hand. It often heals with difficulty and if it remains ununited the proximal fragment may collapse due to an inadequate blood supply. This complication is called *avascular necrosis* and results in osteoarthritis of the wrist. Diagnosis is by clinical examination of the wrist, for there is pain and tenderness on the radial side. The fracture does not always show up on the first X-ray examination, but if a scaphoid fracture is suspected a plaster cast must always be applied. Ten to 14 days later a re-X-ray will demonstrate the break

Fig. 21.26. Fracture of the scaphoid bone.

for the fracture line will be more obvious. A plaster cast is retained initially for 6 to 8 weeks, but if it remains ununited internal fixation with a small screw or bone graft will be necessary.

Fractures of the fingers and thumb

Fractures of the metacarpal necks are common and are nearly always the result of a 'hard punch'. The knuckle may be a little flattened by displacement at the fracture site but union rapidly occurs. A useful axiom in the treatment of fractures of the hand is to 'forget the fracture and exercise the joint' and there is no exception in metacarpal fractures. The fracture-dislocation of the base of the thumb metacarpal is called a *Bennett's Fracture* and a wire piercing the skin and traversing the fracture is frequently required for its fixation (Fig. 21.27).

The phalanges of the fingers are often fractured in crush injuries of the hand. They unite quickly and it is again essential to encourage the early movement of the small joints of the injured digit. A useful method of splinting the finger to avoid the stiffness that a plaster or metal splint would produce is to strap one finger to the next and to encourage movement of both together (Fig. 21.28).

A mallet finger deformity (Fig. 21.29) occurs when the terminal phalanx is stubbed on a cricket ball or other hard object. The extensor tendon is torn from the distal phalanx and frequently a fragment

Fig. 21.27. Bennett's fracture being internally fixed by a percutaneous wire.

of bone is avulsed. To restore active extension to the terminal phalanx a mallet finger splint (Fig. 21.30) should be applied for one month.

FRACTURES AND DISLOCATIONS IN THE LOWER LIMB

Hip joint dislocations

Hip joint dislocations are seen commonly in major car accidents. The most common type is the posterior dislocation which may also be associated with a fracture of the acetabulum. The femoral head may dislocate centrally, fracturing the acetabulum as it enters the pelvis, but only rarely does the femoral head come out anteriorly.

Posterior dislocation of the hip

This is seen in front seat passengers when injured in a car and not wearing safety belts. The knee hits the dashboard and a violent force is transmitted along the shaft of the femur to the hip where the femoral head is forcibly dislocated posteriorly (Fig. 21.31).

Treatment

Under a general anaesthetic strong manipulation is required to reduce the dislocation. If there is a fracture of the acetabular rim

Fig. 21.28. Splintage of two fingers together.

Fig. 21.29. Mallet finger deformity.

Fig. 21.30. Mallet finger splint.

Fig. 21.31. Posterior dislocation of the hip.

making the reduction unstable, internal fixation of the bony fragment may be required. The limb should be immobilised in traction for 6 weeks post-reduction to allow the capsule to heal and to restore and maintain the blood supply to the femoral head.

Central dislocations

Pedestrians struck by a vehicle on the lateral side of the hip region may sustain this injury; the femoral head and neck are driven into the pelvis through the acetabulum. Multiple fractures of the pelvis may be sustained.

Treatment

Strong skeletal traction is required to bring the femoral head back into its original position.

Fractures of the femoral neck

These are common fractures seen in the elderly patient, especially female. It occurs in patients with soft osteoporotic bones and may follow relatively minor trauma. The mortality is high, for the patient is elderly and often has associated general health problems which complicate the treatment. The patient's immobility may lead to early bronchopneumonia, congestive heart failure and pulmonary embolism. With many old people it is not the treatment which is the problem, but the after-care and return to independence. These patients frequently live on their own and after such an injury they require a period of support which a keen and enthusiastic family may be able to give. However, this responsibility may be shunned by relatives and the patient's retention in a geriatric hospital or other rehabilitation unit puts a severe strain and burden on the hospital and social services.

Fractures of the femoral neck are described according to their anatomical position (Fig. 21.32):
1. Subcapital
2. Transcervical
3. Trochanteric
4. Subtrochanteric

It should be noted from Fig. 21.32 that fractures affecting the neck proper occur within the capsule of the hip joint, and the blood supply to the femoral head, which runs along the femoral neck, is disturbed. In neck fractures where there is considerable displacement, this major complication of *avascular necrosis* of the femoral

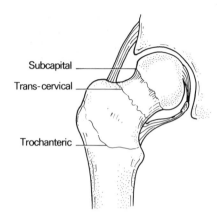

Subcapital

Trans-cervical

Trochanteric

Fig. 21.32. Sites of femoral neck fracture.

head is very high. Avascular necrosis results in collapse of the head and severe osteoarthritis of the hip ensues. This is a disastrous complication (Fig. 21.33).

Fractures affecting the trochanteric and subtrochanteric region are outside the capsule and the blood supply to the femoral head is never interfered with. These fractures, therefore, unite without avascular necrosis.

Some fractures of the femoral neck may unite without operation, but the mortality is high, for the patient may develop pneumonia, urinary tract infection, deep vein thrombosis and pressure sores. It is important, therefore, to stabilise the fracture of the hip joint by appropriate surgical means using internal fixation to allow the patient to get up rapidly and to avoid these severe complications.

Clinical features

Most of these fractures occur in falls in the home and as mentioned previously the trauma involved may be very minor. The elderly patient tripping over a carpet or mat may fracture the femoral neck with the rotary forces applied. The hip is painful and the patient is frequently unable to get up. If the fracture is impacted, reasonable function may be maintained and walking on the hip is possible. In most cases, however, pain and instability is such that the patient has to call for help and is brought to the Accident and Emergency department by ambulance. The affected limb is short, adducted and externally rotated, as shown in Fig. 21.34. Any attempt to move the limb is painful and strongly resisted by the patient. Any elderly patient who has a painful hip following a very minor injury should always be suspected of having this fracture, for although initially it may be impacted and stable, spontaneous loosening at the fracture site may occur and the fragments may become unstable.

Fig. 21.33. Avascular necrosis of the femoral head. Note the densely sclerotic bone.

Fig. 21.34. Position of the leg after left femoral neck fracture.

Treatment

(a) *Subcapital and transcervical fractures (the intracapsular fractures).* If the fracture is impacted and with only very minor displacement internal fixation with a tri-fin nail is undertaken. The correct position is obtained with a guide wire under X-ray control and a Smith–Petersen nail is inserted over this guide wire to immobilise the head on the neck of the femur (Fig. 21.35).

Fractures of the femoral neck which are so displaced as to cause disturbance of the blood supply to the femoral head will be complicated by avascularity of the head with resulting collapse and osteoarthritis of the hip joint.

Fig. 21.35. Nail fixation of a sub-capital fracture.

In most elderly patients the head is excised, the neck trimmed and a replacement prosthesis of a Thompson or Austin Moore type is inserted (Fig. 21.36). The Thompson prosthesis is often seated in acrylic cement in the upper femoral neck and shaft for added stability.

(b) *Trochanteric and subtrochanteric fractures of the femoral neck.* Fractures at this site unite satisfactorily for much of the bone is cancellous with good healing properties and the blood supply to the femoral head is not disturbed. Internal fixation of the fracture is satisfactorily carried out with a pin and plate (Fig. 21.37). The pin is inserted into the femoral neck and head over a guide wire inserted with X-ray control and the plate is attached to the pin by means of a bolt, and to the upper femoral shaft by means of multiple screws.

Fig. 21.36. Thompson replacement of femoral head following sub-capital fracture.

The post-operative management of the patient following hip surgery.

Patients who have had their fractures internally fixed are sat up out of bed the next day if possible. Walking with support—guided by the physiotherapist—is encouraged as soon as the patient is able to co-operate. When a pin or a pin and plate is inserted only partial weight bearing is allowed on the appropriate limb until the fracture has united at approximately the third post-operative month. Until that time frame or crutch support is advised. If the patient has had a prosthetic replacement of the femoral head, rest in bed for two or three days is advisable, with the hip abducted by means of appropriate pillows, or light skin traction. Abduction of the hip is important following this operation for dislocations can occur and this complication is avoided by keeping the legs wide apart during

Fig. 21.37. Pin and plate fixation of a trochanteric fracture.

the initial post-operative period. When muscle control is regained two or three days post-operatively the physiotherapist may get the patient up and walking. The minimal support of sticks is all that is required.

Fractures of the femoral shaft

This is a common fracture seen in all age groups and is sustained in road traffic and industrial accidents and falls from a height. The fracture is frequently associated with other injuries and the patient is often in a shocked state when admitted to the Accident and Emergency department. In the absence of any other injury a fracture of this large bone will produce considerable blood loss. The thigh becomes swollen and tense, and two to three bottles of blood (1.0 l–1.5 l) are lost into the muscles and soft tissues of the thigh. The hypovolaemia resulting from such a fracture may surgically shock the elderly patient and so steps must be taken on admission to restore the blood volume with appropriately cross-matched blood.

Traction is the secret of both reduction and fixation of this fracture. In the child a simple Gallow's traction apparatus (Fig. 21.38) is adequate, and after 4 to 5 weeks the fracture is stable enough for mobilisation to begin.

In the adult strong traction is required to align and reduce the fracture and to keep it fixed in such a position that union will occur. Skeletal traction is required, for weights of between 15 and 20 pounds are not uncommonly necessary. A Steinmann's pin is placed through the upper tibia under a local or general anaesthetic to attach the main traction weight (Fig. 21.39). The body itself acts as a counter-traction with the head end of the bed lowered. The alignment of the fracture and the management of this painful and unstable limb is aided by a Thomas' splint with a knee flexion piece; the whole apparatus being balanced by multiple weights (Fig. 21.40). In many units a simple pillow beneath the thigh is used to maintain the position of the fracture whilst traction is continued, dispensing with the Thomas' splint. Three months in traction are necessary and

Fig. 21.38. Gallow's traction.

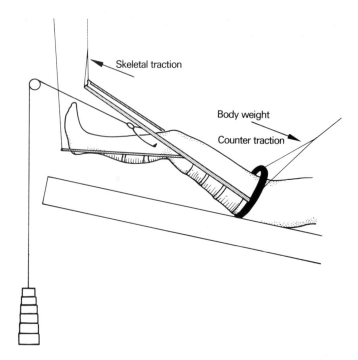

Fig. 21.39. Skeletal traction apparatus for femoral shaft fracture.

Fig. 21.40. Thomas' splint.

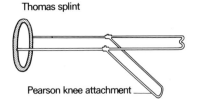

during this time it is vital that the knee is kept mobile. The patient's pressure areas are dealt with adequately and the general exercise and rehabilitation of the patient is started as soon as possible after the accident.

Most femoral shaft fractures are adequately treated by conservative means. If attention is paid to the rehabilitation of the patient and the mobilisation of the knee in particular, no disability will result.

Internal fixation with an intramedullary rod is undertaken in the following circumstances:

1. Where it is impossible to reduce the fracture due to soft tissues and muscle being interposed between the bone ends.

2. In a pathological fracture where metastasis to the femoral shaft has occurred from a carcinoma elsewhere.

3. In multiple injuries, where the tibia, femur and perhaps other bones are fractured. It is impossible to mobilise the knee adequately if multiple fractures in one limb are treated conservatively.

4. If the patient is very elderly and will not tolerate 3 months in traction in bed.

Intramedullary nail fixation of this fracture (Fig. 21.41) has the great advantage of speedy mobilisation and allows full weight bearing, but it should always be remembered that a very small percentage become infected and if an intramedullary nail is present the whole femoral shaft may be involved.

The supracondylar fracture

This is a common fracture in elderly people. It is treated usually conservatively by similar means to the femoral shaft fracture with skeletal traction and an adequate pad beneath the knee to lift up the distal fragment, but again internal fixation with a blade plate (Fig. 21.42) may be necessary.

Fig. 21.41. (LEFT) Intramedullary nail for a femoral shaft fracture.

Fig. 21.42. (RIGHT) Internal fixation of a supracondylar fracture with a blade plate.

Patellar fractures

A transverse fracture is sustained when the knee is struck anteriorly and the pull of the large thigh muscles—the quadriceps—cleanly separates the bone into two fragments. If the fragments can be brought together anatomically they may be fixed by means of a screw (Fig. 21.43) or by an encircling wire. A comminuted fracture with multiple fragments (Fig. 21.44) cannot be replaced and so excision of the patellar portions is undertaken and the surrounding torn capsule is repaired.

Fractures of the tibia

This bone is commonly fractured and as its medial surface is subcutaneous it is most frequently compound fracture seen. It is this latter aspect, together with the relatively poor blood supply of the bone in the lower portions of the tibia, which make it such a difficult injury to treat. In most cases, a simple tibial fracture can be put straight and into good position under a general anaesthetic. The alignment and replacement can be adjusted by manipulation and with a well padded good fitting plaster of Paris cast the fracture will unite satisfactorily in 3 months. The plaster should stretch from the toes to the upper thigh region to adequately immobilise the knee

Fig. 21.43. Patellar fracture fixed by means of a screw.

Fig. 21.44. Comminuted patellar fracture.

and the ankle joints. If the fracture is compound the treatment regimen outlined on page 490 is undertaken. If the tibial fracture is very comminuted and shortened, traction is undertaken with a skeletal Steinmann's pin inserted through the calcaneum.

Many tibial fractures are unstable and this is particularly so in the short oblique fracture, where it is often impossible to stabilise and maintain the position by manipulation. It may be decided in these cases to fix the bone internally with a plate and screws which will hold the position accurately and stably (Fig. 21.12). The stability of internal fixation is increased by a compression plating technique whereby the bone ends are compressed together by the device shown in Fig. 21.45.

POTT'S FRACTURE (Fig. 21.46).

A Pott's fracture is a fracture dislocation of the ankle joint. It is most commonly caused by the patient falling or stumbling, thus rotating the foot externally and forcing it backwards.

Fig. 21.45. Compression plating technique.

Grade I Pott's fracture. The fibula is fractured on the lateral side of the ankle and a spiral break is present. The talus bone, which is retained in the ankle joint mortice by the medial and lateral malleoli, may shift laterally at the time of this fracture dislocation.

Grade II Pott's fracture. With a greater external rotation and posterior force on the foot, the lateral and medial malleoli may both fracture. Frequently the talus shifts and accurate reduction of both bones is necessary. As both sides of the joint are unstable, internal fixation may be required.

Fig. 21.46. Pott's fracture-dislocation of ankle.

Grade III Pott's fracture. The force applied to the ankle joint is sometimes so great that the posterior lip of the tibia is also avulsed. The talus then shifts laterally and posteriorly and the displacement may be so great that the blood supply to the foot is occluded.

Treatment

Grade I Pott's fracture may be treated conservatively by manipulation of the lateral malleolus into a good position. The plaster is applied below the knee with the foot at right angles for 6 to 8 weeks and only in the latter part of this period is weight bearing allowed. In a Grade II fracture, the instability may be such that both the medial malleolus and sometimes the lateral malleolus requires fixation (Fig. 21.47). Grade III fractures always require internal fixation for they are very unstable.

FRACTURES IN THE FOOT

The calcaneum or heel bone is often fractured in falls on to the feet. If the patient falls from a great height not only are the heel bones damaged but frequently a crush fracture of one of the upper lumbar

Fig. 21.47. Internal fixation of a Pott's fracture.

Fig. 21.48. Fracture of calcaneus.

Fig. 21.49. Flexion injury of the neck producing fracture-dislocation. Note the complete transection of the spinal cord.

vertebrae is sustained. The calcaneal fractures which do not involve the subtalar joint are treated by initial plaster cast or by elevation. The foot is mobilised as soon as comfort will allow. Fractures involving the subtalar joint (Fig. 21.48) are more serious for inversion and eversion of the foot will be interfered with, and further operative treatment will be required to arthrodese the joint.

Metatarsal and phalangeal fractures

These injuries are troublesome for they cause great pain on weight bearing. The patients recover faster if weight relief is given by temporary crutches or sticks but the foot must be kept as mobile as possible.

SPINAL INJURIES

Cervical spine

Serious neck injuries are most commonly sustained in road accidents, diving in shallow water and, rarely, in Rugby Football. Head injuries are frequently associated and it is the acute flexion of the neck which does the damage (Fig. 21.49). A patient complaining of a painful and stiff neck after a fall or a road accident of this type should be suspected of having a cervical spine injury, which may be potentially dangerous. If it is possible to lie the patient on his back this will bring the cervical spine into an extended position and this is the safest way to transport him. If, however, the patient is unconscious or there is some other contra-indication to the supine position the neck must be steadied gently by the first aid attendant whilst the patient is transferred to an Accident and Emergency department.

Many cervical spine injuries are stable with the spinous process fractured or the vertebral body crushed. In these instances a simple collar is the only requirement and this together with adequate rest and analgesics will allow the fracture to unite with good restoration of cervical spine movements.

It is the unstable dislocation or fracture-dislocation which is dangerous for the spinal cord may be damaged, producing either death or paraplegia.

Treatment of the unstable cervical fracture dislocation

This fracture, like all others, must be reduced and here again traction in an extended neck position is the answer. Skeletal traction must be used, for any other method of applying a pull to the neck is unsuccessful and extremely uncomfortable. Crutchfield tongs are inserted with spikes which pass through only the outer table of the skull. Traction of 20 to 30 pounds may be required to reduce the fracture dislocation of the cervical spine (Fig. 21.50). Traction for approximately 6 weeks is required and during this time the patient is best nursed on a circle-electric bed (Fig. 21.51) or a Stryker frame which will allow the turning of the patient without disturbing the traction or the position of the cervical spine. If the cervical spine is found to be stable at the end of this 6 weeks' period a plaster collar may be applied for a further 6 weeks. If the cervical spine still remains unstable at the end of the 6 weeks, fusion of the unstable segments should be undertaken by means of either an anterior approach with insertion of graft into the damaged vertebral bodies, or by a posterior approach in which the spinous processes are wired together and strut grafts are applied along the laminae of the vertebrae (Fig. 21.52).

Fig. 21.50. Crutchfield tongs.

Thoracic spine

Thoracic vertebral bodies are frequently crushed in flexion injuries in the elderly osteoporotic patient. There is initial pain and tenderness and there may be some difficulty in rehabilitation of the patient. This fracture is stable and requires no more active treatment than extension exercises and active mobilisation as soon as the patient is comfortable.

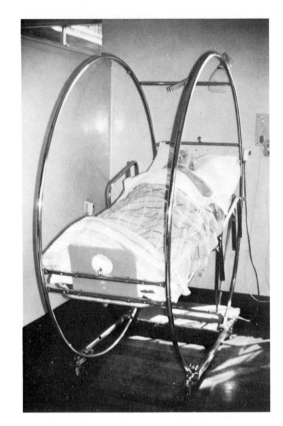

Fig. 21.51. Circle-electric bed.

Fig. 21.52. Posterior cervical fusion.

Lumbar spine

Fractures in this region may again be stable or unstable. If they are stable the same principles apply, with bed rest and analgesics being given until the patient is comfortable. Active mobilisation with particular emphasis on extension exercises are given as soon as possible.

Unstable fracture dislocations of the lumbar spine

This is a serious injury for damage to the cauda equina may occur at time of injury or later if the first aid measures have not prevented further movement at the fracture site. The patient must be treated with great care at the site of the accident and also whilst being transported to the hospital. If he is to be carried on a stretcher it is best to do so lying on his front for the extended position of the spine will tend to prevent further shift and dislocation.

Neurological signs of paralysis and anaesthesia in the lower limbs together with bladder paralysis indicates damage to the nerve roots in the cauda equina. The patient must be nursed as described above on a circle electric bed or a Stryker frame. The nursing areas of particular importance are:

1. Pressure areas. Frequent turning and attention to pressure points must be made.

2. The bladder. Catheterisation is undertaken initially but later regular expression of urine may be made by pressure on the lower abdomen. A urinary antiseptic must be given e.g. sulphadimidine 0.5 gm q.d.s.

3. The chest. The avoidance of chest infection is important. Frequent deep breathing exercises are encouraged.

4. Rehabilitation. When the initial problems of the paralysed patient are over, the nurse will be part of the team which will undertake the rehabilitation programme. The eventual outcome will depend upon the neurological level of paralysis, but with the help of the physiotherapist, physical medicine consultant, appliance maker and social worker the patient should be able to return to a suitable job and lead a reasonably happy and useful life.

Operative treatment

Internal fixation of the unstable fracture dislocation of the lumbar spine may be necessary. The patient who has minor neurological signs but an unstable injury would benefit from this procedure. The spine is explored posteriorly and fixation plates and bolts hold the spinous processes in good position (Fig. 21.53). Bone grafts are laid along the exposed areas and will allow the unstable segments to solidly fuse together.

Bone graft or plate

Bolts through spinous process

Fig. 21.53. Posterior fusion of lumbar spine.

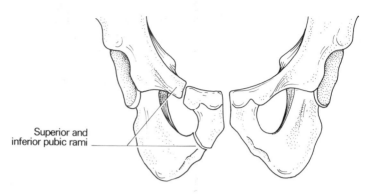

Superior and
inferior pubic rami

Fig. 21.54. Fracture of the pubic
rami.

PELVIC FRACTURES

Fractures of the pelvic ring are common and may be sustained by
both minor falls and by major crushing injuries. Minor fractures of
the pubic rami (Fig. 21.54) occur commonly in the elderly and osteoporotic patients and cause enough pain to prevent walking for a few
days. No specific treatment is necessary but the patient must be
encouraged to be up and mobile at the earliest moment.

Fig. 21.55. Major pelvic ring
fractures.

Crushing injuries which are sustained frequently in road traffic accidents may disrupt the pelvic ring by producing fractures in two or more places (Fig. 21.55). A prolonged period of bed rest is required and often traction to one or both lower limbs is helpful to re-position the fragments.

Complications

1. Haemorrhage. Much of the pelvic bone is cancellous and bleeding from fractured areas may be enormous. Several bottles of blood may be required to restore the blood volume following an injury of this type, and the retroperitoneal haematoma which develops may be equivalent to the size of a 30 week pregnancy.
2. Damage to pelvic viscera. The bladder, and more particularly the urethra, may be damaged by anterior pubic fractures especially in those cases in which a segment is pushed backwards. Any attempt at catheterisation following a pelvic injury must be carried out in the operating theatre if the possibility of urethral or bladder damage is expected (see pages 342 and 347).

Chapter 22. Orthopaedics

Orthopaedics means literally the 'straight child' (orthos and pais in Greek) and the first part of this chapter will be devoted to deformities and diseases of childhood. Orthopaedic surgery covers a wide range of deformities, diseases and ailments of the locomotor system and especially those affecting the limbs, bones, muscles and joints. It is a speciality which is closely connected with the trauma described in Chapter 21 and orthopaedic surgeons usually deal with both injuries and elective orthopaedic problems.

PAEDIATRIC ORTHOPAEDICS

There are many congenital deformities, some single and others complex and multiple, which affect the locomotor system. In most the aetiology is unknown but recent advances in genetics indicate that some are due to abnormalities of the chromosomal composition of the cells. Disease in pregnancy such as rubella may produce abnormalities and the administration of thalidomide to pregnant women during the late 1950s and early 1960s produced a large number of skeletal deformities. Most of the common problems discussed in this section are of unknown aetiology.

CONGENITAL DISLOCATION OF THE HIP (C.D.H.)

This serious abnormality affects girls more frequently than boys (6 : 1) and the incidence in most of the United Kingdom is approximately 3 per 1,000 live births. There is a definite familial incidence and its occurrence is high in certain races such as the North Italians and also the North American Indians. The babies born by breech delivery are especially at risk and the underlying anatomical abnormality is most probably laxity of the hip joint ligaments.

Diagnosis

It is important to diagnose the condition in the early neonatal period for treatment may be fully corrective if started at this early stage. Unstable hips are diagnosed by clinical means and not by X-ray for the joint is too immature skeletally. It is important that the midwife and paediatrician examine the hips of all babies born, for delayed diagnosis may complicate treatment seriously.

If there is a full dislocation the limb will be shorter and abduction of the hip will be limited. Abduction of the hips, as shown in Fig. 22.1 will produce a clunk and a movement of the head of the femur when the hip rides in and out of socket. This is called Ortolani's click test. If the pelvis is steadied with one hand and the suspicious hip manipulated as shown in Fig. 22.2 again a clunk with movement indicates a subluxation or full dislocation of this unstable hip (Barlow's test).

If diagnosis is not made by the medical attendants in the neonatal period then the mother sometimes notices shortening and the absence of full movement of the hip at six months of age. More frequently it is not until the limp is noted at about 16 months that diagnosis is made. By this stage the radiological appearance is very abnormal (Fig. 22.3).

Fig. 22.1. (LEFT) Ortolani's test for hip instability.

Fig. 22.2. (RIGHT) Barlow's test. The pelvis is fixed and the hip is abducted.

Fig. 22.3. Congenital dislocation of the hip. The femoral head is displaced from the shallow acetabulum.

Treatment

In the neonatal period the application of an abduction splint for 6–8 weeks may be all that is necessary (Fig. 22.4). After 3 months of age, abduction of the hips and their retention in this position by a frog-style plaster (Fig. 22.5) allows the normal growth of the acetabulum to deepen the socket around the femoral head.

Fig. 22.4. (left) Abduction splint.

Fig. 22.5. (right) 'Frog' abduction plaster.

Conservative treatment is usually satisfactory until the age of one year but after this time operative treatment is usually necessary. If the hips are tight, abduction traction is applied slowly and increasingly from the neutral position to the fully separated position (Fig. 22.6). A plaster cast will then retain the reduced position and this is maintained until the socket is deepened enough.

Fig. 22.6. Abduction traction.

After the age of one year operative treatment may become necessary to reduce the dislocation. Tight capsular and other obstructing structures are removed to enable the deeper setting of the femoral head. To give greater stability upper femoral osteotomy or pelvic osteotomy (Fig. 22.7) may be necessary. Meticulous follow-up of the child with a congenital dislocation or dysplasia of the hip will be necessary until skeletal maturity occurs.

The untreated or, even worse, the inadequately treated hip dislocation will lead to gross hip deformity and osteoarthritis in later life.

Fig. 22.7. Salter's pelvic osteotomy to deepen acetabular socket.

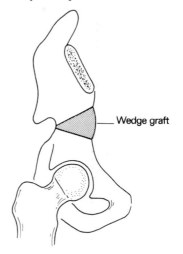

Wedge graft

CONGENITAL CLUB FOOT (Talipes Equino-Varus, T.E.V.)

The term talipes refers to any foot and ankle deformity. The deformed foot is in equinus (plantar flexion), varus (with the soles turned in) and the forefoot is adducted (twisted towards the mid-line). The whole deformity is illustrated in Fig. 22.8.

The club foot is a difficult deformity to treat successfully. It is commoner in boys (3 : 1) and occurs in its full form in approximately 2 per 1,000 live births. Its minor forms are more common.

The club foot deformity may be due to a neurological abnormality such as spina bifida or later acquired in poliomyelitis but most of the babies seen with this abnormality have a congenital talipes equino-varus, of unknown aetiology.

Fig. 22.8. Club foot (talipes-equino-varus).

Treatment

Early treatment is again important, and manipulation should be started by the surgeon or the physiotherapist on the first day of life. The soft tissues later become more contracted and difficult to stretch and eventually a secondary bone deformity develops.

Very regular stretching and manipulation is essential for success. The varus heel must be stretched outwards and the equinus foot must be manipulated upwards to the neutral position. The inturned forefoot is corrected and strapping is then applied to maintain the position (Figs. 22.9 and 22.10).

In approximately half the babies the foot may be corrected without operation. After 6–8 weeks of meticulous manipulation a decision can be reached as to whether conservative treatment will be successful or not. If surgical assistance is necessary it is best to release the deformity at this early stage. Releasing the tight Achilles tendon posteriorly will be sufficient in some but in the others more extensive surgical release will be necessary.

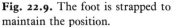

Fig. 22.9. The foot is strapped to maintain the position.

SPINA BIFIDA & MYELOMENINGOCELE

This is a relatively common deformity (2.5 per thousand live births) and occurs when the posterior elements of the spine fail to form and allow the meninges, spinal cord and nerve roots to prolapse through to the body surface (Fig. 22.11). The lumbar region is most commonly involved but it can occur at any spinal level.

Hydrocephalus occurs in 80% of these children and the head swells progressively due to enlargement of the brain ventricles filled with excessive cerebro-spinal fluid under high pressure.

Treatment

Babies with this condition pose a severe moral and ethical problem for the obstetrician and paediatrician. Many of the children will develop severe disturbances of intellect, abnormalities of the urinary tract and paralysis of the lower limbs. The prognosis is worst if the myelomeningocele is high in the spine and covers many segments.

If the defect is not closed many will die of a meningitis. The child with a surgically closed defect will usually require insertion of a

Spitz-Holter valve to drain the cerebro-spinal fluid from the ventricles to the right superior vena cava and right atrium of the heart. This drainage of cerebro-spinal fluid will prevent hydrocephalus from developing (see page 134).

Bladder paralysis and subsequent problems of the urinary tract are often treated by the formation of an ileal loop bladder. Paralysis of the lower limbs is managed by appropriate calipers and braces (Fig. 22.12) but in some children stability and rebalance of musculature is achieved by muscle and tendon transpositions.

The lower limbs may be anaesthetic and the paralysis may be so severe that many children take to a wheelchair in later life.

Fig. 22.10. The completion of successful conservative treatment.

SCOLIOSIS

Scoliosis is a lateral curvature of the spine (Fig. 22.13). The scoliosis may be postural when there is a sciatica and where there is no fixed anatomical abnormality. A true structural scoliosis with a fixed deformity is due to either congenital or acquired causes:

Fig. 22.11. (above) Spina bifida and myelomeningocele.

Fig. 22.12. (left) Caliper and brace to stabilise paralysed lower limbs.

Congenital scoliosis occurs where there are abnormalities of the structure of a vertebral body or a spinal segment.

Paralytic—poliomyelitis or other neurological problems produce imbalance of spinal musculature.

Idiopathic—This is the commonest variety and has no known cause. The curve may increase and may be associated with rotation of the chest cage, producing an unsightly rib hump. The severe scoliosis will produce a decrease in the lung function.

The management

When the skeleton is mature the curve will cease to progress. In children below 10 years of age with a progressive scoliosis a brace must be worn (Fig. 22.14).

Operation is necessary over the age of 10 when the type of scoliosis curve is known to be progressive. A period of stretching in a halo-pelvic traction apparatus may be required pre-operatively (Fig. 22.15) and at operation spinal fusion is carried out, sometimes associated with a Harrington distraction rod (Fig. 22.16).

OSTEOMYELITIS

Bone infection, or osteomyelitis, may affect any part of the skeleton. The child is more frequently affected than the adult but no age is exempt. It may be acute or chronic.

Fig. 22.13. Scoliosis.

Fig. 22.14. Milwaukee brace to hold the scoliotic spine.

Acute osteomyelitis

Pyogenic organisms such as the staphylococcus, streptococcus, pneumococcus, meningococcus, and more rarely the gonococcus and *E. coli* spread by the blood stream from an infected focus, such as a boil, to the metaphyseal area of a bone (Fig. 22.17). Pus soon forms and bursts out through the cortex of the bone to lie beneath the periosteum. The pressure of pus cuts off the blood supply to some areas of the bone; this dead necrotic bone is called a *sequestrum* (Fig. 22.18).

Clinical features

Pain rapidly becomes intense and the child becomes pyrexial and ill. Local signs of inflammation soon become apparent over the infected bone with increased heat, swelling, redness and tenderness. The diagnosis is made from the above symptoms and signs and a blood culture usually grows the infecting organisms. X-rays are not helpful in the first week but during this time it is important to make the diagnosis. Later a periosteal reaction is seen on X-ray and bone destruction in the metaphyseal region becomes apparent. A sequestrum is seen in the later stages as a dense sclerotic area (Fig. 22.19).

Fig. 22.15. Halo-pelvic traction.

Treatment

Antibiotics alone may be successful in the earliest stage. A large dose of cloxacillin and ampicillin together (adult dose 500 mg and 250 mg q.d.s. respectively) is given. When the blood culture is known, the appropriate single antibiotic can then be prescribed. If the temperature and local signs are not reversed within the first 48 hours of this medication operation is indicated.

The bone is exposed at the site of maximum inflammation and the periosteum is incised. Pus is sometimes found beneath the periosteum but failing this the bone is drilled and pus may be found within.

Chronic osteomyelitis

This may follow an acute osteomyelitis with pyogenic organisms. Infection with tubercle bacilli may produce a chronic osteomyelitis and Pott's disease of the spine is a good example (Fig. 22.20). The tubercle bacilli becomes established in the disc space and spread into the vertebral bodies on either side. The wedge-shaped collapse of the vertebral bones produces an angular kyphosis of the spine, usually

Fig. 22.16. Harrington rod correcting scoliosis at the time of spinal fusion.

Fig. 22.17. (LEFT) Osteo-myelitis. Infection arises in the metaphysis of the bone.

Fig. 22.18. (RIGHT) Continued infection produces a necrotic sequestrum.

in the thoracic region. Pus may spread from the bone as a cold abscess compressing the spinal cord (Pott's paraplegia) or it may present in the groin as a psoas abscess.

SEPTIC ARTHRITIS

A joint may be affected with organisms similar to those found in osteomyelitis. Children are again particularly affected and the hip joint is the most common site of neonatal infection (Tom Smith's disease). The infection is blood-borne but in a few cases of septic arthritis of the knee a penetrating wound may be the cause of bacterial entry.

Fig. 22.19. The sequestrum in the fibula shows on X-ray as a dense area.

Clinical features

Pain and loss of function of the infected limb develops at an early stage. The child rapidly becomes ill and feverish and a blood culture may reveal the infecting organism. X-rays may show excessive distention of the joint cavity, and at a later stage erosion of the joint surfaces becomes apparent (Fig. 22.21).

A final diagnosis is made by aspirating the joint with a needle and syringe and if pus is present the joint must be opened and adequately drained under a general anaesthetic. Long-term antibiotics will again be required.

OSTEOARTHRITIS

All joints wear over the years. In some patients however, the wear and tear process is excessive and the joint becomes painful, stiff and eventually deformed. This process is now called degenerative joint disease or osteoarthrosis (osteoarthritis). It should be noted that there is no true inflammation but purely a degeneration of the articular cartilage. Eventually the cartilage wears away completely, leaving bone to articulate with bone. Secondary changes now occur with spurs of new bone forming around the joint margins (osteophytes), thickening of the bone ends (sclerosis), and cysts developing beneath the joint surface (Fig. 22.22).

Aetiology

Joints which have been previously damaged by infection or trauma develop a secondary osteoarthritis at an early stage. Primary or idiopathic osteoarthritis develops as a degeneration of the joint surface but the cause is unknown.

Clinical features

The first symptom is a little pain or ache after exercise in or around the joint affected. The disease is variably progressive and there are frequently exacerbations and remissions in the symptoms. The pain

Fig. 22.20. Pott's disease (tuberculosis of the spine).

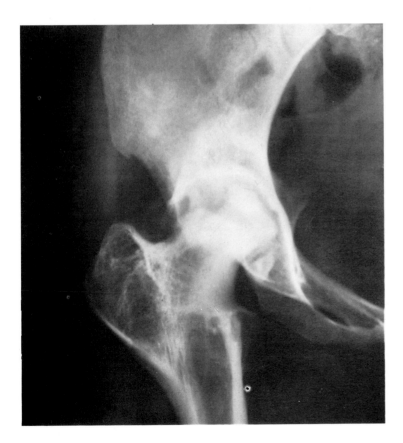

Fig. 22.21. Erosion of the joint surface in a septic arthritis.

may increase and may become particularly troublesome at night. Stiffness increases as the range of joint movement decreases and contractures eventually deform the joint and the limb.

Treatment

Osteoarthritis of the hip is the most common large joint affected and this will be used as an example to illustrate the range of therapy available.

1. *Medication.* Simple aspirin is useful to control the pain. Phenylbutazone 100 mg t.d.s. may be more effective in decreasing pain and stiffness.

2. *Support.* A stick is useful to decrease the weight put upon the affected hip.

3. *Physiotherapy.* Increasing the range of movement and strengthening of the musculature around the joint will always be beneficial. Exercise in a pool (hydrotherapy) may be particularly effective.

4. *Operative treatment.* If the above conservative measures are no longer effective the orthopaedic surgeon may consider one of the following procedures advisable:

(i) *Trochanteric osteotomy*—Pain may be dramatically decreased by dividing the upper femur and repositioning the head and neck as shown in Fig. 22.23. A new articular area is brought into the

Fig. 22.22. Osteoarthritis of the left hip.

Fig. 22.23. Trochanteric osteotomy fixed with a blade plate.

acetabulum and the fracture healing process remodels the diseased bone of the femoral head. The operation is most effective in the osteoarthritic hip joint where there is considerable pain but still a good range of movement. The osteotomy is only successful in relieving the symptoms in two-thirds of the patients operated upon.

(ii) *Total hip replacement arthroplasty*—When the destructive arthritic changes are very severe, replacement of both surfaces of the joint becomes necessary. The head and neck are removed, the acetabular cartilage is excised and the socket deepened. A plastic acrylic cement substance is used to seat firmly the metal or polyethylene components of the new joint. There are many types of total replacement arthroplasty but they fall into two categories: (1) the

Fig. 22.24. McKee Farrar total hip replacement.

Fig. 22.25. Charnley total hip replacement.

metal to metal bearing prosthesis typified by the McKee Farrar model (Fig. 22.24), (2) the metal to high density polyethylene bearing prosthesis of the Charnley type (Fig. 22.25).

These replacement arthroplasties are very successful in returning mobility and comfort to the joint. Complications are few but dislocation may be a problem if the components are not angulated correctly. Infection will always be disastrous and steps must be taken to keep this complication as low as possible.

(iii) *Arthrodesis*—Arthrodesis means the elimination of the joint articulating surfaces and fusion together of the two bones. Arthrodesis produces a painless, stable situation but there is, of course, no mobility. A hip may be arthrodesed in the young person and is usually carried out in the osteoarthritic hip which develops secondary to previous trauma or infection. It is impossible to arthrodese both sides.

RHEUMATOID ARTHRITIS

Rheumatoid arthritis is an inflammatory disease of joints which affects both young and old. There is also a juvenile type called Still's disease.

The first site of this disease is in the synovial membrane lining the joint. This membrane becomes inflamed and thickened and gradually proliferates to eat away the surrounding ligaments and articular cartilage of the joint surfaces. It affects peripheral small joints initially but later the larger weight-bearing joints may become affected.

Treatment

The treatment of rheumatoid arthritis is essentially medical but surgery may have a small part to play. Rest is important in the acute phase and medicines are given to prevent pain and inflammation. Aspirin, 300—600 mg several times each day and phenylbutazone, 100 mg t.d.s. are commonly used. The physiotherapist is an important member of the team treating the patient with this disease for she will help to preserve the mobility and strength of the joints. The occupational therapist will also give good advice as to the aids which may be helpful to the disabled person.

Surgery has a small but important part in the management of the patient with rheumatoid arthritis. Frequently very small surgical procedures have great benefit and such operations as repair of ruptured tendons, release of trigger fingers or release of carpal tunnel syndromes, may help the patient greatly.

Rheumatoid disease may so destroy joints that surgical replacements may become necessary. At the hip the total replacements are very successful. The knee is a difficult joint to replace but a hinge-type prosthesis is indicated in some, and a condylar type replacement of the joint surfaces in others (Fig. 22.26).

Arthrodesis of the knee produces a stable, painless, but fixed joint but again this can only be performed on one side. The hand becomes grossly deformed by rheumatoid disease (Fig. 22.27) but

Fig. 22.26. Westminster condylar replacement of the knee. The femoral surfaces are replaced with metal and the tibial surfaces with polyethylene.

Fig. 22.27. (LEFT) The hand affected by rheumatoid arthritis.

the patients may retain remarkably good function with destroyed joints. There is an indication to replace the metacarpal-phalangeal joints with silastic hinges in some but it should be stressed that the indication for joint surgery of this type is gross limitation of function (Fig. 22.28). The poor appearance of the hand does not constitute an indication for surgical intervention.

Fig. 22.28. Rheumatoid hand with an extremely poor grip.

The toes frequently become very deformed and dislocated on the metacarpals. Excision of the metatarsal heads will restore the shape and comfort of the foot (Fig. 22.29).

BONE TUMOURS

Tumours affecting the skeleton are either benign or malignant. Malignant tumours are primary when they originate in bone or secondary when they have spread to bone from a tumour in another organ. The most common bone tumour which is seen is a secondary deposit (Fig. 22.30). The tumours which particularly spread to bone

Fig. 22.29. The right forefoot has been treated by excision of the metatarsal heads.

Fig. 22.30. A metastasis through the upper humerus (arrowed) showing a pathological fracture. The primary was a carcinoma of the lung.

are carcinomas of the breast in the female and bronchus in the male. The prostate, kidney and thyroid when affected by cancers may all spread to the skeleton.

BENIGN TUMOURS

1. *Osteoma*—this produces a bony lump called an exostosis. It is frequently found in the child as a single lesion but in the condition called diaphyseal aclasis multiple exostoses are seen (Fig. 22.31).

2. *Chondroma*—these cartilage tumours develop within or upon the surface of bone. They frequently present as pathological fractures in the bones of the hand (Fig. 22.32).

3. *Fibroma*—these are frequently seen in X-rays of children's long bones. They usually disappear at the time of skeletal maturity but large areas of fibrous dysplasia may sometimes persist in the bone shaft (Fig. 22.33).

Fig. 22.31. An upper tibial exostosis.

Fig. 22.32. Chondromas of metacarpals and phalanges.

Fig. 22.33. Fibroma.

This is a primary bone tumour which affects the mature skeleton, particularly in the upper tibia and lower femur. The epiphyseal area of the bone is affected and a tumour mass may approach the joint surface. It may remain benign and treatment consists of simply curetting the tumour from the bone. It may be locally recurrent and now more radical measures may have to be undertaken. It may be fully malignant with a production of distant metastases.

Wide local excision of the more aggressive giant cell tumour may be necessary and the neighbouring joint may require replacement with a total prosthesis.

MALIGNANT BONE TUMOURS

1. *Osteosarcoma*—This is a very malignant primary bone tumour which affects young people between the ages of five and twenty-five. It is also seen in the elderly patient and occurs in an area of Paget's disease of bone. Most osteosarcomas develop de novo without known cause but a few may follow radiotherapy to the skeleton.

Clinical features

The osteosarcoma is a very rare tumour and diagnosis is frequently delayed. A lump in relationship to the knee is the most common presenting sign and the swelling may become acutely inflamed and may be mistaken for a bone infection or a joint injury. The X-ray shows much new bone together with bone disruption, as illustrated in Fig. 22.34. The definite diagnosis can only be made on biopsy and a very careful examination of the patient clinically, radiologically, and by bone gamma-scan will be necessary to exclude distant metastases. The tumour rapidly and aggressively metastasises to the lungs and this is the reason for not advising radical amputation of the limb at an early stage.

The tumour is irradiated with a high dose of deep X-rays and then careful follow-up is undertaken over the next 6 months. In many cases metastases will develop during these months but in some no spread will be detected.

At the end of the 6 month period the patient is again carefully reviewed and if there is certainly no evidence of lung or distant metastases then the amputation of the limb will be performed. This treatment programme will eliminate much unnecessary suffering for the amputation of a limb will be avoided in a child who develops metastases after just a few weeks or months. In spite of this treatment regimen the 5 year survival rate still remains at 25%.

Fig. 22.34. Osteosarcoma of the lower femur.

2. *Chondrosarcoma*—This is a malignant cartilage tumour which usually requires radical amputation for its treatment. It is not quite so malignant as the osteosarcoma but the survival rate is again poor.

3. *Ewing's sarcoma*—This is another very malignant tumour affecting the mid-shaft region of the long bones of the child. Radiotherapy is the treatment of choice but the mortality is extremely high.

NEUROLOGICAL CONDITIONS PRODUCING DEFORMITY

1. **Poliomyelitis**

This is now a rare condition in Western countries but it is still seen in less developed areas of the world. A virus infection affects the anterior horn cells of the spinal cord and produces a flaccid paralysis of the limbs.

The principles of treatment are to maintain the stability and balance of the limb by:

(i) using calipers to brace the limb.

(ii) joint stabilisation operation such as foot or wrist arthrodesis.

(iii) tendon transfers to make good use of the remaining muscles in a paralysed area.

2. Hemiplegias

Cerebro-vascular accidents frequently leave the patient with a hemiplegia. The muscles are spastic and the joints become deformed. Full rehabilitation of the patient is necessary and joint abnormalities may be helped by the lengthening or division of tight tendons. Calipers are again often useful for support.

3. Cerebral palsy

Birth trauma may produce a spastic paraplegia. The child may be of normal intelligence but there is often some associated mental handicap. Spasticity of the muscles of the limbs produces gross problems of function and the joints may become deformed. Treatment in a special spastics centre is ideal for there are particular educational needs and the physiotherapist will be able to continue long-term treatment. Surgery has only a very small part to play in the treatment of these disabled children but simple measures such as the lengthening of tendons and the release of contractures may assist the balance and the walking ability.

Fig. 22.35. A thoracic spine kyphosis.

BONE DISEASES

Osteoporosis

A decrease in the protein part of the bone matrix produces a decrease in the bone strength. It occurs especially in the elderly and is associated with the post-menopausal state in the female. It is exacerbated by a poor diet. The decrease in bone strength allows crush fracture to occur in the vertebral bodies and the spine becomes slowly kyphotic (Fig. 22.35). Hip fractures are common in the elderly female suffering from osteoporosis.

Osteomalacia

This occurs when there is a decrease in the mineral content of bone and may be associated with kidney disease and steatorrhoea syndromes. Pathological fractures are common.

Rickets

This is a disease seen in the child and is again characterised by a defect in the mineral content. The most common cause throughout the world is a deficiency of vitamin D in the diet but again kidney and alimentary disease may be responsible. The child affected becomes progressively ill and the bones become bowed and deformed. Growth decreases and the ends of the long bones become widened (Fig. 22.36).

Treatment with extra vitamin D is essential and where there is deformity in the more established case bone division and realignment may be necessary.

Fragilitis osseum (osteogenesis imperfecta)

This is an abnormality of primitive mesoderm tissue. It is characterised by soft bones with multiple fractures (Fig. 22.37) and the sclera of the eyes is frequently blue. There is a congenital type in which multiple fractures are present at birth and a tarda type in which the disease is not so progressive. Deformity follows multiple fractures, and treatment by internal fixation is necessary.

Fig. 22.36. Rickets. The bones become bowed and their metaphyses widened.

Fig. 22.37. Fragilitis ossium. Multiple fractures produce severe deformity.

PERIPHERAL NERVE LESIONS

Carpal tunnel syndrome

The median nerve runs through a closed tunnel at the wrist. The nerve may be compressed by rheumatoid disease or a Colles fracture but in many cases the cause of this nerve compression syndrome is unknown. It frequently affects the middle aged female and produces pain and numbness in the thumb, index and middle fingers. The syndrome sometimes is seen in the pregnant woman where there is swelling and oedema of the extremities.

The symptoms awaken the patient in the early morning and as the compression progresses the muscles of the thenar eminence become wasted and paralysed. The condition is simply treated by dividing the carpal ligament at the wrist, relieving the pressure on the median nerve.

Ulnar Neuritis

The ulnar nerve lies in a groove along the medial side of the elbow where it may be compressed by arthritic changes in the elbow joint. The patient experiences pain and tingling and then numbness in the distribution of the ulnar nerve (i.e. the little and ring fingers). As the compression progresses the small muscles of the hand become paralysed and a claw hand develops (Fig. 22.38). The ulnar nerve must be decompressed by its release from the ulnar groove behind the medial epicondyle at the elbow and its transposition to the anterior aspect of the joint.

PERIPHERAL NERVE INJURIES

Division of the median nerve usually occurs at the wrist and is frequently seen in the child who falls carrying a milk or lemonade bottle. The median nerve laceration produces anaesthesia and muscle paralysis as outlined in the median nerve compression syndrome above. The ulnar nerve is again frequently lacerated at the wrist and produces anaesthesia of the ulnar two fingers and paralysis of all the intrinsic muscles of the hand with the production of a weak claw hand.

The radial nerve is most commonly injured in the mid-arm region where humeral shaft fractures damage the nerve trunk. A wrist drop develops due to paralysis of all the extensor muscles of the wrist.

Treatment

Any wound in which a nerve injury is suspected must be carefully explored. If the wound is clean and there are no other vital struc-

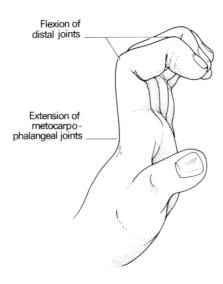

Flexion of
distal joints

Extension of
metocarpo-
phalangeal joints

Fig. 22.38. Claw hand in ulnar nerve paralysis.

tures divided a primary repair of the nerve ends may be undertaken. Very fine suture material is necessary to approximate the nerve sheath and careful splintage of the wrist joint will be necessary to prevent undue tension of the repair site. The recovery of motor and sensory function will be slow for the regenerating nerve grows at a rate of approximately 1 mm per day. If the wound is dirty or tendons are divided then the nerve ends should be tagged with markers and a secondary repair undertaken at a later date.

REGIONAL ORTHOPAEDIC CONDITIONS

THE NECK

Torticollis

Torticollis is a lateral flexion deformity of the cervical spine. It is seen as a neonatal deformity due to a tear and then contracture of the sternomastoid muscle at the time of birth. In most cases simple stretching of the neck is effective, but in some babies the torticollis persists and operative release of the tight sternomastoid muscle is necessary. A torticollis may be acquired later in life and is then accompanied by pain and spasm in the neck. This condition is usually associated with osteoarthritic changes in the cervical spine.

Cervical spondylosis

Osteoarthritis of the cervical spine produces pain, stiffness, and sometimes a torticollis. The pain may radiate to the upper limbs for the nerve roots issuing from the lower cervical region become compressed by the degenerative osteophytes around the joints concerned. Physiotherapy, traction and mobilisation of the neck is helpful and a neck collar may be necessary if the symptoms are acute.

Brachial plexus injuries

Motor cyclists involved in high-speed injuries may damage the shoulder and the neck, avulsing or dividing the roots of the brachial plexus at the base of the neck. Partial division of the nerves will produce patchy paralysis and anaesthesia of the upper limb and recovery will recur to a variable extent. A completely paralysed and anaesthetic arm is a useless member and it may be an advantage to amputate the limb so that a prosthesis may be fitted.

Fig. 22.39. Calcification in the capsule of the shoulder joint.

THE SHOULDER

There are several inflammatory conditions of the shoulder joint and its capsule which produce pain and stiffness:

1. *Acute bursitis.* A minor strain of the shoulder is followed by severe pain and swelling. On X-ray an area of calcification in the capsule develops (Fig. 22.39) and the shoulder becomes progressively stiff. An injection of hydrocortisone into the capsule may give complete relief but sometimes operative release of the tight, calcified plaque is required.

2. *Rupture of the supraspinatus tendon.* A strain of the shoulder may also produce this tendon tear. Abduction of the shoulder is impossible and there is considerable tenderness over the superior aspect of the joint. This condition always spontaneously recovers given time and and there is no indication for operative repair.

3. *Frozen shoulder.* The capsulitis which follows the acute bursitis or a minor tear of the capsule may progress despite treatment. Complete immobility of the shoulder joint may result. It frequently takes 2–3 years to resolve but a good prognosis can always be given to the patient, for full mobility will eventually return.

THE ELBOW

Tennis elbow

Pain and tenderness develops around the lateral epicondyle of the lower humerus at the elbow. Strain of the elbow joint region is usually described by the patient and eventually the pain may become so severe that it is difficult to even raise small objects with the extended wrist. The pain and tenderness is due to an inflammation of the forearm muscle attachment to the bony epicondyle and is treated by a local injection of local anaesthetic and hydrocortisone (xylocaine 4 ml of 1% + 25 mg of hydrocortisone).

Rarely operative release of this extensor tendon from the condyle is necessary in the chronic condition.

Loose bodies

Javelin throwers, fast bowlers and other sportsmen may avulse small portions of bone and articular cartilage from the capitellum and radial head (Fig. 22.40). Osteo-arthritic changes in the elbow may also produce loose bodies which result in an internal derangement of the joint with locking and recurrent painful episodes. Surgical removal of the loose bodies is necessary.

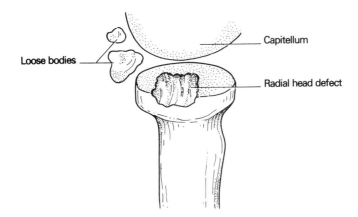

Fig. 22.40. Avulsion of loose bodies from the radial head.

THE WRIST AND HAND

De Quervain's stenosing tenosynovitis (Fig. 22.41)

The extensor tendons to the thumb run over the radial styloid within their own sheaths. At this point the sheath may become inflamed, producing extreme local pain and tenderness locally and there is increasing stiffness of the thumb due to entrapment of the tendon within this sheath. In the early stages an injection of 25 mg of hydrocortisone with xylocaine (1 or 2%) may be helpful, but surgical release is frequently required.

Dupuytren's contracture

This is a common condition in the elderly in which there is fibrosis of the palmar aponeurosis which produces a flexion deformity of the

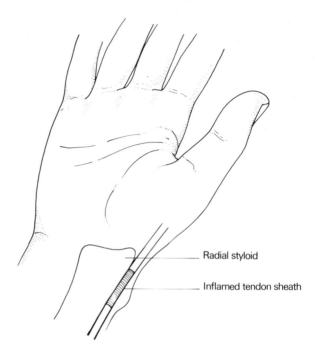

Radial styloid

Inflamed tendon sheath

Fig. 22.41. De Quervain's stenosing tenosynovitis.

finger at the metacarpo-phalangeal and proximal interphalangeal joints, usually starting at the fourth digit and spreading to the fifth and sometimes the third finger. Since the aponeurosis only extends distally to the base of the middle phalanx, the distal interphalangeal joint escapes. The contracture is often bilateral.

Treatment. Mild degrees of contracture are left alone, but if disability is caused the thickened fascia is excised.

Hand infections

Fig. 22.42. Paronychia.

Pus

1. *Paronychia.* This common infection involves the nail-bed and frequently follows a 'hang-nail' (Fig. 22.42). At the early stage antibiotics may be given but after a few days pus develops and surgical evacuation will be required. An incision from the proximal corner of the nail through the infected area is made (Fig. 22.43) and in severe infections a portion of the nail will have to be removed. The whole nail must be removed if the infection has spread to the other side of the finger.

2. *Pulp space infections.* Needle points and other penetrating injuries readily infect the finger or thumb tips. The area becomes painful, swollen and red, and pus develops at an early stage. The

pulp space is divided by fibrous septa into multiple compartments and so surgical drainage must be extensive and complete. An incision on both sides of the pulp space is required and a through-and-through drain remains for twenty-four hours.

Tendon sheath infection. A needle may enter the tendon sheath, infecting the whole length of the tendon in the finger and the palm. The sheath quickly becomes distended with infected fluid or pus and must be drained as soon as possible. Any delay in releasing the infection may result in adhesion of the sheath to the tendon, producing a stiff finger or thumb.

Palmar infections. The palm is divided into three compartments—the thenar compartment on the thumb side, the hypothenar on the little finger side, and the mid palmar space between the two. Penetrating wounds may infect these compartments and drainage will again be necessary. When the mid palmar space is infected the whole hand becomes extremely swollen and the infection points into the web space where it may be drained by a surgical incision.

In all hand infections, surgical drainage is combined with immobilisation, elevation and antibiotic therapy.

Fig. 22.43. Paronychia drained by an incision.

Tendon injuries

Lacerations affecting the dorsum of the hand and wrist in which the extensor tendons are divided present no real problem. The extensor tendons must be carefully sutured and the hand and wrist splinted in extension for three weeks. They always heal satisfactorily and function should return to normal.

The flexor tendons on the anterior aspect of the hand, however, constitute a much more difficult repair problem. Following their division, repair is very likely to produce adhesions to other tendons and surrounding tissues with a result that the hand or finger becomes stiff. In the proximal part of the hand and wrist direct repair of the divided tendon may be undertaken with an end-to-end suture (Fig. 22.44). If the wound is dirty or the wound exploration is extremely delayed then it is preferable to close the skin and to allow the wound to heal. Tendon suture is undertaken secondarily at a later date. If the wound is clean and it is within 6 hours of injury then primary repair of the tendon may be undertaken with antibiotic cover.

Laceration of the fingers affecting the flexor tendons within their tight flexor tendon sheath produce specific problems of adhesion and finger stiffness. In most cases it is better to cut out the lacerated tendons and insert a tendon graft which is taken from either

Fig. 22.44. Tendon repair by an end-to-end suture.

palmaris longus in the forearm or one of the toe extensor tendons. This graft is attached distally to the distal phalanx of the finger and proximally to the flexor tendon in the palm or the wrist (Fig. 22.45). The hand should be completely immobilised for 3 weeks post-operatively with the fingers in flexion and then a prolonged course of physiotherapy is undertaken to mobilise the hand and the affected fingers.

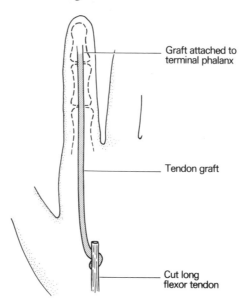

Graft attached to terminal phalanx

Tendon graft

Cut long flexor tendon

Fig. 22.45. Tendon graft.

THE SPINE

Backache

There are many causes of pain in the spine and these include infection, rheumatoid diseases, abnormalities of the retroperitoneum and posterior abdominal wall, and, most commonly, mechanical abnormalities. These mechanical derangements of the spine may be classified into (i) acute back strain, (ii) intervertebral disc syndromes, (iii) instability syndromes, (iv) chronic back strains.

1. *Acute back strain.* This condition is commonly seen in the nurses on the ward. When lifting a heavy patient pain may be experienced in the low lumbar region and there is tenderness where the paraspinal muscles insert onto the iliac crest. Acute pain and stiffness develops but resolve satisfactorily after adequate rest. An injection of local anaesthetic (xylocaine, 1%) into the tender area may be helpful.

2. *Intervertebral disc syndromes.* A prolapsed intervertebral disc produces low lumbar pain together with sciatica (pain radiating into

the leg). There is often a history of a heavy lift or injury and the pain may become very severe. The spine becomes curved with a scoliosis or a tilt (Fig. 22.46). Straight leg raising on the affected side is limited and neurological abnormalities may develop when the lumbar roots are compressed within the spinal canal. An x-ray may reveal a decreased disc space at the affected level.

The essential feature of the treatment of this condition is rest in bed. The mattress must be firm and the nurse should make sure that fracture boards are inserted beneath the mattress. Adequate sedation and analgesia is required and in most cases resolution of pain and the sciatic symptoms occurs over the next few weeks. If neurological signs such as weakness of the muscle group or complete anaesthesia persist, or if the bladder becomes affected by compression of the cauda equina in the spinal canal then there is an indication for operation. A myelogram is usually performed at this stage to confirm the site of the disc prolapse. Dye is injected into the subarachnoid space and its flow is altered by a disc prolapse. A laminectomy is performed to remove the posterior elements of the spinal canal and the disc is removed from around the nerve root.

3. *Instability syndromes.* A spondylolysis is a condition where a defect or fracture through the posterior elements of the vertebra occurs (Fig. 22.47). A spondylolisthesis—a slip of one vertebral body forwards on the next—may follow (Fig. 22.48). Chronic degenerative changes in one disc space may also produce a minor slip of one vertebra on the next. The symptoms of low lumbar spine pain and sciatica are controlled by a lumbar supportive corset and the strengthening effect of physiotherapy. If the slip continues or symptoms become severe in spite of this conservative treatment

Fig. 22.46. Sciatic scoliosis.

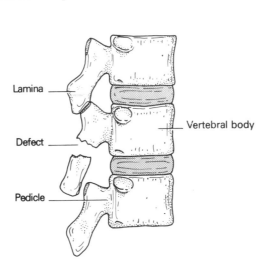

Lamina

Defect

Pedicle

Vertebral body

Fig. 22.47. Spondylolysis.

Fig. 22.48. Spondylolisthesis—
a slip of one vertebral body
forward on the next.

operation may be required to stabilise the segment. Fusion of the
spinal vertebra will be required.

4. *Chronic back strain.* This is a common problem and frequently
seen in the housewife who is required to undertake heavy housework and the frequent lifting of children. Pain is experienced in the
low lumbar region and is aggravated by exercises. The pain sometimes radiates to the buttocks and thighs but true sciatica is not
experienced. On X-ray there is usually no abnormality, but minor
chronic degenerative changes may later develop. The physiotherapist
will be very helpful to this patient, and a supportive corset is
advisable when undertaking housework etc.

Osteomyelitis of the spine

Pyogenic organisms such as those seen in osteomyelitis (page 528)
may travel via the blood stream to the vertebrae and produce
infection within a disc space. Infection rapidly spreads to adjacent
vertebral bone, which may collapse and produce a large paraspinal
abscess. Pain is extremely severe. The spine develops extreme spasm
and the patient becomes ill very rapidly with a high fever, raised
white count, and a high E.S.R. The organisms may be identified on
blood culture and appropriate antibiotics are given. The spine must
be put at rest and to allow this to be as complete as possible the
patient is confined to a plaster bed (Fig. 22.49), or alternatively

Fig. 22.49. Patient being nursed on a plaster bed.

nursed on a circle electric bed. This apparatus is very satisfactory from the nursing point of view and immobilises the spine to allow satisfactory resolution of the infection.

Tuberculous infection of the spine (Pott's disease) (Fig. 22.19)

The disc space and adjacent vertebral bodies are similarly affected. The abscess which develops may distend the psoas muscle sheath on either side of the vertebral column and sometimes may compress the spinal cord producing a paralysis of the lower limbs (Pott's paraplegia).

The infection is treated by appropriate rest and anti-tuberculous drugs. Exploration of the spine through the chest or abdomen may be necessary to eradicate the abscess cavity and to allow bone healing. Bone grafting may be required if a large cavity is present.

THE HIP

Perthes' disease (Fig. 22.50)

This an avascular necrosis of the femoral head and occurs in the child between the ages of 5 and 10 years. The cause of this avascularity is unknown but there is some evidence that the high pressure of synovial fluid within the hip joint may be responsible. There is obstruction of the vessels which supply the femoral head of the developing child with blood. The child limps and pain is experienced in the thigh and knee region (rarely in the hip and groin area). X-rays

Fig. 22.50. Perthes' disease of the right hip.

reveal a sclerotic, fragmented and squashed femoral head and, if this poor shape persists, early osteoarthritis of the hip joint may result.

The *treatment* to be given depends on the extent of the avascularity. In many minor instances no treatment at all is required and the parents can be reassured that the hip will return to a normal functional state and a very good hip shape will be retained. Severe cases of Perthes' disease may require operation. An osteotomy of the upper femur is undertaken to contain the squashed mushroom-shaped head of the femur in a better position within the acetabulum.

Slipped femoral epiphysis

This occurs in children between the ages of 10 and 15 and produces symptoms and signs very similar to the sub-capital femoral neck fractures described on page 502. The children are frequently affected by endocrine abnormalities. They are frequently Fröhlich-like, grossly overweight and with poorly developed secondary sex characteristics. The slip of the epiphysis from the neck may occur suddenly and acutely (Fig. 22.51) or it may occur slowly in a chronic fashion. In the acute type the femoral head must be manipulated back on to the neck and internally fixed with fine pins (Fig. 22.52). In the chronic slip internal fixation with pins must be undertaken before the slip becomes too displaced.

THE KNEE

Internal derangements of the knee

Cartilage Tears. Rotational injuries of the knee most commonly occur on the football or athletics field but similar injuries to the joint may occur in men who have to crouch and work in confined spaces.

Fig. 22.51. Slipped femoral epiphysis.

Pain is experienced immediately and the medial side of the joint is most commonly affected. The footballer has to go off the field and swelling in the joint develops usually that evening or the next day. The joint may remain locked if a 'bucket-handle tear' of the cartilage is sustained with one segment of the meniscus being displaced into the centre of the joint (Fig. 22.53).

Alternatively the joint may spontaneously unlock and the symptoms gradually settle. Recurrent episodes of pain, swelling, locking and 'giving way' are characteristic of the torn meniscus. Repeated mechanical derangements will eventually produce joint surface damage and it is important to remove the torn meniscus.

When the diagnosis is definite, meniscectomy is advised. If the symptoms and signs are not so clear-cut a course of physiotherapy must be given to build up the knee musculature and to await events.

Fig. 22.52. The epiphysis has been repositioned and internally fixed with pins. ▶

Fig. 22.53. Bucket handle torn meniscus. ▼

Some help may be given by the introduction of dye and air into the joint so that X-rays may be taken with the cartilage outlined: this technique being called arthrography (Fig. 22.54).

A small endoscope may be passed into the knee joint and with this instrument the internal structures can be visualised and tears of the cartilage actually seen. This instrument—the arthroscope—has improved the accuracy of diagnosis very greatly in the last few years. *Ligament Tears.* The knee joint is stabilised by the medial and lateral collateral ligaments together with the anterior and posterior cruciate ligaments (Fig. 22.55). The medial collateral ligament is the most commonly torn, and strains of this structure are seen in soccer and skiing injuries.

A partial tear of this ligament will require treatment in a plaster cast with the knee immobilised for 6 weeks. Gross tears of the medial collateral ligament are often associated with anterior cruciate ligament tears and injuries of the meniscus. Conservative treatment of this injury with plaster will be unsatisfactory, for continued instability will result and will usually prevent a sportsman from returning to his games.

Operative treatment of the collateral ligament must be undertaken and the cartilage derangement must be treated. It is sometimes possible to repair the anterior cruciate ligament if it removes a small piece of bone from either end, but if the ligament is shredded, repair is ineffective. The stability of the joint then depends on the quality of the quadriceps muscle.

Loose Bodies. Osteochondritis dissecans is responsible for most of the loose bodies seen in the knee joint in a young person (Fig. 22.56). It is due to a fracture through the articular cartilage and underlying bone and the fragment may either remain in its crater causing symptoms of pain and instability or it may loosen and form a separate loose body which intermittently locks the joint.

Osteoarthritic changes may be the cause of a loose body in the elderly. Loose bodies which are repeatedly deranging the knee must be removed.

Fig. 22.54. Arthrography of the knee showing a cartilage tear (arrowed).

Cruciate ligaments

Lateral collateral ligament

Medial collateral ligament

Fig. 22.55. The knee joint ligaments.

Fig. 22.56. Osteochondritis dissecans.

THE ANKLE

Sprains

Ankle sprains are due to a partial tear of the lateral collateral ligament. An inversion twisting injury of the ankle joint will rupture the front band of this ligament (Fig. 22.57) causing swelling, bruising, and local tenderness. If no fracture is detected on x-ray the essential treatment is rest and elevation of the ankle. After a day or two active exercises are started to return the muscle control of the ankle to normal as soon as possible. If the tear of the lateral collateral ligament is complete producing gross instability, a below-knee plaster is applied for 4 to 6 weeks.

Achilles tendon tears

The large Achilles tendon above the heel bone may rupture in sportsmen who are leaping to reach a ball. The unfit person who is performing strenuous, unaccustomed exercise may also be affected. There is a sharp, sudden episode of pain above the heel and the patient often describes the situation when he feels he has been 'shot in the heel'. Swelling and bruising rapidly develops and a gap in the Achilles tendon can be detected. The patient is unable to stand on tip-toes but simple plantar flexion of the foot is still possible for the other ankle flexors are intact.

If the tear is left untreated the patient's gait will be poor. It is advisable to operate and repair the tendon at this early stage.

Fragment on medial condyle

Fig. 22.57. Sprained ankle. Partial rupture of the lateral ligament.

Following operation 6 weeks immobilisation in a plaster cast will be necessary. If operation is contra-indicated a satisfactory result will be obtained if a below-knee plaster is applied with the foot in full plantar flexion.

THE FOOT

Hallux valgus

The great toe becomes displaced at the metatarso-phalangeal joint (Fig. 22.58). This condition is often inherited and is aggravated by

Fig. 22.58. Hallux valgus.

the use of inappropriate footwear. A bunion may develop due to the formation of an exostosis at the head of the metatarsal, and the second toe may become displaced at the metatarso-phalangeal joint. Pain and discomfort may be due to the bunion and if it persists the exostosis is removed.

A full correction of the deformity may be undertaken by arthrodesing the great toe metatarso-phalangeal joint. The proximal part of the great toe phalanx is removed in the Keller's operation and this will also straighten the deformity and remove the discomfort.

Metatarsalgia

Pain below the forefoot may be due to prominence of the metatarsal heads in the sole musculature. It may also be due to a pain from a neuroma between the metatarsal heads; this condition being called a Morton's metatarsalgia. A simple insole to redistribute the weight beneath the foot together with strengthening exercises of the intrinsic muscles will alleviate the symptoms in most cases. A neuroma must be removed surgically.

Hammer toes

The deformity shown in Fig. 22.59 may be corrected by fusion of the proximal joint.

Plantar fasciitis

Pain beneath the heel is a common condition and is due to inflammation of the plantar ligament where it is inserted into the calcaneum. A calcaneal spur may develop and treatment consists of injection of local anaesthetic and hydrocortisone. A moulded soft heel pad is helpful.

Dorsal callosity

Fig. 22.59. Hammer toe.

Chapter 23. Transplantation

Introduction

Transplantation of human tissues has been a topic for popular discussion for a little over a decade now, mainly because of the use of organs such as kidneys, liver, heart or lungs taken from people who have recently died. But it should not be forgotten that transplantation has been undertaken for longer than this. Skin grafting has been a successful technique for many years as a means for obtaining cover for areas of skin surface denuded by burns.

Types of transplant

If a tissue is taken from one area of the body and is placed in another, this is known as an *autograft*. Examples of autografts are skin grafts, bone chips taken from the iliac crest to fill in bone spaces and the use of the long saphenous vein to bypass a block in the femoral artery. These types of graft will not be discussed further in this chapter.

A tissue taken from one individual in a species and placed in another of the same species is called an *allograft*. Examples of allografts are renal, liver, cardiac and lung transplants.

If an animal from one species donates an organ to an animal of another species this is known as a *xenograft*. This type of graft has been used in the past, for example baboon kidneys have been placed in humans but the problems posed, which will be discussed later, are too great and xenografting is not now used clinically.

Immunological rejection

In precisely the way that the body recognises and rejects an infecting organism, so it recognises and rejects an allograft and a xenograft.

The body contains protein and has the capacity to recognise 'self' in immunological terms. If a foreign protein (an *antigen*) enters the blood stream, *antibodies* against it are formed. The source of the antibodies are the small lymphocyte cells in the regional lymph nodes. When antibodies recirculate in the patient's blood stream and come into contact with the protein which stimulated their production, they react with this protein, altering its structure and function. This antigen-antibody reaction to foreign protein is the basic mechanism that underlies the immune response.

When skin is applied, as an autograft, from, say, the thigh to the arm in a patient with burns, no immune response occurs because the grafted skin contains precisely similar proteins to the skin which covered the grafted area. However, if skin is taken from one member of a species and is placed on a denuded and vascular area of another member of the same species, that is an allograft, antibodies against the graft form within 7 to 14 days and the graft is rejected. For the first few days the graft will be vascularised normally, but, as antibodies begin to form, the endothelium lining the blood vessels that supply the allograft is progressively destroyed because of the antigen–antibody reaction. This process of *rejection* is accompanied by some of the features of an inflammatory response. There is infiltration of the area with white cells and exudation of tissue fluid into the inter-cellular space. Thus, there are two arms of the rejection process, the first being the release into the circulation of foreign proteins with the formation of antibodies and the second being the recirculation of antibodies with an antigen-antibody reaction.

One interesting exception to the rejection seen in allografts is in the case of *identical twins*. It is possible to take tissue from one twin and to graft it on the other twin without there being any development of antibodies. Thus the grafted tissue is not rejected. This is because both twins arise from the division of one cell and both therefore have an identical genetic make-up.

In the case of a xenograft, the rejection process is more vigorous than in the case of an allograft. It is as if the proteins of a different species are more 'foreign' and produce a more rapid and profound antibody response.

Immunosuppression

It is possible to modify the production of antibodies by suppressing their manufacture. To do this it is necessary to interfere with the metabolism of the small, immunologically competent lymphocytes by means of drugs or it is possible to remove them physically. The drugs that are used to suppress the immune response are azathioprine, which interferes with the use by the lymphocytes of an amino-acid, purine, which is vital to their normal function, together with steroids to reduce inflammatory response. Occasionally other drugs such as actinomycin, which is related to the antibiotics, are used. Another form of drug therapy is the use of antilymphocyte serum. Lymphocytes are first removed from the patient and antibodies against them are raised in horses. These antibodies are concentrated and when injected into the patient the immune response so invoked will result in the destruction of the lymphocytes which were originally used to raise the antibodies. Actual removal of lymphocytes can be achieved by cannulating the thoracic duct and clearing the lymph so obtained of the cells before it is re-injected.

By these means it is impossible to suppress the immunological rejection process to the point where it is possible for an allograft to survive for a considerable length of time. There is, however, one other extremely important method whereby the rejection process is modified and this is by immunological donor-recipient matching.

Donor matching

It is possible to match the donor organ to the immunological type of the recipient with the result that the allograft protected by immunosuppressive therapy will survive for years—the longest survival time for an allograft kidney is now over 10 years. The first part of the matching process is to ensure that the blood groups of donor and recipient are the same. Following this, there are a number of antibodies that are recognised as being important to the rejection process. These antibodies (of the HL-A system) are dependant for their existence on the genetic pattern and can be recognised by testing the lymphocytes of either the donor or the recipient against a number (50 to 60) of different types of serum obtained by the purification of serum from a panel of people whose antibody constitution has become known. It is thus possible to 'type' both a potential donor of organs and a potential recipient. If the donor and recipient have a similar immunological construction then the rejection of the transplanted organ has been clearly shown to be modified.

CLINICAL TRANSPLANTATION

Corneal transplantation

One of the forms of transplantation that has been successfully carried out for the longest time is that of the cornea. The reason for the success of this operation (where the cornea from the eye of a person recently dead is used to replace an opaque cornea) is that the grafted cornea is not revascularised. It is thus a privileged tissue nourished by means of tissue perfusion of nutrients and oxygen.

Renal transplantation

Fifteen years ago this was experimental but now this procedure is carried out in a number of centres throughout the world with good therapeutic results. Kidneys are particularly suitable for transplantation because of the development of the artificial kidney, because of their gross anatomical structure and because they are paired organs.

The artificial kidney means that it is possible to maintain life in the absence of any functioning renal tissue at all. The end-point of gradually deteriorating function is not therefore sudden death of the patient, so that it is possible to maintain a potential recipient in good health until a suitable donor kidney is available.

The gross anatomy of artery, vein and ureter makes it surgically simple to remove a kidney with preservation of the vital structures so that the artery can be re-anastomosed end-to-end to the up-turned internal iliac artery, the vein end-to-side to the common iliac vein and the ureter to the bladder of the recipient. It is usual to place the left donor kidney in the right iliac fossa and vice versa so that the renal pelvis of the donor kidney is always anterior.

The fact that the kidney is a paired organ has meant that it has been possible to remove one kidney from a healthy, live donor. This is probably not an important source of kidneys at the present time but in the development stage of transplantation it meant that kidneys were being transplanted between members of families with the result that a form of automatic tissue typing occurred.

The main problems associated with renal transplantation are, first, the obtaining of preservation of suitable donor organs, second the immunological problems already mentioned and finally cost.

There is no doubt now that kidneys for transplantation have to be obtained in most instances from cadavers. They must be removed from the body of the donor not more than 30 minutes after death. Obviously there are difficulties in obtaining permission for this to be done if this has to be sought from relatives. There are also difficulties in ensuring that there is someone who is competent at cadaveric kidney removal and storage present at the time of death. The ethical problems of permission will be debated in forthcoming years. One side points out the number of young or middle-aged adults who die per year from bilateral renal disease and who would be saved by renal transplantation and generally wish permission to be automatic, the onus being on a person, in life, to

Index

573

adynamic obstruction   208–9
anatomy   196, *196*
congenital atresia   214, *215*
Crohn's disease   202, *203*
dynamic obstruction   209
intussusception   216–8
necrotic   213
physiology   198–9
specific infections   200–2
tumours   207–8
volvulus   214–5, *216*
small vessel spasm   102
Smith-Petersen nail   503
Smith's fracture   498
smoking   84, 108, 180
Snellen's types   420
sodium   174
absorption   316
sodium tetra-decyl-sulphate
119
Souttar's tube   60
spectacles   436–8
spermatic cord   271
torsion   364
spherocytosis
hereditary   294
sphincters
unconcious patient   148
spina bifida   133, 524–5, *525*
spinal fusion   526, *527*
injuries   514–7
tumour   358
vertebra fusion   548
spine
orthopaedic conditions   546–9
osteomyelitis   548–9
tuberculosis   527, 529, 549
Spitz-Holter shunt   134, *135*,
525
spleen   298–300
anatomy   298, *298*
ruptured   299
splenectomy
conditions   299–300
splenic artery   298
splenic vein   298
spondylolisthesis   547, *548*
spondylolysis   547, *547*

sprains
ankle   553, *554*
spurious diarrhoea   264
squint   418, 435–6, *435–6*
concomitant   435
operation   436, *436–7*
paralytic   435
treatment   436
staghorn calculus   329, 334, *334*
stapedectomy   454
stapes   442–3
fixation   453
prosthesis   454, *455*
Staphylococcus albus   403
Staphylococcus aureus   2, 2–3,
200, 389, 407
Starr-Edwards prosthesis   98, *98*
Steinmann pin   489, *489*, 507,
511
stelazine   202
sternomastoid muscle   541
steroid drops   423
steroid secretion   383
steroids
Crohn's disease   206
ulcerative colitis   230
stilboestrol   60, 357
breast cancer   399
Still's disease   532
stomach
anatomy   173–4, *173, 175*
carcinoma   182–5, *184*,
193
erosions   196
tumours   182
ulcer   190, 193
stones
urinary tract   332–8, *334–5*
strangulated hernia   269–70,
270–1
treatment   272–3
strangury   323
stratum corneum of skin   403
Streptococcus viridans   92
streptomycin   17
stress reaction
burns   46
stricture formation   169

stridor   472, 474
string snig
Crohn's disease   205
stroke   146
Stryker frame   515
stye   424, *424*
subacute bacterial endarteritis
92, 94, 104
subarachnoid haemorrhage   159
subarachnoid space   155
subconjunctival haemorrhage
154, *155*
subcutaneous tumours   415
subdural abscess   452
subdural haematoma   156,
158
acute   158
chronic   159
subdural space   155
subluxation   484, *485*
submucous resection   459–60,
460, 463
subphrenic abscess   224, *225*
subphrenic spaces
pus   223
subtalar joint   514
subungual exostosis   409
subungual melanoma   410
succussion splash   193
sucking pneumothorax   75
suction clearance
ear   450
suction drainage   400, *400*
sugar tolerance test   308
sulphadimidine   154
sulphamylon   49
sulphasalazine   230
sulphonamides   2
superficial vein system   114–6
supervoltage therapy   63, 67
supracondylar fracture
femur   509, *509*
humerus   486, *486*, 494–5,
495
suprapubic catheter   348, *349*
suprapubic cystostomy   360
suprapubic region   323
suprarenal glands   381–7